PANCREATITIS – TREATMENT AND COMPLICATIONS

Edited by **Luis Rodrigo Saez**

Pancreatitis – Treatment and Complications
Edited by Luis Rodrigo Saez

Published by InTech
Janeza Trdine 9, 51000 Rijeka, Croatia

Publishing Process Manager Vedran Greblo

Technical Editor Teodora Smiljanic

Cover Designer InTech Design Team

Additional hard copies can be obtained from orders@intechopen.com

Pancreatitis – Treatment and Complications, Edited by Luis Rodrigo Saez
p. cm.
ISBN 978-953-51-0109-3

For EU product safety concerns:
IN TECH d.o.o., Prolaz Marije Krucifikse Kozulić 3, 51000 Rijeka, Croatia,
info@intechopen.com or visit our website at intechopen.com.

Meet the editor

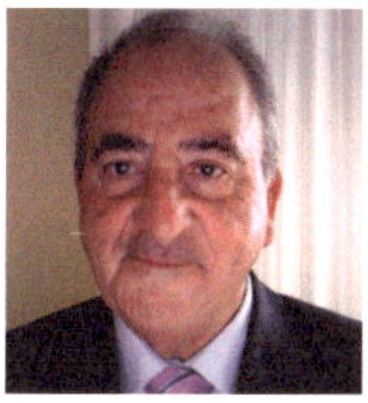

Dr Luis Rodrigo Saez was born in Vitoria, Spain. He studied in the Medical School at the Central University of Madrid, obtaining his graduation as Licensee in Medicine and Surgery, in 1967. In 1975 he obtained his PhD in Medicine in Oviedo, Spain. Dr. Saez was Head of Gastroenterology in the Central University Hospital of Asturias, Spain, from 1996. He was Titular Professor in Medicine at the University of Oviedo, from 1983 until 2009, becoming a Full Professor there in 2010. Over the last 30 years he has helped form a group of around 100 specialists in Gastroenterology within the National Program of Fellowship. He is the main author or co-author of 177 English-language scientific papers and approximately 254 in Spanish. He has written a total of 55 chapters of books on Gastroenterology and five books about treatment in gastroenterological diseases.

Contents

Preface

It is my great pleasure and honor to present this interesting book *Pancreatitis – Treatment and Complications,* written by an international group of experts, doctors, university professors and researchers with great experience in this field.

Pancreatitis may be acute or chronic. Although they can be caused by similar aetiologies, they tend to follow distinct natural histories. Around 80% of acute pancreatitis diagnoses occur as secondary to gallstone disease and alcohol misuse. This disease is commonly associated with the sudden onset of upper abdominal pain radiating to the back that is usually severe enough to warrant the patient seeking urgent medical attention. The onset of pain may be related to a recent alcohol binge or a rich, fatty meal intake. The patient may appear unwell, be tachycardic and have significant tenderness in the upper abdomen.

Overall, 10 to 25% of acute pancreatitis (AP) episodes are classified as severe, leading to an associated mortality rate, of 7 to 30%. Disease severity is best predicted from a number of clinical scoring systems which can be applied at diagnosis in association with repeated clinical assessment, measurement of acute inflammatory markers, and CT. All patients with suspected AP should be referred urgently.

Establishing a biliary etiology in acute pancreatitis is clinically important because of the potential need for invasive treatment, such as endoscopic retrograde cholangiopancreatography. The etiology of acute biliary pancreatitis (ABP) is multifactorial and complex. The passing of small gallbladder stones or biliary sludge through the ampulla of Vater seems to be important in the pathogenesis of ABP.

Infectious complications in severe acute pancreatitis are associated with considerable morbidity and mortality. The course of the disease is often protracted, and patients often stay in hospital for several weeks. Diagnosis of infected pancreatic necrosis is difficult, and the treatment consists of source control and antibiotic treatment. Antibiotic use should be rational in terms of a proper indication, a wide pancreatic penetration and long duration.

Prophylactic antibiotics are ineffective in reducing the incidence of peri-pancreatic infection in patients with severe disease, or even documented necrotizing pancreatitis.

The only rational indication for antibiotics is documented infection. Pancreatitis is one of the most frequent complications of endoscopic retrograde cholangiopancreatography (ERCP). The placement of a prophylactic pancreatic stent after ERCP can help prevent post-ERCP pancreatitis (PEP).

Recurrent acute pancreatitis is a common clinical problem. Most cases of pancreatitis are identified by a careful history and physical examination. Despite advanced evaluation, the cause is not apparent in about 10% of cases.

Increased intra-abdominal pressure (IAP), also referred to as intra-abdominal hypertension (IAH), affects organ function in critically ill patients and may lead to abdominal compartment syndrome (ACS). Its diagnosis and treatment are clearly described in this book.

Although most cases of acute pancreatitis are uncomplicated and resolve spontaneously, the presence of complications has significant prognostic importance. Necrosis, hemorrhage, and infection convey rates of up to 25%, 50%, and 80% mortality, respectively. Other complications such as pseudocyst formation, pseudoaneurysm formation, or venous thrombosis increase morbidity and mortality to a lesser degree. The presence of ascites and pleural effusion and emphysematous pancreatitis, are less commonly found. We have reviewed in several chapters the computed tomographic findings of complications associated with acute pancreatitis with emphasis on their prognostic significance and impact on clinical management, for their early detection and proper follow-up.

Inflammation of the pancreas has many presentations in children and adolescents. The etiology is often elusive, with a great number of cases being idiopathic. However, there have been a number of recent advances in the areas of cell biology, genetics and imaging technology, which should be highlighted. This book provides the reader with a review, with particular emphasis on some of these newer advances.

I want to thank all of the authors for their excellent contributions and to the InTech editorial team, especially to Mr Vedran Greblo, for his continuous support and superb and ongoing help when it was needed.

Prof. Luis Rodrigo Saez
Head of Gastroenterology Service, University Hospital Central of Asturias,
Full Professor of Medicine, Oviedo University,
Spain

Part 1

Etiology

1

Acute Pancreatitis – The Current Concept in Ethiopathogenesis, Morphology and Complications

B. Suresh Kumar Shetty[1], Ramdas Naik[2], Adithi S. Shetty[3], Sharadha Rai[4], Ritesh G. Menezes[5] and Tanuj Kanchan[1]

[1]*Department of Forensic Medicine and Toxicology Kasturba Medical College, Mangalore, Manipal University,*
[2]*Department of Pathology, Kasturba Medical College, Mangalore, Manipal University,*
[3]*Department of Obstetrics & Gynaecology, K. S. Hegde Medical Academy, Mangalore, Nitte University,*
[4]*Department of Pathology, Kasturba Medical College, Mangalore, Manipal University,*
[5]*Department of Forensic Medicine and Toxicology, Srinivas Institute of Medical Sciences & Research Centre, Mangalore,*
India

1. Introduction

This chapter is a comprehensive approach on etiology, patho-phyosiological and complications of acute pancreatitis and its review will aid in evaluation of acute pancreatitis in-toto. Pancreatitis is the inflammation of the exocrine pancreas which results from injury to the acinar cells. It may be classified as either acute or chronic. Acute pancreatitis is the reversible injury to the pancreatic parenchyma associated with inflammation and is characterized by a recurrent episode of abdominal pain and elevated serum amylase and lipase levels.

2. Etiopathogenesis of acute pancreatitis

2.1 Etiology

Acute pancreatitis is relatively common. Among the numerous causes, two factors which account for about 70 -80% of cases of acute pancreatitis are **biliary tract disease** and **alcoholism.** The male-to-female ratio is 1: 3 in the group with biliary tract disease and 6: 1 in those with alcoholism.

2.1.1 Important causes are

Alcohol and pancreatitis: Alcohol-induced acute pancreatitis usually develops in patients who consume large quantities of alcohol for 5-10 years before the first attack. However, it may occur with the consumption of a small quantity of alcohol also (two drinks/day). Environmental factors like smoking and high-fat diet may also contribute to the development of acute pancreatitis in alcoholics. There are three possible different mechanisms of alcoholic pancreatitis.

- **Obstruction of small ductules by proteinaceous plugs**: Chronic alcohol ingestion results in the **secretion of protein-rich pancreatic fluid**, which may result in **inspissated** protein plugs and obstruction of small pancreatic ducts.
- **Abnormal spasm sphincter of Oddi:** Alcohol transiently increases pancreatic exocrine secretion and abnormal **contraction of the sphincter of Oddi** (the muscle at the ampulla of Vater),
- **Direct toxic effects:** Metabolic byproducts of alcohol have **direct toxic effects** on the acinar cells.

METABOLIC FACTORS
• Alcoholism • Hyperlipoproteinemia/hypertriglyceridemia • Hyperparathyroidism • Hypercalcemia • Drugs (e.g., furosemide, azathioprine, cyclosporine, tacrolimus)
GENETIC
Mutations in the cationic trypsinogen (*PRSS1*) and trypsin inhibitor (*SPINK1*) genes
MECHANICAL

• Gallstones
• Trauma and injury
    • Blunt abdominal trauma
    • Iatrogenic injury
    • Operative injury: Endoscopic procedures with dye injection(retrograde cholangiopancreatography)
• Obstruction of the pancreatic duct
    • Periampullary neoplasms (e.g., carcinoma of pancreas)
    • Parasites (e.g., *ascaris lumbricoides* and *clonorchis sinensis*)

VASCULAR/ISCHEMIC INJURY
• Shock • Atheroembolism • Vasculitis
INFECTIONS
• Mumps

Table 1. Etiologic Factors in Acute Pancreatitis

Gallstones and pancreatitis

- The frequency of acute pancreatitis is inversely proportional to the size of gallstones. Persistence of stones in the bile duct or the ampulla of vater is associated with more severe disease. An impacted gallstone may allow the reflux of bile into the pancreatic duct or occlude the duct's orifice.

Pancreatic Obstruction

- It is a less common cause of acute pancreatitis. Sphincter of Oddi dysfunction and carcinoma of the pancreas are associated with acute pancreatitis and is usually of the mild type.

Genetic Factors

- About 10% to 20% of patients with acute pancreatitis have no known associated etiological processes. Though these are termed idiopathic, the evidence suggests that some may have a genetic basis.
- Hereditary pancreatitis is characterized by recurrent attacks of severe pancreatitis usually developing in childhood. Most of these are caused by germline (inherited) mutations in the cationic trypsinogen gene (also known as PRSS1). In patients with these mutations, tryspin is inappropriately activated in the pancreas, which in turn activates other digestive proenzymes.
- The serine protease inhibitor Kazal type 1 (SPINK1) gene codes for a pancreatic secretory trypsin inhibitor. This inhibits trypsin activity and prevents autodigestion of the pancreas by activated trypsin. Mutation in the SPINK1 gene leads to loss of function of the inhibitor gene and causes pancreatitis.

The other etiological factors for acute pancreatitis are shown in the Table.**1.**

2.2 Pathogenesis

The changes of acute pancreatitis are due to autodigestion of the pancreatic substance by inappropriately activated pancreatic enzymes.

2.2.1 Mechanism of activation of pancreatic enzymes (Figure.1)

- *Pancreatic duct obstruction:* Any lesion which narrows the lumen of pancreatic ducts or impairs the flow of exocrine secretions can increase intraductal pressure and cause back-diffusion. This results in the accumulation of enzyme-rich fluid in the interstitium and inappropriate activation of proenzymes. Gallstones is one of the main cause of pancreatic duct obstruction.
- *Defective intracellular transport of proenzymes within acinar cells*: In normal acinar cells, the proenzymes and lysosomal hydrolases are transported in separate pathways. Inappropriate delivery of pancreatic proenzymes to the intracellular compartment containing lysosomal hydrolases may activate proenzymes. This mechanism may be responsible for injury due to alcohol or duct obstruction.
- *Primary acinar cell injury:* Acinar cells may be directly damaged by certain viruses (e.g., mumps), drugs, alcohol, trauma to the pancreas, ischemia and shock.
- *Hyperstimulation of pancreas:* This may be seen in association with consumption of alcohol or fat diet.
- *Reflux of bile:* Infected bile or duodenal content may regurgitate into the pancreatic duct due to disruption of sphincter Oddi (e.g., gallstones).

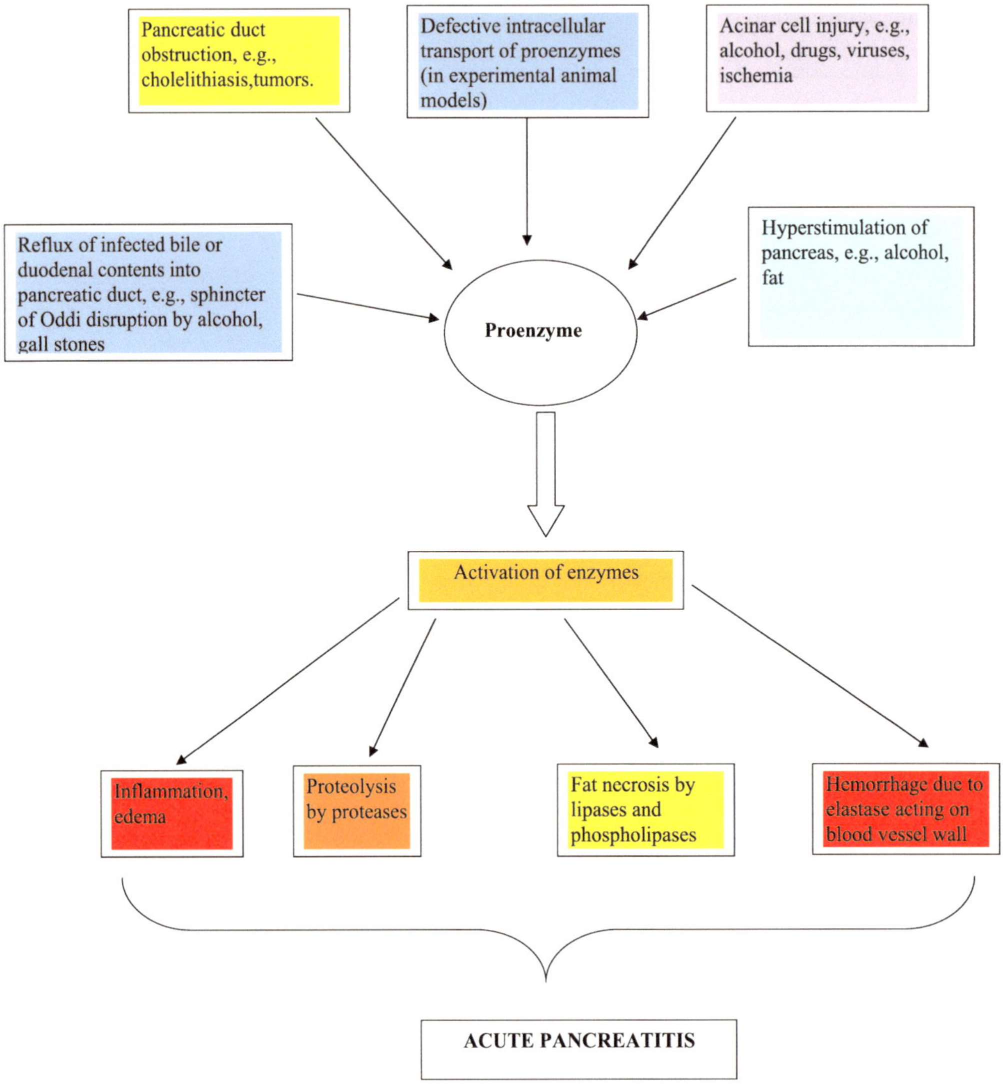

Fig. 1. Diagram Of Mechanism Of Activation Of Pancreatic Enzymes

2.2.2 Pancreatitis evolves in three phases

- **Initial phase**: It is characterised by premature activation of zymogen granules releasing active enzymes which cause acinar cell injury, digestion of the pancreas and surrounding tissue. The hyperstimulation of the pancreas may result in the fusion of lysosome and zymogens within large vacuoles. Lysosomal hydrolase namely cathepsin B, is capable of activating trypsinogen to trypsin.
  - *Inappropriate activation of trypsinogen:* The inappropriate activation of trypsinogen is an important triggering event in acute pancreatitis. Pancreatic enzymes (including trypsin) are synthesized in an inactive proenzyme form. When trypsin is inappropriately activated, it in turn activates other proenzymes like

prophospholipase and proelastase into active forms. The actived enzyme lipase degrade fat cells and elastase damage the elastic fibers of blood vessels. Trypsin also activates kinin system, Hageman factor (factor XII), coagulation and complement systems.

- **Second phase:** It involves the activation, chemoattraction and sequestration of neutrophils into the pancreas, resulting in an intrapancreatic inflammatory reaction of variable severity. Leukocyte release cytokines which is responsible for local inflammation and interstitial edema. Edema may decrease the local blood flow and cause further ischemic damage to acinar cells
- **Third phase:** It is due to the effects of activated proteolytic enzymes and cytokines, released by the inflamed pancreas, on distant organs. Activated proteolytic enzymes, especially trypsin, not only digest pancreatic and peripancreatic tissues but also activate other enzymes such as elastase and phospholipase. The active enzymes protease digest cellular membranes and cause parenchymal cell necrosis. The activated lipase cause fat necrosis and the elastase disrupt the vessel wall leading to hemorrhage. Cell injury and death result in the liberation of bradykinin, vasoactive substances and histamine which produce vasodilation, increased vascular permeability, and edema with effects on many organs. Thus it may lead to systemic inflammatory response syndrome (SIRS) and acute respiratory distress syndrome (ARDS) as well as multiorgan failure.

2.2.3 Safety mechanism

The pancreas has many safety mechanisms to prevent autoactivation of zymogens. One of the known mechanism is the pancreatic secretory trypsin inhibitor (PSTI), which is found in secretory granules. It inhibits trypsin activity.

2.3 Morphology

The normal pancreas has a poorly developed capsule and lies close to adjacent structures, which includes the common bile duct, duodenum, splenic vein and transverse colon. Due to this, in acute pancreatitis these are also commonly involved in the inflammatory process. The morphological feature of acute pancreatitis varies from minimal inflammation and edema to severe extensive necrosis and hemorrhage. **[Figure.2]**

2.3.1 Microscopic features: Important features of acute pancreatitis are

- **Leakage of blood vessels causing edema:** Microvascular leakage results in leakage of plasma into the interstitum of pancreas resulting in edema.
- **Acute inflammation: Leukocytes are seen in the interstitial connective tissue of pancreas along with inflammatory fluid exudates.**
- **Enzymatic fat necrosis:** It is produced due to action of lipolytic enzymes-lipase.
- **Proteolytic destruction of pancreatic parenchyma:** It is brought out by the action of protease.
- **Destruction of blood vessels:** The elastase causes destruction of blood vessels and subsequent interstitial hemorrhage.

Depending on the extent of severity of inflammatory reaction, acute pancreatitis -

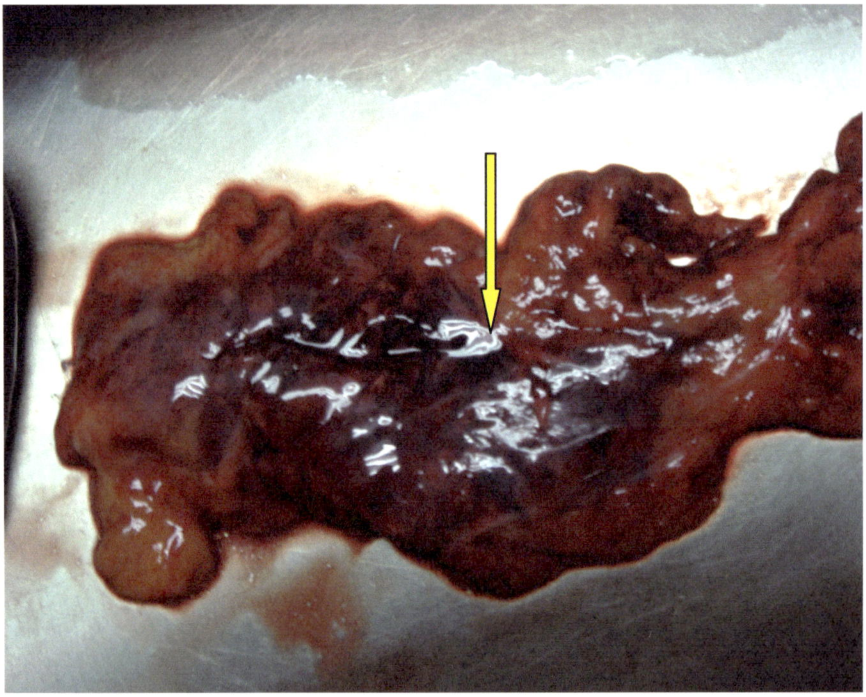

Fig. 2. The Morphological Feature Of Acute Pancreatitis

2.3.2 They are classified into three types

2.3.2.1 Acute interstitial or edematous pancreatitis:

It is a mild and reversible form of acute pancreatitis. It is usually managed medically.

Microscopy: It shows interstitial edema and mild infiltratation of polymorphonuclear leukocytes, without any necrosis or hemorrhage. There may be focal areas of fat necrosis in the substance of the pancreas and in peripancreatic fat. Fat necrosis is due to the action of lipase on triglycerides which releases fatty acids from the fat cells. These fatty acids combine with calcium and form insoluble salts and this process is known as saponification. The insoluble salts impart a granular blue appearance to the involved fat cells.

2.3.2.2 Acute necrotizing pancreatitis

It is the severe form of **acute pancreatitis** in which the acinar, ductal tissues and islets of Langerhans show necrotic changes **[Figure.2.]**

Hemorrhage: Vascular injury due to the enzyme elastase can lead to hemorrhage into the parenchyma of the pancreas, which shows areas of red-black areas of hemorrhage in the substance of pancreas.

Fat necrosis: Foci of fat necrosis is seen both in the pancreatic and extra-pancreatic fat. The extra pancreatic tissue which may show fat necrosis includes: omentum, mesentery of the bowel and outside the abdominal cavity (subcutaneous fat). As a result of deposition of calcium in the area of fat necrosis (saponification), the blood calcium level may be decreased, sometimes to the level of causing neuromuscular irritability.

Peritoneal cavity: In majority of cases, the peritoneal cavity contains a serous, slightly turbid, brown-tinged fluid in which globules of fat (derived from the action of enzymes on adipose tissue) can be seen **[Figure.3].**

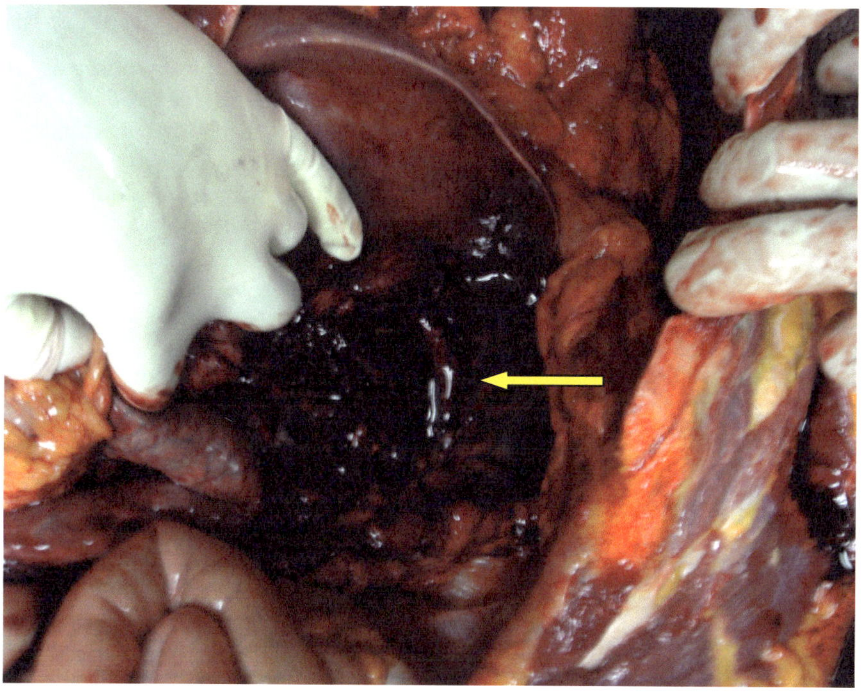

Fig. 3. Peritoneal Cavity In Acute Pancreatitis

- Microscopy:
  - Edema: It is due to leakage through microvasculature.
  - Acute inflammation
  - Enzymatic fat necrosis: It appears granular blue with ghost outlines.
  - Proteolytic destruction of pancreatic parenchyma: Acinar and ductal tissues as well as the islets of Langerhans are necrotic.
  - Destruction of blood vessels (elastase) and subsequent interstitial hemorrhage.

2.3.2.3 Acute hemorrhagic pancreatitis

It is the most severe form of acute **pancreatitis. It u**sually occurs in the **middle aged** and is associated with **high morbidity and mortality**. Microscopically, it shows **extensive parenchymal necrosis** accompanied by **hemorrhage** within the pancreas.

The above features linked with the clinical features, laboratory findings and recent investigative procedures help in diagnosing acute pancreatitis with ease. The effective treatment modalities in recent years will insist on efficient interpretation of patho-physiology in acute pancreatitis so as to ensure a speedy recovery from the cause.

2.4 Clinical features

Abdominal pain is the major manifestation of acute pancreatitis. The pain may vary from mild and tolerable to severe, constant and incapacitating distress. Characteristically, the pain is steady and intense, located in the epigastrium and periumbilical region. It often radiates to the upper back as well as to the chest, flanks, and lower abdomen . Anorexia, nausea, vomiting and abdominal distention due to gastric and intestinal hypomotility and chemical peritonitis also frequently accompany the pain.

Full-blown acute pancreatitis usually present with sudden calamitous onset of an "acute abdomen" and is a medical emergency. Many of the systemic features of severe acute pancreatitis are due to release of toxic enzymes, cytokines, and other mediators into the circulation and activation of the systemic inflammatory response. These mediators result in leukocytosis, hemolysis, disseminated intravascular coagulation, fluid sequestration, acute respiratory distress syndrome, and diffuse fat necrosis. Peripheral vascular collapse and shock with acute renal tubular necrosis may also occur.

2.5 Laboratory findings

Marked elevation of serum amylase levels during the first 24 hours, followed within 72 to 96 hours by a rising serum lipase level.

Hyperglycemia is common and is due to multiple factors, including decreased insulin release, increased glucagon release, and an increased output of adrenal glucocorticoids and catecholamines. Glycosuria occurs in 10% of cases.

Hypocalcemia may result from precipitation of calcium soaps in necrotic fat; if persistent, it is a poor prognostic sign.

Hypertriglyceridemia occurs in 15 to 20% of patients, and serum amylase and lipase levels in these individuals are often spuriously normal.

Direct visualization of the enlarged inflamed pancreas by radiography is useful in the diagnosis of pancreatitis.

2.6 Complications of pancreatitis

Complication	Mechanism
Local pancreatic complications	
Necrosis	Inflammation
Abscess	Localised collection of necrotic material
Pseudocyst	Disruption of pancreatic ducts
Pancreatic ascites	Disruption of pancreatic ducts
Systemic complications	
Acute respiratory distress syndrome (ARDS)	Hypoxia due to microthrombi in the pulmonary vessels.
Hypocalcemia	Sequestration of calcium in fat necrosis
Hyperglycemia	Disruption of islets of Langerhans with altered insulin/glucagon release
Gastrointestinal complications	
Upper GI bleeding	Gastric /duodenal erosions
Duodenal obstruction	Compression by pancreatic mass/pseudocyst
Obstructive jaundice	Compression by pancreatic mass/pseudocyst

2.7 Treatment

In the majority of patients (85–90%) acute pancreatitis is self-limited and subsides spontaneously, usually within 3–7 days after treatment is started. About 5% with severe acute pancreatitis die from shock during the first week. Acute respiratory distress syndrome and acute renal failure are dangerous complications

The key to the management of acute pancreatitis is "resting" the pancreas by total restriction of oral intake and by supportive therapy. Conventional mode of treatment include

1. Analgesics for pain,
2. Intravenous fluids and colloids to maintain normal intravascular volume, and
3. No oral alimentation.

The nasogastric suction has no clear-cut advantages in the treatment of mild to moderately severe acute pancreatitis. Therefore, it must be considered elective rather than mandatory. The drugs which block pancreatic secretion have not found to be of any benefit. For this and other reasons, anticholinergic drugs are not indicated in acute pancreatitis.

Role of antibiotics: The benefit of antibiotic prophylaxis in the treatment of necrotizing acute pancreatitis remains controversial. It was observed that there is no benefit of antibiotic prophylaxis with regard to the risk of developing infected pancreatic necrosis.

3. Conclusion

These features linked with the clinical features, laboratory findings and recent investigative procedures will help in diagnosing acute pancreatitis with ease. The effective treatment modalities in recent years will insist on efficient interpretation of patho-physiology in acute pancreatitis so as to ensure a speedy recovery from the cause.

4. References

[1] Hruban RH, Iac0buzio-Donahue C: The pancreas, In Kumar V, Abbas AK, Fausto N, Aster JC; Robbins and Cotran Pathologic Basis of Disease, 8th ed. Philadelphia: WB Saunders, 2009.

[2] Frossard JL, et al: Acute pancreatitis. Lancet 371:143, 2008.

[3] Mitchell RM, et al: Pancreatitis. Lancet 361:1447, 2003.

[4] Cappell MS: Acute pancreatitis: etiology, clinical presentation, diagnosis and therapies. Med Clin North Am 92:889, 2008.

[5] Carroll JK, et al: Acute pancreatitis: diagnosis, prognosis, and treatment. Am Fam Physician 75:1513, 2007.

[6] Granger J, Remick D: Acute pancreatitis: models, markers, and mediators. Shock 24:45, 2005.

[7] Sand J, et al: Alcohol consumption in patients with acute or chronic pancreatitis. Pancreatology 7:147, 2007.

[8] Vonlaufen A, et al: Molecular mechanisms of pancreatitis: current opinion. J Gastroenterol Hepatol 23:1339, 2008.

[9] Kanchan T, Shetty M, Nagesh KR, Khadilkar U, Shetty BSK, Menon A, Menezes RG, Rastogi P. Acute haemorrhagic pancreatitis- a case of sudden death. J Forensic Leg Med. 2009 ;16(2):101-3

[10] Shetty BS, Boloor A, Menezes RG, Shetty M, Menon A, Nagesh KR, Pai MR, Mathai AM, Rastogi P, Kanchan T, Naik R, Salian PR, Jain V, George AT.Postmortem diagnosis of acute haemorrhagic pancreatitis. Journal of Forensic and Legal Medicine. 2010; 17: 316-320.

2

Acute Biliary Pancreatitis

Morgan Rosenberg[1], Ariel Klevan[2] and Eran Shlomovitz[1]
[1]*University of Toronto,*
[2]*University of Miami,*
[1]*Canada*
[2]*USA*

1. Introduction

More than 220,000 patients are admitted to hospital each year with acute pancreatitis in the United States alone.[1] The most common etiology of acute pancreatitis is gallstones. This chapter will focus on diagnostic and management issues related to acute biliary pancreatitis (ABP). Differentiating gallstone-induced acute pancreatitis from other etiologies (alcohol, medication induced, hypertriglyceridemia) should be prioritized in the initial investigation of acute pancreatitis as ABP has its own specific management considerations.

2. Epidemiology

Cholelithiasis, or gallstones, are present in up to 10% of the general population. Risk factors for developing gallstones include female sex, advancing age, ethnicity and genetics, obesity and the metabolic syndrome, rapid weight loss, high fat low fiber diet, pregnancy, and certain disease states such as cirrhosis and Crohn's disease.[2] Gallstones are present in 35-75% of all patients with acute pancreatitis in developed nations.[3,4] Up to 8% of patients with symptomatic gallstones will develop biliary pancreatitis due to migration into the bile duct, and ABP may be the initial presentation of gallstones in up to 40% of previously asymptomatic patients.[5] The yearly incidence of ABP is estimated at 4.9-80.0 cases per 100,000 population in the United States. Although most cases of ABP are mild and self-limited, case fatality rates as high as 15% have been reported in severe cases.[6] Risk factors for ABP include female gender with a ratio of 2:1 over males, age, with an incidence of ABP

---

[1] Whitcomb DC. Clinical practice. Acute pancreatitis. *NEJM*. 2006;354:2142-2150.

[2] Shaffer SA. Epidemiology of gallbladder stone disease. *Best Practice and Research Clinical Gastroenterology* 2006;20:981-996.

[3] van Geenen EJM, van der Preet DL, Bhagirath R, et al. Etiology and diagnosis of acute biliary pancreatitis. *Gastroenterology & Hepatology*. 2010;7:495-502.

[4] Agrawal S, Jonnalagadda S. Gallstones, from gallbladder to gut. Management options for diverse complications. *Postgraduate Medicine*. 2000;108:143-153.

[5] van Erpecum KJ. Complications of bile-duct stones: acute cholangitis and pancreatitis. *Best Practice & Research Clinical Gastroenterology*. 2006;20:1139-1152.

[6] Kaw M, Al-Antably Y, Kaw P. Management of of gallstone pancreatitis: cholecystectomy or ERCP and endoscopic sphincterotomy. *Gastrointestinal Endoscopy*.2002;56:61-65.

over 3 times higher at age 75 compared with age 20, and ethnicity, with increased incidence in those of white and Hispanic backgrounds.[7]

3. Pathogenesis

The exact pathogenesis of acute biliary pancreatitis is unclear. Several structural and genetic explanations are supported in the current literature.

3.1 Structural

One mechanism involves obstruction of the common bile and pancreatic ducts as gallstones migrate down and become impacted in the ampulla of Vater. Classic observational studies revealed gallstones may be retrieved from the stool of patients with biliary pancreatitis in >90% of cases as compared to approximately 10% of patients with symptomatic gallstones in the absence of pancreatitis, and in no patients with alcohol induced pancreatitis.[8,9] The precise mechanism of how the gallstones passing through the ampulla initiate and sustain pancreatic inflammation is unknown. It seems just the passage of material through the ampulla of Vater without overt obstruction may be enough to initiate pancreatitis as in the case of sludge containing microlithiasis. In this situation, passage of material through the ampulla may lead to spasm or local edema of the sphincter of Oddi resulting in temporary obstruction. Episodes of recurrent acute pancreatitis caused by microlithiasis may be significantly reduced by cholecystectomy or endoscopic sphincterotomy (ES).

A second mechanism involves reflux of infected bile into the pancreatic duct. The inflammation associated with cholangitis may extend as far as the pancreas initiating the episode of acute pancreatitis. Normal pressures in the pancreatic duct are well above pressures in the common bile duct (CBD), preventing reflux of bile into the pancreatic duct under physiologic conditions. With ampullary obstruction secondary to passing gallstones, pressure gradients may shift, allowing flow of bile and pancreatic juice back into the pancreatic duct. Studies have shown sterile refluxate does not cause acute pancreatitis, however infected bile (especially with *Escherichia coli*) or mixtures of bile and pancreatic juice can lead to acute pancreatitis.[10]

Gallstone-related factors have also been implicated as they relate to the number and frequency of gallstones that pass into the common bile duct and through the ampulla of Vater as well as the likelihood of obstruction. These factors include small size (<2-5mm), higher number (>20) of gallstones in the gallbladder, irregular surface of the gallstones, good emptying of the gallbladder with meals, and cystic duct width over 5mm. Next, bile duct anatomy including an enlarged CBD (>1.3mm), a wide angle between the CBD and pancreatic duct, and a common pancreaticobiliary channel may also predispose to acute

[7] van Geenen EJM, van der Preet DL, Bhagirath R, et al. Etiology and diagnosis of acute biliary pancreatitis. *Gastroenterology & Hepatology*. 2010;7:495-502.
[8] Acosta JM, Ledesma CL. Gallstone migration as a cause of acute pancreatitis. NEJM. 1974;290:484-487.
[9] Acosta JM, Rossi R, Ledesma CL. The usefulness of stool screening for diagnosing cholelithiasis in acute pancreatitis. A description of the technique. *American Journal of Digestive Diseases*. 1977;22:168-172.
[10] van Geenen EJM, van der Preet DL, Bhagirath R, et al. Etiology and diagnosis of acute biliary pancreatitis. *Gastroenterology & Hepatology*. 2010;7:495-502.

biliary pancreatitis. Patients with a history of ABP were found to be twice as likely to have a common pancreaticobiliary channel when compared to those with choledocholithiasis and cholelithiasis without a history of pancreatitis.[11]

3.2 Genetic

Genetic variations and mutations have been well described in idiopathic pancreatitis, and it appears that genetics may play a role in selected circumstances of biliary pancreatitis as well. Marschall et al. recently published a review of the genetic basis for gallstone formation and symptomatic gallstone disease including the development of biliary pancreatitis.[12] Using data from 43,141 mono- and dizygotic twins born between 1900 and 1958, they calculated that genetics account for up to 25% of the phenotypic variation among twins. As cholesterol stones account for over 90% of all gallstones, metabolic pathways involved in the formation of cholesterol stones have been studied. Bile is made up of water and three lipid components, namely cholesterol (4%), phospholipids (24%), and bile salts (72%). Genes encoding for transport proteins have been identified for each of these components with varying significance for the risk of ABP.

One such susceptibility locus is the D19H variant of *ABCG8*, a cholesterol transport protein. This allele increases the *ABCG5/8* mediated transfer of cholesterol into bile, resulting in biliary cholesterol hypersaturation, a necessary pre-requisite for cholesterol stones. Marschall et al. determined an odds ratio of 2.5 (95% CI 1.3-4.8) for the formation of symptomatic gallstones disease in 341 Swedish twins with at least one D19H allele.

Cases of recurrent ABP have been associated with a mutation in the *ABCB4* gene, which encodes for multidrug resistant p-glycoprotein MDR3, a protein involved translocation of phospholipids from the inner to the outer leaflet of the canalicular membrane of hepatocytes. Point mutations in *ABCB4* have been associated with low phospholipid-associated cholelithiasis syndrome, which is characterized by early gallstone disease (<40 years old), intrahepatic sludge and microlithiasis, and recurrent biliary disease after cholecystectomy. Mutations in *ABCB4* have also been associated with several other hepatobiliary diseases including intrahepatic cholestasis of pregnancy, progressive familial intrahepatic cholestasis type 3, and adult biliary cirrhosis.[13,14]

Bile salts are the third lipid component with several susceptibility loci identified. The *ABCB11* gene, encoding the bile salt export pump (BSEP), has been found as a rare cause of cholesterol stones with less than 2% of young adults being heterozygous for functionally relevant mutations. Expression of ABC transporters *ABCB11* and *ABCB4* are induced by the farnesoid X receptor (FXR), a bile acid sensor that regulates hepatic bile acid synthesis, uptake, and excretion genes, as well as other genes involved with turnover of cholesterol

---

[11] van Geenen EJM, van der Preet DL, Bhagirath R, et al. Etiology and diagnosis of acute biliary pancreatitis. *Gastroenterology & Hepatology*. 2010;7:495-502.

[12] Marschall HU, Katsika D, Rudling M, Einarsson C. The genetic background of gallstone formation: an update. *Biochemical and Biophysical Research Communications*. 2010;396:58-62.

[13] van Geenen EJM, van der Preet DL, Bhagirath R, et al. Etiology and diagnosis of acute biliary pancreatitis. *Gastroenterology & Hepatology*. 2010;7:495-502.

[14] Marschall HU, Katsika D, Rudling M, Einarsson C. The genetic background of gallstone formation: an update. *Biochemical and Biophysical Research Communications*. 2010;396:58-62.

and glucose homeostasis. The reduction in bile acid synthesis that results is associated with increased cholesterol gallstone formation. The A105G variant of the *SLC10A2* gene, encoding the apical sodium-dependent bile acid transporter (ASBT) was also identified as a risk factor for cholesterol stones with an odds ratio of 2.04 (95% CI 1.19-3.55).[15]

4. Diagnosis

The presentation of acute pancreatitis may be quite similar whether the etiologic basis is biliary or non-biliary in origin. This makes distinguishing acute biliary pancreatitis from other etiologies somewhat challenging. Certain clues may exist on history and physical examination, however laboratory investigations and abdominal imaging are often required for a more definitive diagnosis.

4.1 Clinical presentation

Abdominal pain, classically severe epigastric pain radiating to the back that is worse in the supine position, is a hallmark of acute pancreatitis of any etiology. The abdominal pain may worsen over the course of several hours and may be associated with nausea and vomiting. Patients may also report worsening of their pain following meals. Due to the significant inflammatory process and release of cytokines, fever is another common manifestation. Still, most patients will have a mild, self-limited course of their biliary pancreatitis. In one early series of 153 patients with ABP, only twenty-two (14%) were febrile and thirty (20%) were volume depleted. Eighty-one (53%) had right upper quadrant tenderness, and seventy-one (46%) had mid-epigastric tenderness. Notably, twenty-one (14%) had completely benign abdominal examinations, and only nine patients (6%) had diffuse peritonitis.16

During an episode of acute pancreatitis, pancreatic enzymes, vasoactive materials such as kinins, and other toxic substances extravasate from the pancreas into surrounding areas resulting in chemical irritation and contribute to third space losses that may lead to hypovolemia, tachycardia, and hypotension. In this situation, the abdomen may also become distended and tympanic due to paralytic ileus. When toxic mediators reach the systemic circulation, the corresponding systemic inflammatory response syndrome (SIRS) may be severe and result in end-organ damage including acute respiratory distress syndrome (ARDS) and acute kidney injury. Hemorrhagic pancreatitis may lead to the classic Cullen's sign, with ecchymosis in the periumbilical region, and Grey Turner's sign, with ecchymosis of the flank.

History of known gallstones, especially symptomatic gallstone disease such as biliary colic may indicate a biliary etiology, although it cannot rule out other etiologies of acute pancreatitis, nor can the absence of gallstones rule out a biliary source, as pancreatitis can be the first presentation of gallstone disease, and sludge and microcalculi are still a possibility. The absence of other associated etiologies including significant alcohol intake, initiation of medications known to be associated with pancreatitis, recent endoscopic retrograde cholangiopancreatography (ERCP), and known hypertriglyceridemia or hypercalcemia may

[15] Marschall HU, Katsika D, Rudling M, Einarsson C. The genetic background of gallstone formation: an update. *Biochemical and Biophysical Research Communications*. 2010;396:58-62.
[16] Frel G, Frel V, Thirlby R, McClelland R. Biliary pancreatitis: clinical presentation and surgical management. *American Journal of Surgery* 1986;151:170-175.

also lead to the diagnosis of ABP. Scleral icterus or overt jaundice may be associated with acute pancreatitis in select cases due to edema of the head of the pancreas or an obstructing stone in the case of biliary pancreatitis. History and physical examination should also aim to rule out mimickers of pancreatitis including acute cholecystitis, perforated duodenal ulcer, intestinal obstruction, mesenteric ischemia, or ruptured aneurysm amongst other etiologies.

4.2 Biochemistry

The diagnosis of pancreatitis of any etiology is classically made with elevations in serum amylase and lipase. Enzyme levels tend to rise within 4 - 8 hours of onset, peak around 24 hours, and return to normal between 2 - 14 days after onset of acute pancreatitis. Lipase has a longer half-life, up to 12 hours, compared to a half-life of only 2 hours for serum amylase, and thus lasts several days longer in the bloodstream. Most would consider elevations in amylase and lipase upwards of three times the upper limit of normal significant in the diagnosis of acute pancreatitis. However, in one retrospective study of 284 patients with a first episode of acute pancreatitis, over 30% of patients had amylase levels below three times the upper limits of normal and 18% had lipase levels below three times the upper limit of normal.[17] They did show that patients with a biliary origin of their acute pancreatitis were significantly ($p = 0.007$) more likely to have elevations in serum amylase over three times the normal limit compared to non-biliary etiologies. This study also determined that there was no association between level of elevation of enzymes and severity of disease looking at factors such as development of pseudocysts, renal impairment and need for dialysis, ICU admission requiring ventilatory support, need for surgery, and overall mortality.[18]

It is important, however, to remember that a long differential diagnosis exists for elevations in serum amylase and lipase. Other pancreatic diseases, acute cholecystitis or cholangitis, post-ERCP, trauma, bowel obstruction or ischemia, and medications may lead to elevations in both serum amylase and lipase. Additionally, renal impairment, penetrating peptic ulcer disease, salivary disease, several solid tumors and multiple myeloma, and gynecologic disease can raise serum amylase but not serum lipase, making lipase a more specific serum marker.

With a diagnosis of acute pancreatitis made, biliary etiology may be determined using several serum markers, especially serum alanine aminotransferase (ALT). As with serum amylase and lipase, elevations over three times the upper limit of normal are considered significant, however, up to 15% of patients with biliary pancreatitis will have normal liver enzymes.[19] There is also a differential diagnosis for elevations in ALT, most significantly alcohol (the second leading cause of acute pancreatitis in Western countries), viral hepatitis, and non-alcoholic fatty liver disease.

There have been several studies looking at the diagnosis of biliary pancreatitis through the use of ALT, either alone or in combination with other serum markers. Early studies looked

---

[17] Lankisch PG, Burchard-Reckert S, Lehnick D. Underestimation of acute pancreatitis: patients with only a small increase in amylase/lipase levels can also have or develop severe acute pancreatitis. *Gut.* 1999;44:542-544.

[18] Lankisch PG, Burchard-Reckert S, Lehnick D. Underestimation of acute pancreatitis: patients with only a small increase in amylase/lipase levels can also have or develop severe acute pancreatitis. *Gut.* 1999;44:542-544.

[19] van Geenen EJM, van der Preet DL, Bhagirath R, et al. Etiology and diagnosis of acute biliary pancreatitis. *Gastroenterology & Hepatology.* 2010;7:495-502.

at using multiple serum and urine biomarkers and occasionally clinical data to distinguish biliary from non-biliary etiologies. One such study developed a scoring system using seven variables including serum and urine amylase, serum AST and ALT, ALP, lipase/amylase ratio, and erythrocyte mean corpuscular volume (MCV) to differentiate biliary from alcoholic pancreatitis.[20] Each parameter was given a single point, and a score of 4 or greater out of 7 was significantly correlated to a biliary etiology of pancreatitis ($p < 0.0001$), and a score below 4/7 correlated with alcoholic etiology with a sensitivity of 92% and specificity of 94%. On the other hand, Davidson et al. argued against multi-factor systems in their study that compared test characteristics of a one-, three-, and five-factor test for biliary pancreatitis.[21] The one-factor test used serum ALT and aspartate aminotransferase (AST) alone, the three-factor test used alkaline phosphatase (ALP) and bilirubin in addition to transaminases, and the five-factor test included clinical data such as age and female sex, as well as amylase, alkaline phosphatase, and transaminases. In their study, the one- and three-factor tests performed slightly better than the five-factor test, and thus using serum transaminases alone were recommended for simplicity.

More recent studies have lent support for single-factor systems. One study looked at serum ALT ≥ 80 (U/L) in a cohort of 68 patients with acute pancreatitis, of which 44 (65%) had a biliary etiology.[22] They demonstrated that serum ALT ≥ 80 (two times the upper limit of normal) had a sensitivity of 91%, specificity of 100%, positive predictive value (PPV) of 100% and negative predictive value (NPV) of 86%. Combined with abdominal ultrasound, test characteristics improved somewhat with a sensitivity of 98%, specificity of 100%, PPV of 100% and NPV of 96%. A subsequent study looked at a cohort of 213 patients, of which 62% had ABP confirmed with endoscopic ultrasound (EUS), and found serum ALT levels over two times the upper limit of normal had a sensitivity of 74%, specificity of 84%, PPV of 88%, and NPV of 66% for predicting a biliary etiology, whereas serum ALT levels over three times the upper limit of normal had a sensitivity of 61%, specificity of 91%, PPV of 92%, and NPV of 59%.

4.3 Abdominal imaging

The contribution of medical imaging to the diagnosis and evaluation of pancreatitis has evolved substantially. Early plain film description of the effects of pancreatic inflammation on the intra-abdominal bowel gas pattern has emerged over 50 years ago. Despite today's widespread use of modern imaging technology including MRCP, these alterations in bowel gas patterns remain an occasional useful adjunct in the diagnosis of pancreatitis.

Various abdominal film patterns have been described and may be occasionally seen in the setting of pancreatitis. One of the better described is the "colon cutoff sign". In this pattern a dilated transverse colon appears to be abruptly cutoff occasionally simulating the appearance of colonic obstruction. This pattern is likely related to inflammation of the phrenicocolic ligament causing spasm or occasionally actual mechanical narrowing in the

---

[20] Stimac D, Lenac T, Marusic Z. A scoring system for early differentiation of the etiology of acute pancreatitis. *Scandinavian Journal of Gastroenterology* 1998;33:209-211.

[21] Davidson BR, Neoptolemos JP, Leese T, Carr-Locke DL. Biochemical prediction of gallstones in acute pancreatitis: a prospective study of three systems. *British Journal of Surgery* 1988;75:213-215.

[22] Ammori BJ, Boreham B, Lewis P, Roberts SA. The biochemical detection of biliary etiology of acute pancreatitis on admission: a revisit in the modern era of biliary imaging. *Pancreas* 2003;26(2):e32-e35.

region of the splenic flexure. This appearance is further accentuated on the background of an adynamic colon. Additional imaging findings may include a mottled appearance of the peripancreatic region secondary to fat necrosis or peripancreatic gas in the setting of suppurative pancreatitis. Numerous other non-specific signs in the setting of pancreatitis have been described including ascites, left sided pleural effusion and diaphragmatic elevation. Needless to say all these signs require additional imaging modalities, clinical and biochemical correlation for to establish the diagnosis.

4.3.1 Ultrasonography

Despite its dependence on operator skill and patient's body habitus ultrasonography has become a mainstay in the imaging of suspected biliary pancreatitis. In the setting of acute inflammation the pancreas may appear focally or diffusely enlarged, as well as relatively hypoechoic secondary to parenchymal edema. This is a reversal of the normal pattern in which the pancreas is echogenic relative to the adjacent liver. The main utility of sonography however is in its ability to image the biliary system in the search for cholelithiasis/choledocholithiasis as the etiology in order to guide further management. The widespread availability, sensitivity and relatively low cost of ultrasonography makes it particularly suitable for this role. Biliary stones typically appear as echogenic foci with posterior clean shadowing (Figure 1). Small stones and sludge however may not demonstrate posterior shadowing. Stones are more easily appreciated in the setting of biliary dilatation although distal CBD stones may remain obscured by overlying bowel gas.

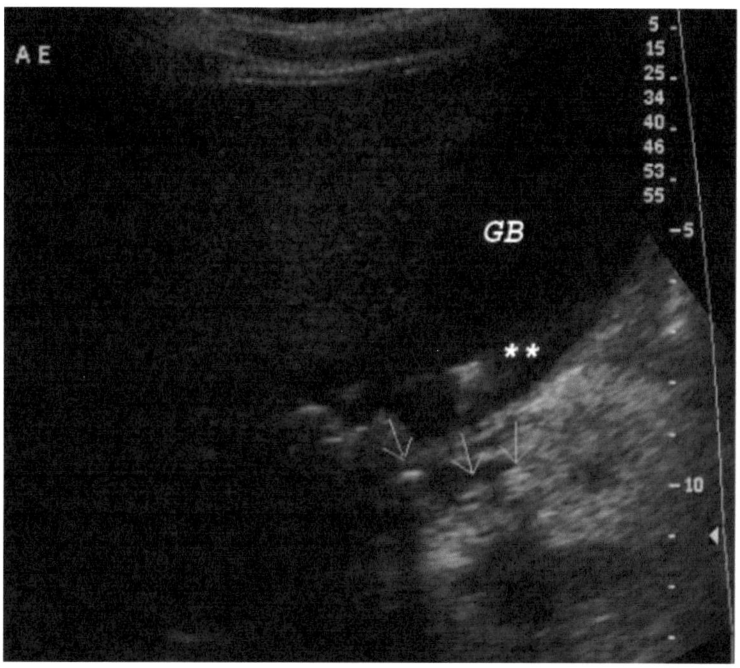

Fig. 1. Sonographic image demonstrating the typical appearance of CBD stones. Three stones (arrows) are visualized within a mildly dilated distal CBD. The stones appear as echogenic foci with posterior shadowing (best appreciated in the most proximal stone). Layering sludge and stones (asterisks) are also appreciated within the gallbladder (GB).

4.3.2 Computed tomography

Computed tomography (CT) has unique advantages in the evaluation of pancreatitis. It is relatively cheaper, non-invasive and more available as compared to ERCP and its sensitivity does not depend on the sonographer or the patient's body habitus as is the case with ultrasound. An inflamed pancreas may appear enlarged and heterogeneous with surrounding inflammatory changes. CT is also particularly useful is the evaluation of pancreatic necrosis, pseudocyst formation or other secondary complications of pancreatitis.

In the evaluation of a biliary cause of pancreatitis, CT however does have a significant weakness as up to 25% of biliary stones may be isodense to bile and therefore poorly visualized. Visible CBD stones may appear as a dense intraluminal mass with the so called "target sign" (Figure 2). As with other modalities, CBD dilatation may signal an underlying obstructing stone or mass and may require further evaluation with other methods in order to elucidate the underlying cause.

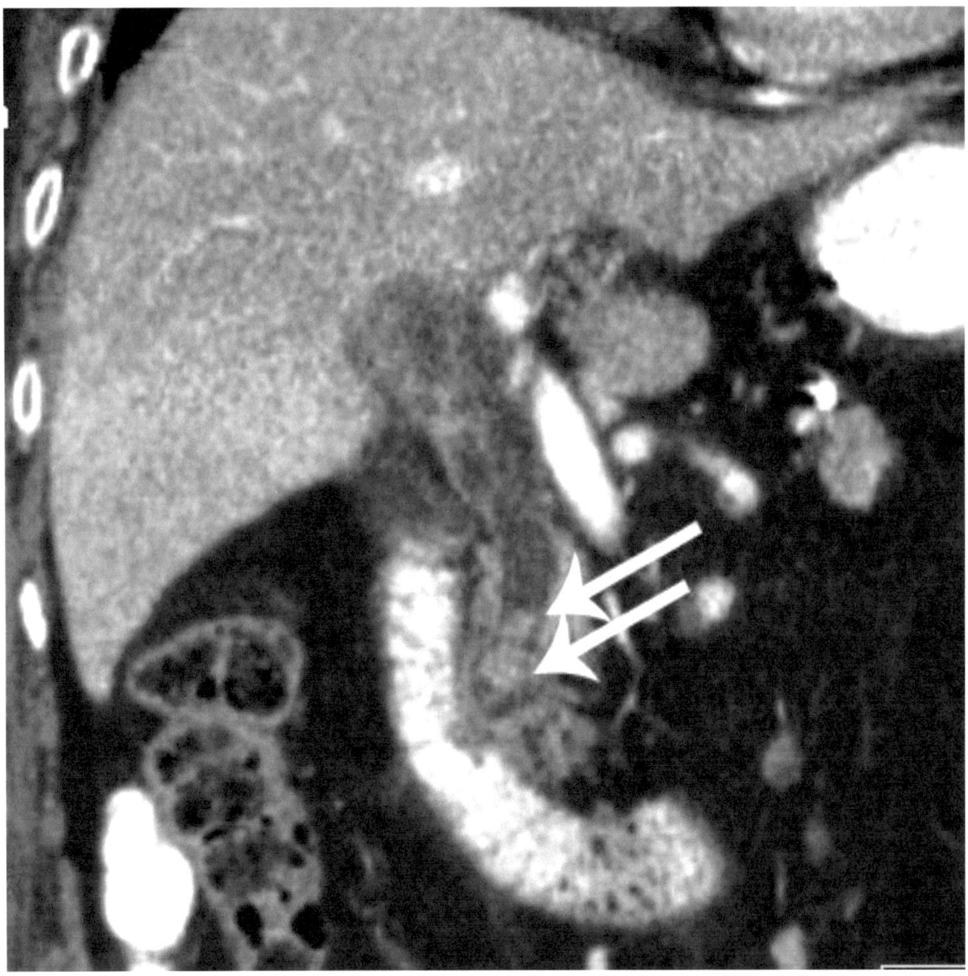

Fig. 2. Coronal reformatted CT centered on the distal CBD. Two dense stones(arrows) are noted in the distal CBD. The CBD is dilated secondary to the obstructing stones.

4.3.3 Magnetic resonance cholangiopancreatography

Magnetic resonance cholangiopancreatography (MRCP) is the most sensitive and specific non-invasive method of assessing the biliary system for choledocholithiasis as an underlying etiology for pancreatitis. MRCP uses a heavily T2 weighted sequence which highlights the biliary ducts due to their high water content. The signal of the surrounding soft tissues saturates out, thus allowing for exquisite visualization of the bright bile ducts in the background of low intensity surrounding soft tissues (Figure 3). In this setting biliary duct stones appear as dark signal voids within the bright bile fluid (Figure 4).

MRCP is comparable to ERCP with respect to its sensitivity in the detection of choledocholithiasis (Table 1). Although MRCP has lower special resolution as compared to ERCP and therapeutic interventions cannot be performed, it does afford several advantages. MRCP is non-invasive, it is less operator dependent, does not use ionizing radiation, and allows for visualization of the surrounding tissues when combined with additional MR sequences. Major disadvantages of MRCP include increased cost, decreased availability in many centers, and it requires a compliant patient to lie still and flat for 30-60 minutes, which may be difficult in the setting of acute pancreatitis when patients are in a significant amount of pain that may be worsened by a supine position.

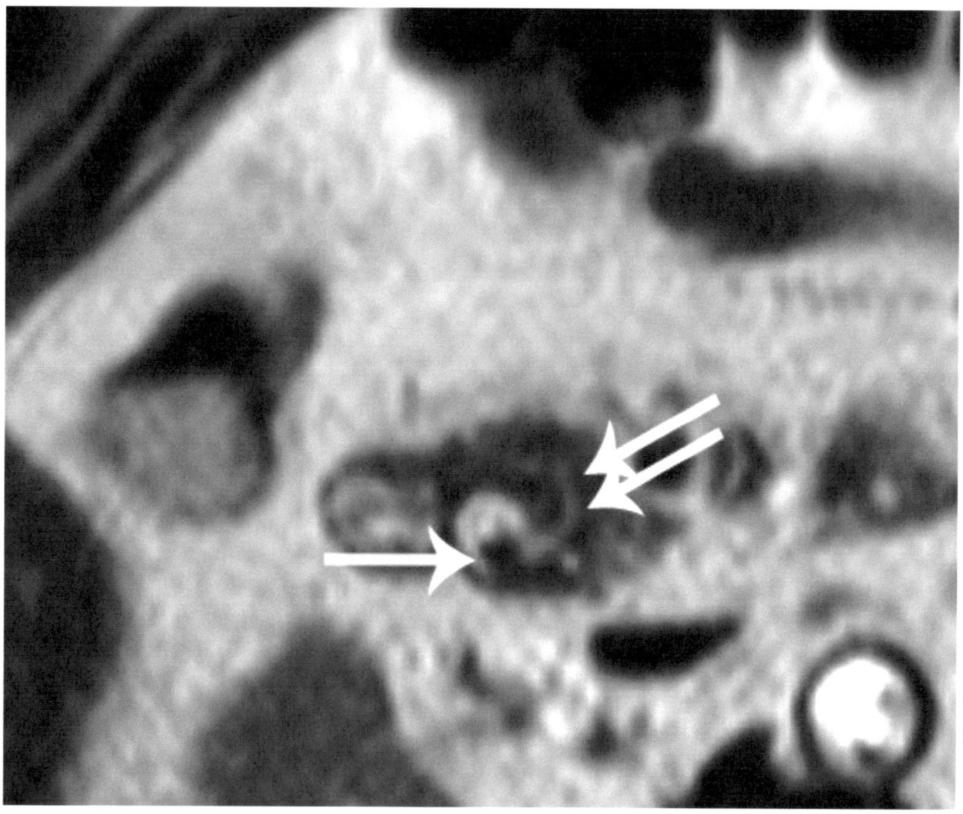

Fig. 3. Axial T2 image obtained as a part of the MRCP study demonstrating a stone at the distal CBD (arrow). The insertion point of the pancreatic duct into the distal CBD near the ampulla is also well visualized (double arrows). *Courtesy of Dr. Y. Krakowsky.*

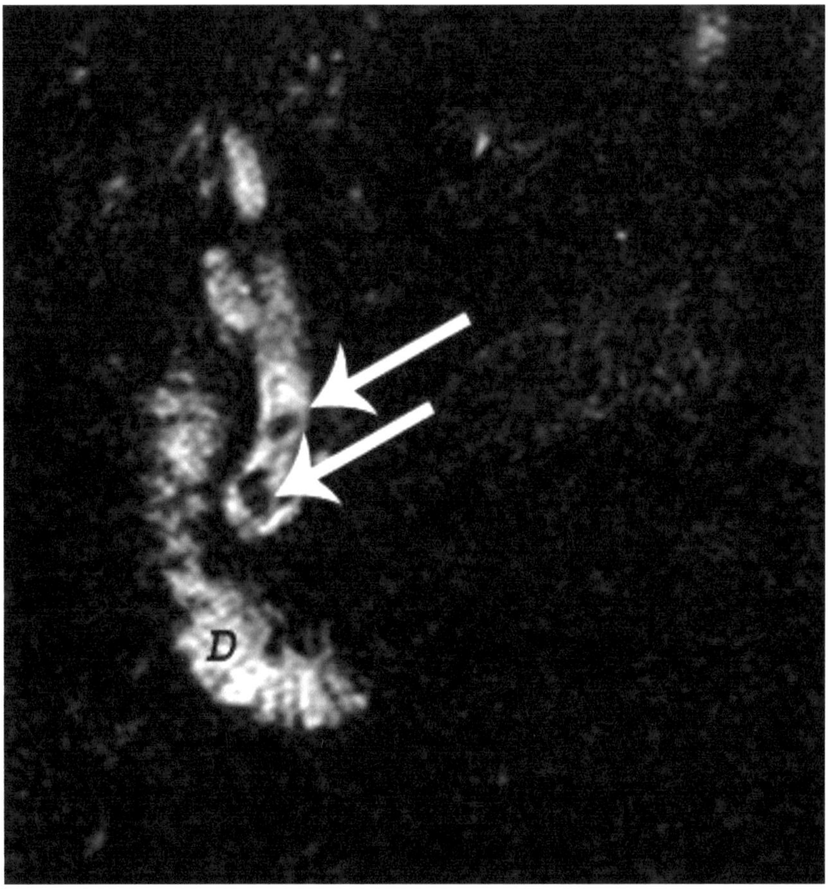

Fig. 4. Coronal MRCP image in the same patient at Figure 2. Image demonstrates two signal voids (arrows) on the background of the high intensity bile in the dilated CBD. The high water content intraluminal fluid in the duodenum (D) is also well appreciated.

4.3.4 Endoscopic retrograde cholangiopancreatography

Endoscopic Retrograde Cholangiopancreatography (ERCP) is a highly sensitive and specific test for assessing the biliary tree and in particular looking for choledocholithiasis (Table 1). Using a side-viewing endoscope, the ampulla is identified and cannulated, after which dye is injected into the biliary tree. Stones in the common bile duct show up as a filling defect on fluoroscopic imaging (Figure 5). During ERCP, endoscopic sphincterotomy (ES) may be performed to allow for improved passage of sludge and stones into the duodenum.

ERCP is the only imaging modality that can also be used therapeutically for removing CBD stones and sludge from the common bile duct. However, the major disadvantage to using ERCP for the initial diagnosis of a biliary etiology of pancreatitis is the potential for exacerbating the acute episode of pancreatitis, and therefore this modality should only be used in conjunction with endoscopic sphincterotomy for treatment of impacted stones in jaundiced patients, those with signs and symptoms of biliary sepsis or potentially in severe ABP.

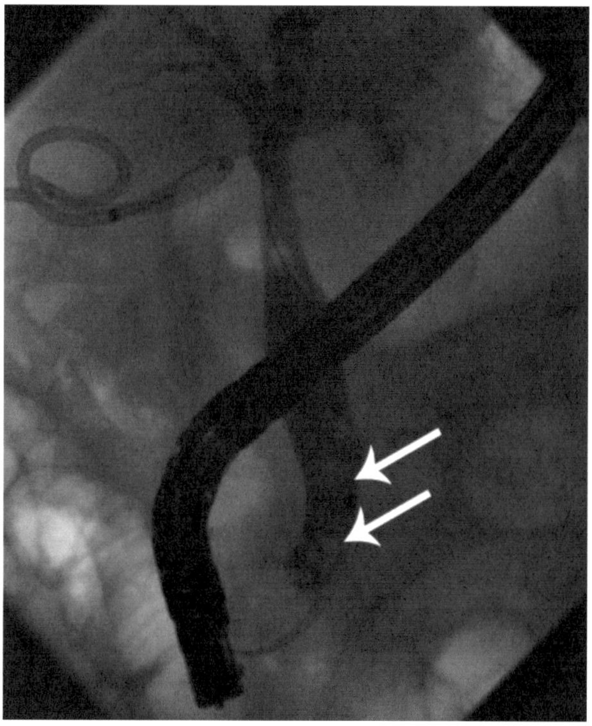

Fig. 5. Fluoroscopic image demonstrating a dilated common bile duct and several common bile duct stones seen as filling defects (arrows) at the time of ERCP.

4.3.5 Endoscopic ultrasound

Endoscopic ultrasound (EUS) has the highest sensitivity and specificity of any imaging modality for the identification of choledocholithiasis (Table 1). It is also a very sensitive technique for visualization of pancreatic lesions, pseudocysts, and elucidating pancreatic ductal anatomy. Like transabdominal ultrasound, EUS is somewhat operator dependent, and access to EUS may be limited in some centers.

Imaging Modality	Sensitivity (%)	Specificity (%)	PPV (%)	NPV (%)
U/S - Gallstones	67-87	93	100	75-80
U/S - CBD Stones	20-50	83	67	39
CT	40	92	89	48
MRCP	80-100	83-98	89	71-100
ERCP	90-100	92	95	85
EUS	91-100	85-100	92-98	88-92

PPV = positive predictive value, NPV = negative predictive value, U/S = ultrasound, CBD = common bile duct, CT = computed tomography, MRCP = magnetic resonance cholangiopancreatography, ERCP = endoscopic retrograde cholangiopancreatography, EUS = endoscopic ultrasound

Table 1. Test characteristics of the common abdominal imaging modalities

5. Assessment of severity

Determining whether a given case of acute pancreatitis is mild or severe has important management and prognostic implications. Those with severe disease (up to 20% of ABP) may require admission to a monitored setting as they have morbidity rates of 30-50% and mortality rates up to 10-30% despite ICU management.[23] Several scoring systems exist, including Ranson's score, which combines 11 clinical data criteria, 5 from the first 24 hours, and the remaining 6 at 48 hours (Table 2). Each criterion is assigned 1 point, with scores ≥3 points representing severe pancreatitis, correlating with a 15% mortality rate, and scores more than 6 points carrying a mortality rate upwards of 50%.

	Non-biliary Pancreatitis	**Biliary Pancreatitis**
On Admission		
Age	>55	>70
WBC (mm^3)	>16,000	>18,000
Blood glucose (mg/dl)	>200	>220
LDH (U/L)	>350	>400
AST (U/L)	>250	>250
48 Hours		
Fall in hematocrit (%)	>10	>10
Rise in BUN (mg/dl)	>5	>2
Calcium (mg/dl)	<8	<8
PaO_2 (mmHg)	<60	<60
Base deficit (mEq/L)	>4	>5
Fluid sequestration (L)	>6	>4

WBC = white blood cell count, LDH = lactate dehydrogenase, AST = aspartate amino-transferase, BUN = blood urea nitrogen, PaO_2 = arterial partial pressure of oxygen

Table 2. Ranson's Criteria of severity for non-biliary and biliary origin of pancreatitis

A second scoring system validated for use in acute pancreatitis is the Acute Physiology and Chronic Health Evaluation (APACHE-II), calculated by adding 12 individual variable points, age points, and chronic health points. A score over 8 represents severe pancreatitis, and a score below 8 is unlikely to result in a fatal outcome. Although the APACHE-II score is cumbersome to calculate, its benefit over Ranson's score is that it can be repeated over the course of illness, whereas Ranson's score applies only to the initial 48 hours after presentation. Another commonly used scoring system is the CT severity index (CTSI), which combines CT grade with extent of necrosis to assign a score that reliably correlates with morbidity and mortality rates (Table 3). A score of 3 or above represents severe pancreatitis with scores 3-6 corresponding to a 35% morbidity and 6% mortality rate, and scores 7-10 corresponding to morbidity and mortality rates of 92% and 17% respectively.[24]

---

[23] Howard T. (2008) Management of gallstone pancreatitis, In: *Current surgical therapy, 9th ed.* Cameron J. pp. 477-480. Mosby Elsevier Inc., ISBN: 978-1-4160-3497-1, Philadelphia.

[24] Howard T. (2008) Management of gallstone pancreatitis, In: *Current surgical therapy, 9th ed.* Cameron J. pp. 477-480. Mosby Elsevier Inc., ISBN: 978-1-4160-3497-1, Philadelphia.

CT Grade	Points	Necrosis (%)	Points	Total CTSI score
A	0			0
B	1	0	0	1
C	2	<30	2	4
D	3	30-50	4	7
E	4	>50	6	10

Grade A = normal pancreas, B = pancreatic enlargement, C = inflammation of the pancreas and/or peripancreatic fat, D = single peripancreatic fluid collection, E = two or more peripancreatic fluid collections and/or retroperitoneal air.

Table 3. CT Severity Index (CTSI).

6. Management

Initial management of biliary pancreatitis is mainly directed at supportive care, limiting complications, and prevention of infection in the case of pancreatic necrosis. All patient are treated with bowel rest, fluid resuscitation, as well as appropriate analgesia and anti-emetics. Attempts should be made to re-institute oral nutrition, preferably post-pyloric with a jejunal nasoenteric feeding tube, however if oral nutrition is to be withheld for more than 5-7 days on the basis of ongoing fever, tachycardia, nausea, vomiting, severe abdominal pain, or leukocytosis, nutritional support with parenteral nutrition should be considered. Severe pancreatitis or development of systemic complications should be managed in a monitored setting such as the intensive care unit. There may be a role for urgent ERCP in select situations with patients who present jaundiced or have evidence of biliary sepsis.

Unique to a biliary origin of pancreatitis is the requirement for definitive removal of the etiologic trigger with cholecystectomy (or ERCP/ES). In severe cases of pancreatitis, cholecystectomy should be delayed at least 3 weeks to minimize the risk of infecting the pancreatic necrosis at the time of surgery. Also, in patients with evidence of large peripancreatic fluid collections, cholecystectomy may be delayed up to 6 weeks to allow for the maturation of a pseudocyst that can be drained at the time of surgery. In a study by Kelly and Wagner, 165 patients presenting with ABP were randomized to early surgery within 48 hours after admission or delayed surgery after 48 hours. The early surgery group was associated with higher rates of morbidity and mortality when compared to the late group with 83 versus 48% for morbidity and 18 versus 12% for mortality.[25]

In the case of mild biliary pancreatitis, practice guidelines from several international societies have recommended early cholecystectomy, but the definition of early has not been clearly defined and varies between the different guidelines. The International Association of Pancreatology has recommended cholecystectomy should be ideally performed prior to discharge from the initial hospitalization for pancreatitis.[26] The UK Working Party on Acute Pancreatitis have recommended that cholecystectomy not be delayed more than two weeks

[25] Kelly T, Wagner D. Gallstone pancreatitis: a prospective randomized trial of the timing of surgery. *Surgery* 1988;104:600-605.

[26] Uhl W, Warshaw A, Imrie C, et al. IAP Guidelines for the surgical management of acute pancreatitis. *Pancreatology* 2002;2:565-573.

after discharge from the index admission,[27] whereas the American Gastroenterological Association guidelines allow for 2-4 weeks after discharge.[28] Guidelines from the American College of Gastroenterology state early cholecystectomy should be performed, but do not define a particular target.[29] Perhaps the reason for the lack of consensus is due to that evidence for these recommendations is largely based on single-center observational studies and not large randomized clinical trial data. Studies done to date have demonstrated a risk of recurrent biliary pancreatitis from 25 to 63% when cholecystectomy was delayed until after discharge from the index hospitalization.[30,31,32]

In a retrospective observational study of 281 patients with ABP, Ito et al. demonstrated gallstone-related complications in 33% of patients who did not have index cholecystectomy, with recurrent ABP found in 13.4% of patients (versus no recurrences in the index cholecystectomy group). Of note, almost one third of recurrences occurred within 2 weeks after discharge, and half of recurrences occurred within 4 weeks.33 They also looked at ERCP with ES as definitive treatment in 42 out of the 119 patients who did not have index cholecystectomy. A significant reduction in recurrence of ABP was noted in the ES group compared to no intervention group with rates of 4.8 versus 18.2% respectively. However, rates of biliary complications such as acute cholecystitis, jaundice, and cholangitis did occur with greater frequency in the ES group versus no intervention group. This trend of decreased recurrence of ABP but increased biliary complications has been replicated in several other studies, and as such, ERCP with ES should not be used in place of cholecystectomy for definitive treatment except in the case of patients who are deemed to be poor surgical candidates.[34]

Other than reduced recurrence rates, several benefits have been identified with early cholecystectomy during index hospitalization. A recent randomized prospective study has suggested that early cholecystectomy may actually reduce length of index hospitalization. This study looked at 50 patients who were admitted with mild ABP, with half randomized to the early group where cholecystectomy was performed within 48 hours of admission regardless of whether abdominal pain had subsided or laboratory values had normalized. They found that hospital length of stay was shorter for the early cholecystectomy group with an average of 3.5 days as compared to the control group with an average stay of 5.8

---

[27] UK Working Party on Acute Pancreatitis. UK guidelines for the management of acute pancreatitis. *Gut* 2005;54(Suppl 3):iii1-9.

[28] Forsmark CE, Baillie J. AGA Institute technical review on acute pancreatitis. *Gastroenterology* 2007;132(5):2022-44.

[29] Banks PA, Freeman ML. Practice guidelines in acute pancreatitis. *American Journal of Gastroenterology* 2006;101(10):2379-400.

[30] Uhl W, Muller CA, Krahenbuhl L, Schmid SW, Scholzel S, Buchler MW. Acute gallstone pancreatitis: timing of laparoscopic cholecystectomy in mild and severe disease. *Surg Endo* 1999;13:1070-1076.

[31] Ranson JH. The role of surgery in the management of acute pancreatitis. *Ann Surg* 1990;211:382-393.

[32] Ranson JH. The timing of biliary surgery in acute pancreatitis. *Ann Surg* 1979;189:654-663.

[33] Ito K, Ito H, Whang E. Timing of cholecystectomy for biliary pancreatitis: do the data support current guidelines? *Journal of Gastrointestinal Surgery* 2008;12:2164-2170.

[34] Kimura Y, Arata S, Takada T, et al. Gallstone-induced acute pancreatitis. *Journal of Hepatobiliary Pancreatic Sciences* 2010;17:60-69.

days (p=0.0016).[35] Of note, they did not find any statistically significant differences in the need to convert to open cholecystectomy or peri-operative complications between the two groups. Previous observational studies have also shown similar results. One of the largest series is that of 281 patients, of which 162 underwent cholecystectomy during index admission, where length of stay was 5 days for the early group compared to 7 days for the post-discharge cholecystectomy group. This difference was exaggerated further by the fact that 33% of the post-discharge cholecystectomy group required at least one other pre-cholecystectomy admission for gallstone-related events, resulting in an average of 3 additional days in hospital.[36]

Despite the decrease in biliary complications, reduced length of stay, and reduced readmissions, several studies have shown that most jurisdictions are still not following guidelines for early cholecystectomy. One retrospective study looked at 100 consecutive patients admitted with ABP and found only 40 had surgery within the index admission, with another 38 who were discharged for interval cholecystectomy. Two of the 38 were re-admitted while waiting for surgery with biliary complications.[37] Nguyen et al. explored whether lack of resources was a contributing factor to low compliance with guidelines, and they demonstrated that the rate of cholecystectomy during index admission increased at centers with the highest annual volume of cholecystectomies, decreased at centers with the highest volumes of acute pancreatitis, and decreased in centers with the highest volumes of ERCP.[38] These results confirm the hypothesis that resource intensification may be necessary to more consistently meet international guidelines.

7. References

Aboulian A, Chan T, Yaghoubian A, et al. Early cholecystectomy safely decreases hospital stay in patients with mild gallstone pancreatitis: a randomized prospective study. *Annals of Surgery* 2010;251(4):615-19.

Acosta JM, Ledesma CL. Gallstone migration as a cause of acute pancreatitis. *NEJM* 1974;290:484-487.

Acosta JM, Rossi R, Ledesma CL. The usefulness of stool screening for diagnosing cholelithiasis in acute pancreatitis: a description of the technique. *American Journal of Digestive Diseases* 1977;22:168-172.

Agrawal S, Jonnalagadda S. Gallstones, from gallbladder to gut. Management options for diverse complications. *Postgraduate Medicine* 2000;108:143-153.

Ammori BJ, Boreham B, Lewis P, Roberts SA. The biochemical detection of biliary etiology of acute pancreatitis on admission: a revisit in the modern era of biliary imaging. *Pancreas* 2003;26(2):e32-e35.

---

[35] Aboulian A, Chan T, Yaghoubian A, et al. Early cholecystectomy safely decreases hospital stay in patients with mild gallstone pancreatitis: a randomized prospective study. *Annals of Surgery* 2010;251(4):615-619.

[36] Ito K, Ito H, Whang E. Timing of cholecystectomy for biliary pancreatitis: do the data support current guidelines? *Journal of Gastrointestinal Surgery* 2008;12:2164-2170.

[37] Sanjay P, Yeeting S, Whigham C, et al. Management guidelines for gallstone pancreatitis. Are the targets achievable? *Journal of the Pancreas* 2009;10(1):43-7.

[38] Nguyen GC, Boudreau H, Jagannath SB. Hospital volume as a predictor for undergoing cholecystectomy after admission for acute biliary pancreatitis. *Pancreas* 2010;39:e42-e47.

Banks P, Freeman M. Practice guidelines in acute pancreatitis. *American Journal of Gastroenterology* 2006;101:2379-2400.

Davidson BR, Neoptolemos JP, Leese T, Carr-Locke DL. Biochemical prediction of gallstones in acute pancreatitis: a prospective study of three systems. *British Journal of Surgery* 1988;75:213-215.

Forsmark CE, Baillie J. AGA Institute technical review on acute pancreatitis. *Gastroenterology* 2007;132(5):2022-44.

Frel G, Frel V, Thirlby R, McClelland R. Biliary pancreatitis: clinical presentation and surgical management. *American Journal of Surgery* 1986;151:170-175.

Howard T. (2008) Management of gallstone pancreatitis, In: *Current surgical therapy, 9th ed.* Cameron J. pp. 477-480. Mosby Elsevier Inc., ISBN: 978-1-4160-3497-1, Philadelphia.

Ito K, Ito H, Whang E. Timing of cholecystectomy for biliary pancreatitis: do the data support current guidelines? *Journal of Gastrointestinal Surgery* 2008;12:2164-2170.

Kaw M, Al-Antably Y, Kaw P. Management of gallstone pancreatitis: cholecystectomy or ERCP and endoscopic sphincterotomy. *Gastrointestinal Endoscopy* 2002;56:61-65.

Kelly T, Wagner D. Gallstone pancreatitis: a prospective randomized trial of the timing of surgery. *Surgery* 1988;104:600-605.

Kimura Y, Arata S, Takada T, et al. Gallstone-induced acute pancreatitis. *Journal of Hepatobiliary Pancreatic Sciences* 2010;17:60-69.

Lankisch PG, Burchard-Reckert S, Lehnick D. Underestimation of acute pancreatitis: patients with only a small increase in amylase/lipase levels can also have or develop severe acute pancreatitis. *Gut* 1999;44:542-544.

Marschall HU, Katsika D, Rudling M, Einarsson C. The genetic background of gallstone formation: an update. *Biochemical and Biophysical Research Communications* 2010;396:58-62.

Nguyen GC, Boudreau H, Jagannath SB. Hospital volume as a predictor for undergoing cholecystectomy after admission for acute biliary pancreatitis. *Pancreas* 2010;39:e42-e47.

Ranson JH. The role of surgery in the management of acute pancreatitis. *Annals of Surgery* 1990;211:382-393.

Ranson JH. The timing of biliary surgery in acute pancreatitis. *Annals of Surgery* 1979;189:654-663.

Sanjay P, Yeeting S, Whigham C, et al. Management guidelines for gallstone pancreatitis. Are the targets achievable? *Journal of the Pancreas* 2009;10(1):43-7.

Shaffer SA. Epidemiology of gallbladder stone disease. *Best Practice & Research Clinical Gastroenterology* 2006;20(6):981-996.

Stimac D, Lenac T, Marusic Z. A scoring system for early differentiation of the etiology of acute pancreatitis. *Scandinavian Journal of Gastroenterology* 1998;33:209-211.

Uhl W, Muller CA, Krahenbuhl L, Schmid SW, Scholzel S, Buchler MW. Acute gallstone pancreatitis: timing of laparoscopic cholecystectomy in mild and severe disease. *Surgical Endoscopy* 1999;13:1070-1076.

Uhl W, Warshaw A, Imrie C, et al. IAP Guidelines for the Surgical Management of Acute Pancreatitis. *Pancreatology* 2002;2:565-573.

UK guidelines for the management of acute pancreatitis. *Gut*. 2005;54(S3):iii1-iii9.

van Erpecum KJ. Complications of bile-duct stones: acute cholangitis and pancreatitis. *Best Practice & Research Clinical Gastroenterology* 2006;20:1139-1152.

van Geenen E, van der Peet D, Bhagirath P, et al. Etiology and diagnosis of acute biliary pancreatitis. *Gastroenterology and Hepatology* 2010;7:495-502.

Whitcomb DC. Clinical practice. Acute pancreatitis. *NEJM* 2006;354:2142-2150.

3

Childhood Pancreatitis

Ali E. Abdelbasit
Department of Paediatric Surgery, Soba University Hospital,
University of Khartoum,
Sudan

1. Introduction

Most of the available English literature on pancreatitis is adult based. The last few decades have witnessed increasing interest in childhood pancreatitis and attention to research into the subject. Many recent published works have focused on various aspects of pancreatitis. The incidence of childhood pancreatitis is a rare event though it appears to be increasing. Despite its rarity, pancreatitis in children deserves special attention because of the significant morbidity and mortality associated with it. The management of childhood pancreatitis has also witnessed remarkable development in the last few decades. The improvement in the imaging resolutions, biochemical tests, endoscopic procedures and the intensive care facilities have resulted in better outcome.

This chapter aims at providing an up-to-date review of childhood pancreatitis. It includes the aspects of aetiological factors, pathophysiology, classification, typical and atypical clinical presentation with abdominal and extra-abdominal manifestations of the disease and its complications, applicability of severity scores, the diagnostic and prognostic investigations, various methods of medical and surgical treatment - with indications thereof - touching on the pros and cons of the different methods, and the overall prognosis.

2. Aetiology

2.1 Acute pancreatitis

The causes of acute pancreatitis in children are diverse (Table 1) and unlike in the adults where the majority of the cases are due to alcoholism or gallstone disease, most of the cases in children are due to pancreaticobiliary tract anomalies, biliary tract stones, trauma, drugs and a plethora of systemic diseases. In a considerable proportion of up to 25% of the patients, no aetiological factor is identified and is therefore labeled as idiopathic (Haddock et al., 1994; Uretsky et al., 1999; Mehta & Gittes, 2005; Hebra et al, 2009; Werlin, 2003).

2.1.1 Pancreaticobiliary anomalies

Pancreaticobiliary malunion (PBMU) accounts for approximately 6-33% of cases of pancreatitis in children. PBMU is used synonymously with common pancreaticobiliary channel, anomalous pancreaticobiliary channel, pancreaticobiliary maljunction, anomalous pancreaticobiliary ductal union or long common pancreaticobiliary channel, with or without a choledochal cyst or common bile duct (CBD) dilatation. PBMU is complicated by bile reflux into the pancreatic duct predisposing to pancreatitis. Common channel and pancreatic duct obstruction by protein plugs, biliary stones or sludge may result in pancreatitis or jaundice. Presence of a choledochal cyst may produce pancreatitis by direct mechanical pancreatic duct compression (Miyano, 2006).

Pancreas divisum is a persistence of the developmental pancreatic ductal system due to failure of fusion of the dorsal (Wirsung) and the ventral (Santorini) ducts. As a result, the exocrine drainage of the pancreatic body and tail is impaired due to the narrow minor duct and its papilla. The resultant flow impediment may cause recurrent episodes of acute pancreatitis. The anomaly is encountered in approximately 4-11% of patients and, as such, is one of the most common congenital anomalies of the pancreas (Miyano, 200; Mehta & Gittes, 2005). Annular pancreas was reported to cause recurrent acute pancreatitis in children (Hwang et al 2010, Ohno & Kanematsu, 2008).

2.1.2 Biliary stone disease

Choledocho- or cholcystolithiasis are uncommon in children; however, when they exist they cause pancreatitis secondary to transient pancreatic duct obstruction. Biliary stones may result from haemolytic disorders such as hereditary spherocytosis, B thalassemia and sickle cell disease. Occasionally, biliary stones may complicate obesity or cholestasis due to biliary dyskinesia or prolonged use of total parenteral nutrition (TPN) (Mehta & Gittes 2005).

2.1.3 Trauma

Trauma is a major cause of pancreatitis in children. By virtue of the position of the pancreas against the lumbar spine, accidents or violent acts leading to blunt abdominal trauma in children and adolescents - typically as in bicycle handle bar injuries- may cause acute pancreatitis. The severity of the trauma influences the onset of symptoms, severity of clinical manifestations and course of the disease. In cases of ambiguity of the history, child abuse must be taken into consideration. Iatrogenic pancreatitis may be experienced following pancreatic injury that occur during the course of abdominal surgery or may complicate endoscopic retrograde cholangiopancreatography ERCP (Miyano, 2006; Mehta & Gittes, 2005; Uretsky et al., 1999; Ibrahim et al., 2011).

2.1.4 Systemic infections

Infection with viruses including Mumps, Rubella, Coxsackie B and Rotavirus can be incriminated in the aetiology of pancreatitis. Also, generalised bacterial sepsis may cause pancreatitis (Mehta & Gittes, 2005).

2.1.5 Systemic diseases and metabolic abnormalities

Including hypercalcaemia, hyperlipidaemia, hypertriglyceridaemia, Reye syndrome and Kawasaki's disease, may be associated with cases of acute pancreatitis. Cystic fibrosis with inspissation of pancreatic secretions within the pancreatic ducts may cause recurrent acute pancreatitis (Uretsky et al., 1999; Mehta & Gittes, 2005).

2.1.6 Drugs

Use of a wide range of drugs, including corticosteroids, HIV therapeutic agents, immunosuppressants and cytotoxic drugs, has been associated with incidents of acute pancreatitis accounting for 8-25% of cases (Miyano, 2006).

Pancreatitis may be induced by the administration of corticosteroids and valproic acid. Perhaps young children are more commonly affected when valproic acid is incriminated. Bai found that there was a higher frequency of valproic acid-associated pancreatitis in children younger than 11 years of age (Bai et al., 2011).

Didanosine (Nucleoside analogue) and Zalcitabine used in the treatment of human immunodeficiency viral (HIV) infection were incriminated as causative agents of acute pancreatitis (Ridout & Lakhoo, 2011). Butler et al found that pancreatitis developed in 7% of 95 children with HIV who received the reverse transcriptase inhibitor Dideoxyinosine (ddI) at 60 to 540mg/m2 per day for a mean of 56 weeks. They also noted that pancreatitis occurred only in patients who received the highest dose levels and resolved in all of the affected children upon withdrawal of the drug (Butler et al, 1993).

Immunosuppressive drugs such as Azathioprine and Mercaptopurine were incriminated as causative factors in approximately 5% of cases. The causative effect of Immunosuppressants can be reversed by early use of high doses of the synthetic protease inhibitor gabexate mesylate (Miyano, 2006).

The use of the cytotoxic drug L asparaginase in leukaemia regimens was associated with a marked increase in acute pancreatitis in childhood oncology clinics (Nydegger et al., 2006). Ifosfamide used in the treatment of paediatric solid tumours is known to have serious adverse effects, including acute pancreatitis as a rare complication of therapy (Garg et al., 2010). Tetracycline, erythromycin, metronidazole and nitrofurantoin are among other drugs reported to induce acute pancreatitis (Kuhls, 2004).

Alcohol abuse is an uncommon cause of acute pancreatitis in children, however, it was reported to be implicated in older children and adolescents (Camp et al., 1994; Uretsky et al., 1999).

2.1.7 Miscellaneous

Acute pancreatitis can be caused by hypovolaemia. The disease was related to hypovolaemia in one third (33%) of 21 children following cardiopulmonary bypass or severe GI bleeding (Berney, 1996).

Liver transplantation was recently reported as a possible cause for acute pancreatitis, with an incidence of 1.9% and a mortality rate of 43% (Miyano, 2006).

Early antenatal destruction of pancreas, Shwachman Diamond syndrome, is an autosomal recessive disorder recently mapped to the centromeic region of chromosome 7. Children suffering from this condition have pancreatic insufficiency at birth, generally with very low serum trypsinogen levels, indicative of nearly total exocrine pancreatic atrophy by birth (Miyano, 2006). Hereditary pancreatitis may present with acute recurrent pancreatitis (Aamarapurkar, 2001).

Congenital anomalies of the biliary system:		Choledochal cyst
		Pancreatico-Biliary Malunion (PBMU)
		Pancreas divisum
Biliary stone disease:		Cholelithiasis
		Choledocholithisis
Trauma:	Blunt	
	Iatrogenic: Surgery, ERCP	
Infections: Viral and others:		Mumps
		Rubella
		Coxsakie B virus
		Rota virus
		Generalised bacterial sepsis
Chronic inflammatory diseases		
Systemic diseases:		Cystic fibrosis,
		Reye syndrome,
		Kawasaki's disease,
		Hyperlipidaemia,
		Hypercalcaemia
		Hypertriglyceridaemia
Drugs:	Corticosteroids	
	Valproic acid	
	Anti HIV drugs:	
		Didanosine (Nucleoside analogue)
		Zalcitabine
	Immunosuppressive drugs	
		Azathioprine
		Mecaptopurine
	Cytotoxic drugs:	L-Asparaginase
		Ifofamide
		Tetracycline, Pentamidine,
		Sulphonamides, Metronidazole, Nitrofurantoin,
		Ceftriaxone, Furosemide,
		Rifampin, Interferon alpha-2b, Erythromycin
Miscellaneous:		Hypovolaemia
		Liver transplantation
		Early antenatal destruction of pancreas,
		Shwachman Diamond syndrome
		Hereditary pancreatitis
		Hyperactive sphincter of Oddi
		Extracorporeal Shock Wave Lithotripsy (ESWL)
Idiopathic		

Table 1. Aetiological factors of acute pancreatitis in children

2.2 Chronic pancreatitis

In children, the most common causes of chronic and chronic relapsing pancreatitis are trauma, hereditary, systemic disease and malformations of the pancreaticobiliary ductal system such as pancreas divisum and annular pancreas, and choledocholithiasis.

Chronic pancreatitis could either be **calcifying** (commoner) or **obstructive** (less common).

2.2.1 Calcifying chronic pancreatitis

The most common cause of calcifying pancreatitis is hereditary or familial pancreatitis. Comfort and Steinberg gave the first description of hereditary pancreatitis in 1952 (Comfort & Steinberg, 1952). Since then a number of cases of hereditary pancreatitis have been reported. The mode of inheritance strongly suggested was an autosomal dominant trait (Aamarapurkar, 2001). The gene mutations identified in early-onset idiopathic chronic pancreatitis (ICP) are the serine protease inhibitor, Kazal type 1 (SPINK1) gene mutations, and the cystic fibrosis transmembrane regulator (CFTR) gene mutations. Recently, Cationic trypsinogen protease serine 1 PRSS1 gene mutations were detected in "idiopathic pancreatitis" and SPINK1 gene mutations in idiopathic and tropical pancreatitis. It is also very likely that SPINK1 gene mutations are important in tropical calcific pancreatitis (TCP) (see below) (DiMagno M & E., 2003). As many as 10% of patients with "idiopathic pancreatitis" may have hereditary pancreatitis if finding a PRSS1 gene mutation without a family history is considered an acceptable diagnostic criterion (DiMagno M & E, 2003).

The association of CFTR gene mutations and chronic pancreatitis is well known. Even in classic cystic fibrosis (CF) with pancreatic functional preservation, the prevalence of pancreatitis may be 17% or higher because such patients have recurrent, severe abdominal pain that may be due to unrecognized pancreatitis (DiMagno M & E., 2003).

Gene sequencing of the 7q35 chromosome region revealed a strong association of the (p.R122 H) mutation of the PRSS1 gene encoding cationic trypsinogen with hereditary pancreatitis (Teich et al., 2006). Developments in genetics have shown that in the majority of patients, hereditary pancreatitis is usually associated with expression of one of two specific mutations in the cationic trypsinogen PRSS1 gene, specifically R122H or N29I. Further sequencing of the PRSS1 gene in the proband of families without these common mutations revealed R122C and N29T mutations in independent families that segregated with the disease in an autosomal dominant fashion. The R122C mutation eliminates the arginine autolysis site as with R122H mutations. The N29T mutation may also enhance intrapancreatic trypsin activity as has been demonstrated in vitro (Pfutzer et al., 2002). Further mutations of this gene were discovered in patients with hereditary or idiopathic chronic pancreatitis. In vitro the mutations increase autocatalytic conversion of trypsinogen to active trypsin and thus probably cause premature intrapancreatic trypsinogen activation in vivo. The clinical presentation is highly variable, but most affected mutation carriers have relatively mild disease (Teich et al, 2006).

Tropical calcific pancreatitis is a type of pancreatitis seen exclusively in tropics. Though the exact aetiology of tropical chronic pancreatitis is obscure, malnutrition with protein deficiency, cassava toxicity, impaired immune response, viral infection and genetic susceptibility have been considered as various factors in the aetiopathogenesis

(Aamarapurkar, 2001). It is also very likely that *SPINK1* gene mutations are important in tropical calcific pancreatitis (TCP), a disease associated with malnutrition and cassava consumption in Afro-Asian countries that is characterized by onset at an early age and variable familial clustering (DiMagno M & E., 2003).

2.2.2 Obstructive chronic pancreatitis

Encompasses the other causes of chronic pancreatitis in children which include congenital anomalies of the pancreaticobiliary duct system such as pancreas divisum, pancreaticobiliary malunion and annular pancreas. Trauma is also a major cause leading to chronic pancreatitis, particularly when fibrosis complicates pancreatic duct disruption, resulting in pancreatic duct stricture and, consequently, obstructive chronic pancreatitis. Other aetilogical factors include biliary disease, systemic inflammatory and metabolic diseases (table 2). Hypertriglyceridaemia and hyper parathyroidism, though rare, were reported to cause chronic pancreatitis in children (Aamarapurkar, 2001).

Idiopathic fibrosing pancreatitis is a rare condition that affects children and adolescents. It can be a cause of recurrent abdominal pain and obstructive jaundice (Harb & Naon, 2005).

Biliary disease		
	Congenital anomalies of the biliary system:	Pancreas divisum
		PBMU
		Choledochal cyst
	Biliary stone disease:	Cholelithiasis
		Choledocholithisis
Hereditary pancreatitis		
Systemic and metabolic diseases:		Hyperlipoproteinaemia
		Hyperparathyroidism
		Hypercalcaemia
		Hypertriglycaedaemia
		Cystic fibrosis
		Inborn errors of metabolism
		Systemic lupus erythematosus
		Haemophilia
		Shwachman Diamond Syndrome
Infection		
Chronic inflammatory diseases		
		Crohn's disease
		Ulcerative colitis
		Chronic fibrosing pancreatitis
		Juvenile tropical pancreatitis
		Tropical calcific pancreatitis
		Idiopathic chronic pancreatitis
		Idiopathic fibrosing pancreatitis

Table 2. Aetiological factors of chronic pancreatitis in children:

3. Pathophysiology

The pancreas matures after birth and by 2 years of age it is functioning in the same way as an adult pancreas. Due to its excellent reserve, the immature pancreas does not seem to affect the healthy children significantly, however, it can have a major impact on very ill or malnourished children (Durie, 2011).

3.1 Acute pancreatitis

3.1.1 Acinar cell injury

Acute pancreatitis originates from acinar cell injury due to factors such as trauma, drugs, metabolic disorders and infection which lead to premature intraductal activation of proenzymes, specifically trypsinogen to trypsin. The resultant autodigestion of the pancreatic tissue and accompanying aggressive immune response cause the pathological process of pancreatitis and subsequent complications (Uretsky et al.,1999; Nydegger et al., 2006)

3.1.2 Proenzyme activation

Inappropriate, premature proenzyme activation in the pancreas, and consequently autodigestion of pancreatic tissue, may occur due to either ductal flow obstruction (structural) with extravasation of enzyme rich ductal fluid into the parenchyma of the pancreas, reflux of duodenal enterokinase into the pancreas or failure in feed-back control (hereditary).

3.1.3 Inflammatory mediators

Once activated, elastase, phospholipase A2 and superoxide free radicles in addition to release from the pancreas of other active mediators including cytokines such as tumour necrosis factor-alpha; and vasoactive substances such as histamines, prostaglandins, kinins and kallikreins, are thought to play an important role as mediators of tissue damage (Weber & Adler, 2003; Mehta & Gittes, 2005).

Along with premature activation of digestive enzymes, disturbances of intracellular calcium, and activation of transcription factors such as NF-κB characterize the initial phase of acute pancreatitis. Depending on the severity of pancreatic injury, the impact may not be confined to the pancreas. Pancreatic enzymes can cause damage at distant sites either by vascular dissemination or by the release of proinflammatory mediators and the recruitment of immune cells which may expand the local disturbances to a systemic inflammatory response associated with diffuse tissue damage throughout the body and failure of distant organs such as lungs or kidneys, a form of multiple system organ failure (MSOF). Patients with severe acute pancreatitis are, therefore, likely to have a high incidence of refractory sepsis and death (Weber & Adler, 2003; Mehta & Gittes, 2005).

3.1.4 Role of cytokines

Cytokines themselves do not induce pancreatitis but rather mediate the progression of pancreatitis. Cellular immune responses are the major determinants of severity. The most important step for the development of severe pancreatitis appears to be the activation of the

T helper cell type 1 (Th1) response. Pancreatic production of proinflammatory cytokines such as TNF-alpha, interleukin IL-1B, IL-6 and IL-8 modulates local injury, systemic inflammatory response and distant organ failure. This modulation, coupled with pancreatic necrosis, determine the outcome from acute pancreatitis. The TNFa, IL1B, IL6 & IL8 released from granulocytes and macrophages also reach the liver through the portosystemic circulation and act on Kupffer cells that produce more cytokines and acute phase proteins. Other factors determining the severity of pancreatitis include free radicles, pancreatic glutathione, ischaemia, chemokines and neurokines. Because the onset of cytokines action follows immediately after the onset of pancreatitis and peaks after 36-48 hours, cytokine antagonists therapy represent a potential therapeutic target and therefore is of intense interest (Nydegger et al, 2006; Berney et al, 1999).

3.2 Chronic pancreatitis

Chronic pancreatitis is an inflammatory disorder that results in anatomical changes that include chronic inflammatory cell infiltration and gland fibrosis, with loss of exocrine function (malabsorption) and endocrine function (diabetes mellitus). In susceptible children, repeated episodes of acute inflammation may lead to chronic pancreatitis, the so called necrosis-fibrosis hypothesis of Comfort et al. and, accordingly, it is likely that there is significant overlap in the underlying pathophysiology of these conditions (Nydegger et al, 2006).

Whitcomb has proposed a sentinel acute pancreatitis event SAPE which acts as a priori step toward the development of chronic pancreatitis. The acute injury must be sufficiently severe to attract monocytes and to cause infiltration, differentiation and proliferation of pancreatic stellate cells. For fibrosis to occur there must be recurrent acinar injury resulting in chemocytokine release that then stimulates stellate cells (Whitcomb 1999, 2004).

Genetics: Cationic trypsinogen gene Protease Serine 1 (*PRSS1*) gene accounts for 65% of trypsinogen and is one of the most abundant molecules produced by acinar cells. In chronic pancreatitis, it has been suggested that mutations of the cationic trypsinogen *PRSS1* gene lead to an alteration in the trypsin recognition site that prevents deactivation of trypsin within the pancreas. Consequently, autodigestion occurs resulting in pancreatitis. The genetic mutations responsible for hereditary pancreatitis have been isolated to chromosome 7q35. The most common hereditary pancreatitis causing mutations in *PRSS1* gene are R122H and N29I (Pfutzeret al., 2002; Teich et al, 2006; Nydegger et al., 2006). These two mutations in the cationic trypsinogen gene appeared to allow prematurely activated trypsinogen to cause acinar cell auto-digestion and acute pancreatitis. Chronic pancreatitis in these patients certainly arises from recurrent acute pancreatitis (Aamarapurkar, 2001). Several other mutations in the *PRSS1* gene have been identified including mutations in codons 16, 22, 23 and 122. This discovery of genetic mutations associated with hereditary pancreatitis support the hypothesis that intrapancreatic activation of pancreatic zymogens is crucial to the pathogenesis of acute pancreatitis. The mutant trypsin in hereditary pancreatitis is resistant to lysis, remains active and causes auto-digestion of the pancreas and episodes of acute pancreatitis. Median age at onset of disease is 11 years in patients with the N29I mutation and 10 years in those with the R122H. Approximately half of patients with hereditary pancreatitis develop chronic pancreatitis (Nydegger et al., 2006).

Trypsin can exert a negative feed-back, self inactivation to protect the pancreas from auto-digestion. The serine protease inhibitor SPINK1 produces a similar pancreas sparing effect by inhibition of prematurely activated trypsinogen. This gene may have a role in tropical pancreatitis, an idiopathic form of pancreatitis seen in southern Asia and parts of Africa and probably related to malnutrition, together with cassava intake. SPINK1 mutations were also shown to be associated with a subtype of tropical pancreatitis, fibrocalculous pancreatic diabetes. SPINK1 mutations alone probably do not cause pancreatitis but act as disease modifier. The SPINK1 mutations are relatively common, being present in approximately 2% of the general population. However, the frequency of SPINK1 mutations in populations with idiopathic chronic pancreatitis is markedly increased, approximately 25%, an evidence that an association exists between the SPINK1 mutations and pancreatitis (Nydegger et al., 2006).

Cystic fibrosis transmembrane regulator (CFTR): An association between idiopathic chronic pancreatitis and CFTR gene mutations was reported. Several mild CFTR mutations were found to be associated with idiopathic pancreatitis. Available data suggest that patients with two severe mutations have classical cystic fibrosis (CF), those with a single mutation are carriers and those who are compound heterozygotes with one severe and one mild mutation are at risk of developing pancreatitis (Ridout & Lakhoo, 2011; Nydegger, 2006).

4. Classification

Pancreatitis can be classified as:

- Acute pancreatitis: Simple
  Necrotizing
  Haemorrhagic
- Acute recurrent pancreatitis
- Chronic pancreatitis: Calcific or Obstructive
- Chronic relapsing pancreatitis

5. Clinical presentation

5.1 Acute pancreatitis

Diagnosis is based on symptoms and signs accompanied by a three fold increase in either amylase or lipase. Presentation is variable in children and symptoms may range from mild abdominal pain to severe systemic involvement, metabolic disturbances and shock. **Abdominal pain, anorexia, nausea and vomiting** are the most frequent symptoms (Hebra et al., 2009; Mehta & Gittes, 2005). The pain can be of a sudden or insidious onset with slow and gradual progression with increasing intensity. Although the pain is usually epigastric in origin, right and left upper abdominal quadrants are infrequently involved. Central and lower abdominal pain may also be encountered (Uretsky et al, 1999). The typical radiation of pain to the back observed in adults is not a common feature in children. Food intake exacerbates pain and vomiting (Haddock et al, 1994) while drawing the knees up to the chest relieves the pain (Uretsky et al, 1999). Extracellular fluid losses can be enormous (Mehta & Gittes, 2005).

On examination, the child may be ill, irritable, quiet or a combination of these. Movement aggravates the abdominal pain, therefore children typically tend to assume a still, supine position, or they may lie on their side or doubled up with the hips and knees flexed (Hebra et al, 2009). Tachycardia, mild fever, hypotension, jaundice and abdominal signs such as diffuse tenderness, rebound tenderness, guarding, distension and decreased or absent bowel sounds may be elicited (Nydegger et al., 2006, Hebra et al., 2009, Ibrahim & Gabr, 2011). Parotid enlargement may be observed occasionally (Haddock et al, 1994). In severe cases of necrotizing or haemorrhagic pancreatitis, haemorrhage may dissect from around the pancreas along the abdominal wall tissue planes appearing as discoloration either in the flanks (Grey Turner's sign) or at the umbilicus (Cullen's sign). These echymoses may take 1-2 days to develop (Mehta & Gittes, 2005). These signs of haemorrhagic pancreatitis are seldom present in children (Nydegger et al, 2006). Evidence of pleural effusion or dyspnoea, with or without acute respiratory distress syndrome, may be found on examination of the chest (Uretsky et al, 1999, Ali et al, 2010). Recurrent acute pancreatitis is seen in 10% of children after the initial acute episode. It is more likely in children with structural anomalies, idiopathic and familial causes (Nydegger et al, 2006).

5.2 Chronic pancreatitis

Unlike acute pancreatitis in which complete reversal of the inflammatory changes occurs upon resolution of the episodes, chronic pancreatitis is characterised by permanent structural changes in the pancreas associated with varying degrees of pancreatic dysfunction and, accordingly, increased risk of developing pancreatic insufficiency, adenocarcinoma, and pancreatic pseudocysts. Patients with this disease typically present with chronic or recurrent upper abdominal pain with significant morbidity. The pain is most commonly described as epigastric, deep or radiating towards the back and accompanied by nausea and vomiting. It is often relieved by sitting and leaning forward and may increase following meal. It may commence as intermittent attacks with periods of well-being and then become more continuous, others may have little or no pain. Common other associated clinical features include weight loss and diabetes mellitus. Paediatric data on prevalence and incidence of exocrine and endocrine failure are limited, however, steatorrhea and weight loss will not occur until pancreatic exocrine function has been reduced to around 2% of the normal output. Because insulin and glucagons secreting cells are destroyed in chronic pancreatitis, the diabetes in these patients can be particularly refractory to treat (Nydegger et al, 2006; Mehta & Gittes 2005).

Tropical calcific pancreatitis is characeritized by recurrent episodes of abdominal pain, severe malnutrition, and ketosis resistant diabetes. Ten per cent of patients with tropical calcific pancreatitis develop pancreatic cancer. Almost one third of patients with tropical calcific pancreatitis get recurrent episodes of pain in childhood and may develop diabetes in childhood (Aamarapurkar, 2001).

6. Investigations

6.1 Acute pancreatitis

Serum amylase levels are usually, but not invariably elevated. Normal levels do not exclude the diagnosis of acute pancreatitis. Also, the degree of serum amylase elevation does not correlate with severity of the disease. Goh found that serum amylase levels were elevated in all the 11 patients in his study. Their serum amylase levels ranged from 190 to 1370 U/L

(Median 512.5). One third of them had amylase levels lower than 4 times the upper limit of normal, ie. 440 U/L. (Goh et al., 2003). Amplified elevations of serum amylase are suggestive of development of a pseudocyst or other complications of pancreatitis.

Amylase is excreted in the urine when the level of hyperamylasemia exceeds the tubular reabsorptive capacity. Therefore, moderately elevated levels of serum amylase may not be detectable in the urine. It is important to note that other conditions may cause hyperamylasemia or hyperamylasuria. These include salivary inflammation or trauma, intestinal disease including perforation, ischaemia, necrosis or inflammation, renal failure and macroamylasemia (Mehta & Gittes, 2005). To differentiate the likely underlying cause, a three fold, or more, elevation of serum amylase concentration is strongly in favour of the diagnosis of acute pancreatitis. The half life of amylase is approximately 10 hours and the value frequently becomes normal after 2-5 days.

Initial serum amylase level does not correlate with the severity of pancreatic injury. Schmittenbecher noted a longer lasting elevation of serum amylase in patients with traumatic pancreatitis (Schmittenbecher et al., 1996).

Elevated level of pleural effusion fluid-amylase in children with respiratory symptoms secondary to pancreatitis is a useful diagnostic test (Segura, 2004). Thoracic pancreatic pseudocyst as a complication of traumatic pancreatitis has been reported (Ali et al, 2010).

Lipase: Unlike amylase, lipase is produced only in the pancreas and its measurement is particularly helpful for distinguishing pancreatic trauma from salivary trauma. In children with acute pancreatitis, the serum lipase level is usually elevated for many days. Therefore, lipase levels have been proposed as a more specific test of pancreatic tissue damage. An important caveat to note here is that the degree of lipase elevation has little correlation with the extent of the pancreatitis and that intestinal perforation does cause an elevation of lipase through reabsorption via the peritoneum. Urinary lipase levels may remain elevated for a few days longer than serum levels (Mehta & Gittes, 2005).

Calcium and Glucose: Hypocalcaemia was reported in 10-15% of children with pancreatitis (Goh et al., 2003; Uretsky et al., 1999) while hypoglycaemia was noted in 25% of cases during the acute attack (Uretsky et al., 1999).

The blood glucose level measurement is a key investigation when chronic pancreatitis is suspected. Persistently elevated blood glucose level indicates significant pancreatic endocrine-reserve impairment.

Haematological: Elevated total white blood cell counts (with increased band counts) are usually present (Goh et al., 2003). An increased haematocrit secondary to haemoconcentration that occurs after volume depletion may be found.

Genetics: The majority of pancreatic diseases are associated with genetic polymorphism. Early use of genetic testing is likely to play a critical role in early diagnosis and prognosis of pancreatic diseases (Whitcomb, 2004).

The levels of cationic trypsinogen gene and SPINK1 mutations are said to be a more sensitive early marker of pancreatic inflammation (Uretsky et al., 1999).

Gene testing for CFTR gene is helpful in the diagnosis of pancreatitis in cases thought to be related to cystic fibrosis.

Imaging: plain abdominal radiographs may reveal obscured psoas margins, a sentinel loop of a dilated duodenum and a gasless segment of mid transverse colon. The latter is caused by local spasm with proximal dilatation known as colon cut-off sign due to inflammation of the adjacent pancreas. Pancreatic calcifications suggest chronic pancreatitis. In cases of tropical calcific pancreatitis, dense calcification is seen in pancreatic parenchyma (Mehta & Gittes, 2005).

Plain chest x rays should be performed in all patients with acute pancreatitis to look for evidence of pleural effusion and pulmonary oedema (Mehta & Gittes, 2005). One fifth of children show evidence of pleural effusion (Uretsky et al., 1999).

Ultrasound Scan (US): is one of the most useful imaging tools in childhood pancreatitis (Haddock et al., 1994). Abdominal US may show pancreatic swelling or a decrease in pancreatic echogenicity due to oedema or peri-pancreatic fluid collection. These findings *per se* are not sufficient to coin the diagnosis of acute pancreatitis or estimate its severity. The main use of US is to demonstrate gallstones as a possible cause of pancreatitis and to follow up the treatment by serial observation of improvement in oedema or peripancreatic fluid collection (Mehta & Gittes, 2005).

Abdomominal CT scan: provides images of the pancreas superior to those obtained by US scan in as far as determining the size of the pancreas, the degree of oedema and the presence of fluid collection is concerned. Due to the much better resolution, the size and anatomy of the pancreatic duct can often be delineated much more accurately with CT than with US. The presence of complications such as pancreatic abscess or pseudocyst may also be determined. Dynamic CT pancreatography, using an intravenous bolus of contrast with rapid scanning in fine cuts through the pancreas, has the advantage of differentiating perfused from non-perfused (necrotic) pancreas. It has the ability to provide a precise assessment of the percentage of and distribution of pancreatic perfusion. Furthermore, CT scan can be used for interventional procedures for diagnosis or drainage of fluid collections (Mehta & Gittes, 2005).

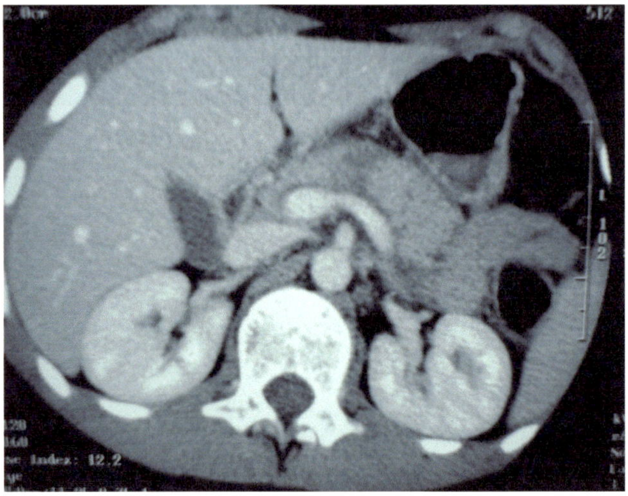

Fig. 1. An abdominal CT scan of a 10 year old child with blunt abdominal trauma. Note the radiolucency at the neck of the pancreas indicating parenchymal disruption

ERCP: although the literature suggest that the complication rates with ERCP are higher in children than in adults, ERCP is being used increasingly in children. ERCP can provide detailed information on the pancreatic duct. It is particularly helpful for its diagnostic and therapeutic roles in the management of children with acute obstructive biliary pancreatitis. ERCP and pancreatic duct stenting can also be beneficial in trauma patients in whom a ductal injury is suspected or a pancreatic pseudocyst has formed (Mehta & Gittes, 2005, Ali et al., 2010). In cases of pancreas divisum, however, cannulation of the minor papilla is possible in less than half of the cases because of its small size and the angle at which it meets the duodenum (Miyano, 2006).

MRCP: the magnetic resonance cholangio-pancreatography is a useful, non invasive diagnostic tool for evaluating the biliary tree and the pancreatic duct. This technique precludes the risk of complications encountered with ERCP. The study is cheaper and employs no radiation or administration of contrast media which is routinely performed with ERCP. MRCP is not without disadvantages. As an essentially diagnostic study, it does not facilitate therapeutic intervention and it has a tendency to overestimate the stenosis of the main pancreatic duct in patients with pancreatitis. Despite the recognized disadvantages, MRCP is now the initial imaging study of choice in the evaluation of pancreatic ductal anatomy in children with unexplained or recurrent pancreatitis (Mehta & Gittes, 2005).

6.2 Chronic pancreatitis

In children with suspected **chronic pancreatitis** the following investigations are suggested:

- Sweat test and gene testing for CFTR
- Testing for cationic trypsinogen and SPINK1 mutations
- Assessment for autoimmune causes
- Biochemical investigations for diabetes mellitus, lipase, electrolytes and stools for evidence of malabsorption
- Imaging to exclude structural (congenital or acquired) abnormalities. In children with chronic pancreatitis, changes on imaging studies are usually encountered
- Pancreatic biopsy, considered to be a gold standard for diagnosis in adults, is rarely if ever required in children (Nydegger et al., 2006).

7. Severity scores

Many scoring systems were used to assess the severity of acute pancreatitis in adults, however, there is no widely adopted robust severity scoring system that is specifically targeting children (Nydegger et al., 2006). The applicability of adult scoring systems such as Ranson's and the Imrie prognostic criteria, the Glasgow and modified Glasgow scores and the Acute Physiology and Chronic Health Evaluation (APACHE) II score have not been validated in children. An alternative severity scoring system has been suggested by other researchers. This group has compared a scoring system designed specifically to paediatric patients with selected adult scoring systems (DeBanto et al., 2002). This system compares eight variables to predict severe outcome and mortality during an episode of acute pancreatitis. An episode of pancreatitis is considered to be severe if the patient died, had surgery on the pancreas, developed a pseudocyst or abscess or infected necrosis, or met criteria for multiple organ dysfunction. The admission criteria considered are:

- Age <7 yrs
- Weight <23Kg
- WBC (Admission) >18.5/cmm
- LDH (Admission) >2000 IU/L
- 48hr trough albumin <2.6mg/dl
- 48hr trough calcium <8.3mg/dl
- 48hr fluid sequestration >75ml/kg/48hrs
- 48hr rise in blood urea nitrogen >5mg/dl

Each factor is allocated a score of 1 point and higher total scores are associated with an increased chance of severe pancreatitis and mortality.

Scores of 5-7 points showed 80% severe outcome and 10% mortality

2-4 points showed 38.5 severe outcome and 5.8% mortality

0-2 points showed 8.6% severe outcome and 1.4% mortality

When the cutoff for predicting severe outcome was set at 3 criteria, this new system had a sensitivity of 70%, a -ve predictive value of 91%, a specificity of 79% and a +ve predictive value of 45%. The system probably performs better in identifying those patients who are at risk for severe pancreatitis than the existing systems used in adults (DeBanto et al., 2002). When compared with the Ranson's and Glasgow systems used in adult patients with pancreatitis, this system showed a better sensitivity (70%) versus Ranson (30%) and Glasgow (35%) scores and a better negative predictive value (91% vs 85% and 85% respectively) (DeBanto et al., 2002). In trauma, the grade of pancreatic injury was an independent predictor of both pancreatic complications (Kao et al., 2003).

Some researchers associated the severity of pancreatitis to the aeiology. Haddock found that severe pancreatitis was most commonly associated with systemic disease (22 of 51; 43.1%) and trauma (13 of 51; 25.4%), beside associated factors such as significantly higher body weight, higher frequency of dyspnoea and pleural effusion, and lower serum calcium and albumin levels (Haddock et al., 1994; Chang et al., 2011).

Many classification systems were adopted for grading of disease severity based on various factors. Examples of these classification systems include:

- Marseille classification which relies on grading of biopsy specimens.
- Cambridge classification with more emphasis on imaging to provide grading and severity scoring, Computed tomography (CT) was more accurate than ultrasound in evaluation of the severity of pancreatitis.
- TIGAR-O system: more recently, the Toxic, Idiopathic, Genetic, Autoimmune, Recurrent severe associated chronic pancreatitis and Other systems has been developed and allows multiple risk factors to be assessed in an individual patient either as a risk factor or as an aetiology (Nydegger et al., 2006).
- Atlanta criteria: though this is still controversial with lack of consensus (Berney et al., 1999; Bollen et al., 2007).

Overall, it is relevant to state that up till now commonly used scoring systems have limited ability to predict disease severity in children and adolescents with acute pancreatitis.

Careful and repeated evaluations are essential in managing these patients as they may develop major complications without early signs (Lautz et al., 2011).

8. Treatment

8.1 Acute pancreatitis

8.1.1 Conservative treatment

Treatment of acute pancreatitis is primarily and essentially supportive. It aims at limiting exocrine pancreatic secretion and monitoring for acute and long term complications. Key features in the empirical therapeutic regimen commonly used in treating patients with acute pancreatitis are: aggressive **IV fluid administration** to replace the profound fluid deficit and to maintain a good hydration as indicated by adequate urine output (2ml/kg/hr), usually measured with the aid of an indwelling urinary catheter. **Pain control** should be achieved with parenteral analgesia. Adequate analgesia is critical to minimize the additional stress from pain. Meperidine (Demerol) is thought to be a better analgesic in pancreatitis because morphine is well known to cause spasm of the sphincter of Oddi which in turn is known to increase pancreatic duct pressure and potentially worsen the pancreatitis (Mehta & Gittes, 2005). It is also important to be certain of the diagnosis of pancreatitis before giving the patient significant doses of narcotics because the ability to diagnose serious non-pancreatic problems, such as intestinal ischaemia or perforated ulcer, may be lost. It is imperative to have a very low threshold for transferring the patient to an **intensive care unit** and provide constant monitoring to avoid development of profound hypovolemia. Initially, bowel should be kept at rest with **NG suction**. Most mild to moderate cases will settle if food and drink is withheld for a few days. **Proton pump inhibitors** (PPI) or **H2 receptor antagonists** administration helps to prevent exposure of the duodenal secretin producing cells to gastric acid, which is a potent stimulator of pancreatic secretion. These antagonists also may help prevent stress ulceration seen in patients with pancreatitis. While clinical trials have shown improved outcome in acute pancreatitis by using long acting **somatostatin analogues** octreotides, controversy still exists concerning the use of **prophylactic antibiotics**. In general, mild to moderate cases probably do not benefit from antibiotics. More severe cases of pancreatitis, however, may benefit because of the high rate of sepsis. Prophylactic antibiotics are indicated when there is pancreatic necrosis or when infection is either suspected or documented in severe acute pancreatitis. Studies have related prophylactic antibiotic administration for 10-14 days in adult patients with severe acute pancreatitis and proven pancreatic tissue necrosis with decrease in superinfection of necrotic tissue and mortality (Nydegger et al., 2006; Mehta & Gittes, 2005; Miyano, 2006)). Some advantages have been demonstrated with the use of imipenem with reduction in the incidence of pancreatic sepsis in patients with necrotizing pancreatitis. Because the onset of cytokine action follows immediately after the onset of pancreatitis and peaks after 36-48 hours, **cytokine antagonist therapy** represents a potential therapeutic target and therefore is of intense interest (Nydegger et al., 2006). In children with relapsing attacks of pancreatitis we would advocate similar management and also include investigations to exclude structural, metabolic and hereditary pancreatitis (Nydegger et al., 2006). **Nutrition** is a crucial factor in the management of patients with pancreatitis. Early positive nitrogen balance has been shown to improve survival rates. This need for aggressive nutrition should come in the form of early TPN administration. The TPN should include lipid formulations. To minimise the causal association of hyperlipidaemia and pancreatitis, it is recommended that serum lipid levels should be monitored to maintain triglyceride levels no greater than 500 mg/dl (Mehta & Gittes, 2005).

The results of several controlled studies in adult patients with acute pancreatitis, support enteral nutrition. It costs less than TPN by approximately 1/4. Total enteral nutrition moderates the acute phase response and improves disease severity and clinical outcome despite unchanged pancreatic imaging findings (Windsor et al., 1998; Nydegger et al., 2006). Although there are sparse paediatric data, enteral feeding has been widely adopted. Perhaps a nasojejunal feeding with high protein and low-fat formula through a tube inserted under radiological or endoscopic guidance can be implemented until the child is ready to commence oral intake (Nydegger et al., 2006). Naso-jejunal feeding may be particularly useful in places where TPN availability is considered to be a luxury!.

It is imperative to note that despite the known advantage of nutritional support in facilitating resolution of pancreatitis, quite often early commencement of enteral feeding results in relapse of acute abdominal pain and elevation of amylase levels.

In general, the resumption of enteral nutrition should be cautious, usually after complete resolution of abdominal pain and preferably after normalization of the serum enzyme levels (Mehta & Gittes 2005).

8.1.2 Surgical treatment

Surgery for pancreatic disorders in children is rarely required. Surgical intervention in children with acute pancreatitis is even less practiced. It should be restricted to patients with complications such as severe necrotizing pancreatitis requiring debridement or patients with other complications associated with acute pancreatitis including pancreatic ascites, pancreatic abscess collections not amenable for percutaneous drainage and pancreatic pseudocyst (Rabinovich et al., 2006) (see below).

In traumatic pancreatitis, as most children with a solid-organ abdominal injury can be managed conservatively, the pancreas is no exception. Non-operative management of low grade pancreatic injury is widely accepted. Management of major pancreatic parenchymal or ductal injury in children, however, remains controversial (Haddock et al., 1994; Stringer et al., 2005). Initial nonoperative management of injuries of the proximal pancreatic duct is a common practice and allows for the formation and uneventful delayed drainage of a pseudocyst, rather than the risks of early radical interventions (Jobst et al., 1999). If there is delayed or no response to conservative management, ERCP with sphincterotomy and/or stenting of injured pancreatic duct may be attempted as it has reportedly had a proven efficacy in resolving the symptoms in such patients (Cay et al., 2005; Canty & Weinman, 2001; Ali, 2010). Distal duct injuries are best managed by prompt spleen-sparing distal pancreatectomy (Jobst et al., 1999). Removal of impacted stones in gallstone pancreatitis in children should be performed endoscopically (Mehta & Gittes, 2005).

When discovered incidentally during the course of laparotomy for other suspected causes of peritonitis, it is imperative to palpate the gallbladder (GB) for stones. In the presence of gallstones and mild pancreatitis, cholecystectomy can be performed. However, with severe pancreatitis, cholecystostomy may be the safer option which can provide an access to the biliary calculi later. Cholecystectomy can be done at a later stage when the patient's condition is favourable. If no gallstones are present, but the patient has severe necrotizing pancreatitis, limited debridement and/or leaving large sump drains in place is probably adequate (Mehta & Gittes, 2005).

Overall, early pancreatic lavage, pancreatic drainage, and pancreatic resection have not been shown to improve survival rates in cases of severe pancreatitis (Mehta & Gittes, 2005) and early intervention for pancreatic injury, in the absence of clinical deterioration or major ductal injury, is not recommended either (Keller et al., 1997). There is also an iatrogenic dimension to the problem as the rarity of pancreatic surgery in children caused an unfamiliarity that can be associated with contracting significant morbidity and mortality.

When comparing traumatic and non-traumatic pancreatitis, Schmittenbecher and co-researchers found that more patients with traumatic pancreatitis were operated on in 86% of cases and the rate of pseudocysts reached 61.5% whereas non-traumatic pancreatitis required surgical intervention in 50% and developed pseudocysts in 17% of cases. In non-traumatic pancreatitis it is recommended that surgery should be avoided and reserved for complications. Exceptions are obstructions of the pancreaticobiliary ducts which need early removal to prevent chronicity of the disease and functional loss of the organ (Schmittenbecher, 1996). In their study, Stringer et al summarized the indications for surgery in acute pancreatitis in persistent pseudocysts and treatment of an underlying cause of pancreatitis (Stringer et al., 2005).

Key points in the management of acute pancreatitis

IV Fluids
ICU admission
Pain control
NGT aspiration
PPI or H2 receptor-blockers
Somatostatin analogues
Prophylactic antibiotics
Cytokine antagonists
Adequate nutrition
Endoscopic intervention
Surgical intervention

8.2 Chronic pancreatitis

Management of chronic pancreatitis is directed towards identification of the aetiological factors, diagnosis of the condition and hence implementation of the appropriate therapy. Due to the structural changes associated with chronic pancreatitis, many more surgical indications exist here when compared with acute pancreatitis. As appropriate, conservative management consists of provision of **medications, analgesia, antibiotics and nutrition**. Emphasis should be made on treatment of pancreatic exocrine insufficiency, therefore, digestive problems related to failure of the pancreas require **enzyme replacement therapy** with meals as well as **fat soluble vitamins** supplements (Durie, 2010). Endocrine insufficiency, particularly **diabetes mellitus**, should be **controlled**.

Indications for operative intervention include unsuccessful conservative medical therapy, intractable pain, narcotic addiction, impaired nutrition and poor weight gain.

The goal of surgery in these patients is to relieve pain by provision of adequate analgesia and to preserve the exocrine and endocrine functions of the pancreas through decompression of pancreatic ducts and restoration of adequate pancreatic drainage.

Surgical options include lateral longitudinal pancreaticojejunostomy (Puestow procedure), distal pancreatectomy with Roux-en-Y pancreaticojejunostomy (Duval procedure), ERCP sphincterotomy or operative sphincteroplasty. In cases of intractable and refractory disease, a few pediatric patients with chronic pancreatitis and chronic abdominal pain were successfully treated with total pancreatectomy and islet cell transplantation (Hebra et al., 2009; Bellin et al., 2008).

Surgical intervention is indicated for the management of **congenital anatomic defects,** such as **pancreas divisum.** The primary goal of treatment of **pancreas divisum** associated with pancreatitis is to establish adequate drainage of the duct of Santorini. This can be achieved with accessory papilla sphincteroplasty. Correct use of this procedure demands that intrapancreatic ductal obstruction be ruled out by pancreatography. The progression of disease to **pancreatic insufficiency** can be arrested when the **obstruction** is relieved early.

Endoscopic stenting with or without **sphincterotom**y has been described, however, the technique requires particular skill with the endoscope in cannulation of the small ducts encountered in children. Re-stenosis and recurrence of symptoms have been reported following endoscopic sphincterotomy.

If chronic pancreatitis has developed in the presence of a dilated duct, **longitudinal pancreaticojejunostomy (Puestow)** should be performed. The indication for the use of a **direct ductal decompression** procedure is evidence of **pancreatic ductal ectasia** with multiple intrapancreatic **duct strictures,** particularly when symptomatic (Stringer et al., 2005). An important precautionary measure in any drainage procedure is preservation of existing endocrine function by avoiding major pancreatic resection. Longitudinal pancreaticojejunostomy (Puestow technique) in adults has been successful in eliminating or reducing pain intensity from chronic pancreatitis in 70 to 97% of patients. In children, some authors maintain that the Puestow procedure improves pancreatic function, decreases hospitalization and increases body weight toward ideal. Others have reported that distal pancreatectomy and pancreatico-jejunostomy are effective whereas longitudinal pancreaticojejunostomy is ineffective (Miyano, 2006). Traditionally, these procedures were performed with open surgery. A **minimally invasive** approach to the longitudinal pancreaticojejunostomy using **robotic surgery** in a child has been reported recently (Meehan & Sawin, 2011). Due to this controversy regarding appropriate operative procedures in paediatric cases, further consideration is warranted.

Subtotal or total **pancreatectomy** is associated with considerable morbidity and mortality and is reserved for patients with intractable pain who have diffuse parenchymal damage without ductal dilatation. The procedure is not generally indicated in children.

DuBay et al. reported that in the treatment of complicated **hereditary pancreatitis** (HP) in children, the modified Puestow procedure (longitudinal pancreaticojejunostomy) improves the quality of life by improving pancreatic function, decreasing hospitalizations, and increasing the percentile ideal body weight. Direct pancreatic duct localization during the procedure reduces morbidity rate than localization via distal pancreatectomy. Surgery performed in the early stage of complicated disease may preserve pancreatic function (DuBay et al., 2000). Likewise, surgery for **chronic relapsing pancreatitis** is done to relieve pain, treat complications or both. Adequate surgical decompression, ultimately, can **prevent disease recurrence** (Clifton et al., 2007; Bellin et al., 2008).

In children suffering from **chronic pancreatitis** complicated by **diabetes mellitus**, **pancreatectomy** and **islet autotransplantation** can prevent or reduce the severity of diabetes in about 75% of patients. Furthermore, outcome is noted to be better in younger than older children (Bellin et al., 2008).

Treatment of chronic calcific pancreatitis includes control of diabetes, relief of pain with analgesics, pancreatic enzyme replacements, endoscopic or surgical decompression of dilated ducts and removal of pancreatic calculi (Aamarapurkar, 2001).

The role of laparoscopy: laparoscopy has been reported to be used for common bile duct (CBD) exploration in obstructive recurrent pancreatitis (Shah et al., 1997). The commoner use of laparoscopy is for cholecystectomy when gallstones are incriminated in childhood pancreatitis. Laparoscopy has also been used in the treatment of pancreatic pseudocysts (see below).

Surgery of the pancreas is generally of 3 types,

1. Sphincteroplasty
2. Pancreatic drainage via longitudinal pancreaticojejunostomy (Puestow)
or end to end pancreaticojejunostomy (Duval)
or pancreatogastrostomy (Smith)
3. Pancreatectomy: partial or total

9. Complications

Expected local complications of childhood pancreatitis include necrotizing pancreatitis, haemorrhagic pancreatitis, pseudocyst and pancreatic fistula. While systemically, as cases of severe pancreatitis progress, close monitoring of the patients should be exercised for signs of development of hypovolaemic shock and of multiorgan system failure. Pleural effusion and pulmonary oedema can progress to severe adult respiratory distress syndrome with hypoxia requiring endotracheal intubation. The tense abdominal distention associated with pancreatitis, either due to ileus or ascites, frequently contributes to the hypoventilation. Hypocalcemia, hypomagnesemia, anaemia from haemorrhage, hyperglycemia, renal failure and late sepsis can be seen in these patients and require close monitoring and treatment.

9.1 Acute haemorrhagic pancreatitis

Most of the complications related to acute pancreatitis tend to occur in the first two weeks of onset of pain; and secondary infection and necrosis account for 70-80% of deaths (Munoz &

Katerndahl, 2000). Zhu et al. noted that pancreatic damage or pancreatic necrosis in critically ill children is characterized by acute onset, profound severity, short course and multiple organ failure. It may be asymptomatic in early stage, and can be easily missed (Zhu et al., 2011).

Acute hemorrhagic pancreatitis is a rare event in children. This serious complication of acute pancreatitis may be attended with a mortality rate approaching 50% because of shock, systemic inflammatory response syndrome with multiple organ dysfunction, acute respiratory distress syndrome (ARDS), disseminated intravascular coagulation (DIC), massive gastrointestinal bleeding and systemic sepsis or peritonitis. Clinical manifestations related to hemorrhagic pancreatitis may include Grey Turner sign (bluish discoloration of the flanks) or Cullen sign (discoloration of the periumbilical region) because of blood extravasation in the fascial planes of the abdominal wall. Additional signs include pleural effusions, haematemesis, melaena, and coma (Mehta & Gittes, 2005; Miyano 2006)

9.2 Pancreatic pseudocysts

9.2.1 Definition

Pancreatic pseudocysts are localized collections of pancreatic secretions with no epithelial lining. They develop as a complication of pancreatitis where they were reported to complicate 10-23% of the acute episodes. When associated with abdominal trauma, the frequency rate of pseudocyst identification is higher than 50% (Hebra et al., 2009). The other common causes of pseudocysts in children are pancreatic duct obstruction, infection and, rarely, drug induced acute pancreatitis such as with valproic acid (Miyano, 2006; Mehta & Gittes, 2005).

9.2.2 Pathology

As a result of extravasation of digestive pancreatic enzymes, pseudocysts develop in the lesser sac between the pancreas posteriorly and the stomach anteriorly. The cavity is lined by fibroelastic connective tissue capsule due to inflammatory reaction on the surrounding organs such as the pancreas, stomach, duodenum, colon, small bowel and omentum. An acute pseudocyst develops a thick fibrous wall in 4 to 6 weeks (Mehta & Gittes, 2005). After 6 weeks, a pancreatic pseudocyst is considered mature. Cysts may vary in size and if greater than 6 cm in size, resolution with conservative medical management is doubtful (Yoder et al., 2009). Cyst fluid is clear or straw coloured in most cases and may contain toothpaste-like debris. The amylase level of the cyst fluid is typically higher than 50000 U/mL (Miyano, 2006).

9.2.3 Diagnosis

A pancreatic pseudocyst formation should be suspected in patients with a history of abdominal trauma or pancreatitis followed by clinical or radiological appearance of an upper abdominal mass. Common associated symptoms and signs include persistent abdominal pain, tenderness, abdominal mass, gastric outlet obstruction, anorexia, nausea and vomiting. Occasionally, gastrointestinal haemorrhage, weight loss, jaundice, chest pain, fever and ascites may be encountered (Miyano, 2006; Yoder et al., 2009).

Pseudocysts may be acute or chronic. The acute pseudocyst has an irregular wall on CT scan, is tender and usually follows a recent episode of acute pancreatitis or trauma. Chronic pseudocysts are usually spherical with a thick wall and they are commonly seen in patients with chronic pancreatitis. It is important to distinguish these two types of pseudocysts because 50% of acute pseudocysts resolve without therapy, whereas chronic pseudocysts rarely do (Mehta & Gittes, 2005).

US, CT and MRI are reliable imaging modalities in the diagnosis of pancreatic pseudocysts (Fig 2, a & b). These studies are highly sensitive for evaluating the thickness of the cyst wall and for observing changes in the cyst during the ensuing period of treatment. ERCP is often useful as a diagnostic and a therapeutic tool because it can definitively determine the status of the pancreatic duct and thus guide surgical intervention (Miyano, 2006).

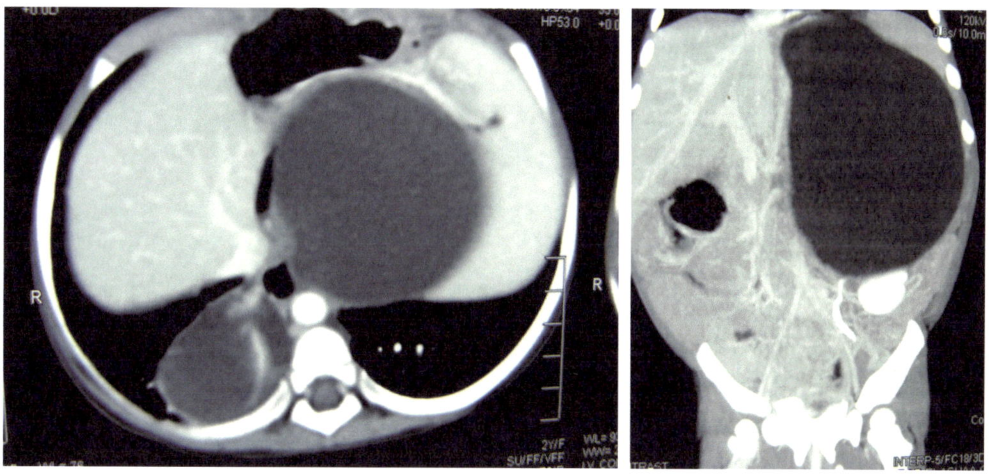

a) b)

Fig. 2. Pseudocyst of the pancreas on a thoracoabdominal CT scan of an 18 month old child. Note the related posterior mediastinal cyst seen on picture film a. (a, transverse section; b, coronal section)

9.2.4 Treatment

Optimal management of pancreatic pseudocysts in children remains controversial. A large proportion of these pseudocysts tend to resolve with medical therapy alone and have a low risk for recurrence. Pseudocysts less than 5 cm in diameter usually disappear without intervention (Mehta & Gittes, 2005). Accordingly, drainage should be performed in patients with pseudocysts that are more than 6 weeks old and have a diameter more than 5 cm. Occasionally, a demonstrable cyst wall thickening sufficient for internal drainage may appear on CT as early as 3-4 weeks from the onset of symptoms (Miyano, 2006). Approximately 60% of pancreatic pseudocysts that are caused by blunt trauma require surgical intervention (Hebra et al., 2009).

Available treatment options range from conservative medical management to surgical drainage. Conventional management involves supportive therapy over a 6-week interval during which time the cyst may either resolve spontaneously or the cyst wall undergoes fibrous maturation, potentially allowing internal surgical drainage to the stomach or jejunum.

Octreotide acetate, a long acting somatostatin analogue, has been shown to be successful in reducing exocrine function and, thereby, helps resolving pancreatic pseudocysts in children (Miyano, 2006; Mehta & Gittes, 2005).

If the patient can not withstand major surgery, has an infected or an immature cyst, percutaneous external surgical drainage is preferred. U/S or CT guided percutaneous drainage is the treatment of choice for infected pseudocysts because these cysts typically have thin, weak walls not amenable to internal drainage. However, when compared with internal drainage, external drainage is generally associated with adverse consequences such as fistula formation and a higher recurrence rate (Miyano, 2006).

Internal drainage, especially transgastric cysto-gastrostomy is widely used. There is significant evidence indicating that it is effective in the treatment of mature pancreatic pseudocysts (Miyano, 2006; Mehta & Gittes, 2005).

Roux-en-Y cysto-jejunostomy is an alternative internal drainage procedure and is associated with less complications and recurrence rates.

Though less commonly used than other operative procedures, contemplating cysto-duodenostomy may be effective when a cyst is intimately adherent to the duodenum.

Either pancreatico-duodenectomy or distal pancreatectomy, as indicated, is effective in treating patients with pseudocysts in selected cases. Pseudocysts in the body or tail of the pancreas or those involving the head and uncinate process of the pancreas that are not amenable to internal drainage are rare and may require distal or proximal pancreatic resection, respectively (Miyano, 2006).

Minimally invasive drainage approaches to pancreatic pseudocysts were reported. Strategies for cysto-gastrostomy include transoesophago-gastric endoscopic cysto-gastrostomy and percutaneous drainage (Mehta & Gittes, 2005). The other minimally invasive technique is laparoscopic transgastric cysto-gastrostomy or laparoscopic cysto-jejunostomy. There are few reports on the use of laparoscopy in the management of pancreatic pseudocysts (Saad et al., 2005; Sietz et al.,2006). In a multi-institutional retrospective review of 13 patients with a mean age of 10.4 years and mean weight of 52.1 kg who underwent laparoscopic cysto-gastrostomy with no conversions, the authors concluded that a laparoscopic approach to pancreatic cysto-gastrostomy for chronic pseudocysts proved to be safe and effective. Techniques varied, but 92% of patients had complete resolution with minimal morbidity and rapid recovery. Laparoscopic cysto-gastrostomy can be adopted as an appropriate first-line treatment for chronic pseudocysts in children (Yoder et al., 2009).

Both endoscopic and laparoscopic drainage approaches are safe, efficient and effective, however, the two procedures should be performed at institutions with significant experience with these techniques to minimize serious potential risks.

Treatment of persistent Pancreatic pseudocysts:

- Internal drainage (preferred)
- Excision (distal pseudocysts only)
- External drainage (infected or immature cysts)

9.2.5 Pseudocyst complications

Untreated pseudocysts may present with persistence of symptoms or become complicated with major haemorrhage, infection or cyst rupture. Haemorrhage can occur as a result of cyst pressure and erosion into an adjacent blood vessel and may be controlled with emergency angiography and embolization. For infected or ruptured pseudocysts, early intervention with external drainage is indicated (Miyano, 2006; Mehta & Gittes, 2005)

9.3 Pancreatic ascites

Pancreatic ascites is uncommon but may follow trauma or pancreatic surgery. Leakage of pancreatic fluid from a damaged major pancreatic duct results in ascites. Treatment is initially conservative and consists of bowel rest, TPN administration and use of long-acting somatostatin analogue. In many cases ascites resolves with this treatment. If not, ERCP or MRCP should be performed to determine the site of the ductal injury and, accordingly, the appropriate course of surgical intervention (Mehta & Gittes. 2005).

9.4 Pleural effusion

Occasionally, pancreatic pleural effusion may develop following severe pancreatitis. A significantly elevated level of pleural fluid amylase/lipase with concentrations higher than those obtained from patient's serum sample, may be encountered following traumatic pancreatitis. Intrathoracic pancreatic pseudocyst has been reported following traumatic pancreatitis where, eventually, persistent pancreatic ductal leak was successfully managed with ERCP stenting of the pancreatic duct (Ali et al., 2010).

9.5 Pancreatic abscess

Infection may complicate necrotic pancreatic tissue or peripancreatic fluid collection resulting in pancreatic abscess. Abscess increases the mortality rate of pancreatitis threefold and is an absolute indication for surgical intervention. Persistence of fever and leukocytosis in a child with pancreatitis for more than 7 days is an indication for CT guided needle aspiration to differentiate pancreatic abscess from an uninfected pancreatic fluid collection. Dynamic CT pancreatography is a useful test in showing pancreatic necrosis which is a likely predisposing factor for the subsequent development of a pancreatic abscess. The definitive therapy for pancreatic abscess entails surgical debridement and adequate abscess cavity drainage (Mehta & Gittes, 2005).

9.6 Pancreatic fistula

Pancreatic fistula develops following surgical procedures in the pancreas. Most low output fistulas close spontaneously but may drain for several months. Long acting somatostatin analogue is beneficial in decreasing the fistula output and accelerating the rate of closure. Fistula closure can be facilitated by adequate nutrition, with TPN if enteral feeding results in high-volume output, and by ensuring that the fistula tract does not become obstructed. In persistent fistulas surgical Roux-en-Y jejunostomy to the leak point is recommended (Mehta & Gittes, 2005).

9.7 Hyperglycaemia

Both hyperglycaemia and diabetes can occur in children with pancreatitis. In a recent study, researchers looked at 176 patients who were up to 21 years of age and who were hospitalized with acute pancreatitis, acute recurrent pancreatitis, and chronic pancreatitis, excluding those with known pre-existing diabetes or cystic fibrosis before presentation with pancreatitis. Severe pancreatitis was associated with hyperglycaemia, and eight patients developed diabetes requiring insulin by the time of discharge. The authors noted that while adults tend to develop diabetes after chronic pancreatitis, children can develop diabetes due to a single episode of acute pancreatitis (Raman et al., 2011).

9.8 Adenocarcinoma of the pancreas

In patients with chronic pancreatitis, it has been reported that there is a 4% life risk of developing pancreatic adenocarcinoma. This risk may be as high as 40% in patients with hereditary pancraetitis (Nydegger et al., 2006).

10. Prognosis

Uncomplicated acute pancreatitis in children usually have excellent prognosis. The outcome also depends on the co-morbid conditions (Werlin 2003). The mortality rate is approximately 10% in mild disease and up to 90% in cases of necrotizing or haemaorrhagic pancreatitis (Uretsky 1999).

11. Conclusion

Pancreatitis in children is an uncommon event, however, it is attended with significant morbidity and mortality. The presentation may range from transient mild symptoms to life threatening, overwhelming sepsis, multiple organ system failure and death. Prompt institution of appropriate diagnostic and therapeutic measures is crucial to achieve good clinical results. Conservative management and minimally invasive surgical and endoscopic procedures are usually sufficient to treat most of the patients. Children rarely need surgical intervention for the treatment of pancreatitis and its complications. Further developments are anticipated in the field of research, diagnostic tools, disease severity scoring and therapeutic methods to improve the outcome.

12. References

Aamarapurkar, D. (2001). Chronic pancreatitis, cited on 15/07/2011, available from www.bhj/journal/2001_4301_jan/sp_76.htm

Ali, A.; Tan, H.; Gent, R.; Davidson, G. & Roberts-Thompson, I. (2010). Intra- thoracic pancreatic pseudocyst. A rare complication of traumatic pancreatitis. *Pediatr Surg Int*, Vol.26, No.8, pp. 859-861

Bai, H.; Ma, M.; Orabi, A.; Park, A.; Latif, S.; Bhandari, V.; Husain, S. Novel Characterization of Drug-Associated Pancreatitis in Children. *J Pediatr Gastroenterol Nutr.* (Jun 2011) 14. DOI:10.1097/MPG.0b013e318228574e. Retrieved on 18/07/2011 from http://pubget.com/paper/21681111

Bellin, M.; Carlson, A.; Kobayashi, T.; et al. (2008) Outcome after pancreatectomy and islet autotransplantation in a pediatric population, *J Pediatr Gastroenterol Nutr*, Vol.47, No.1, (Jul 2008), pp.37-44

Berney, T.; Belli, D.; Bugmann, P.; Beghetti, M.; Morel, P. & LeCoultre, C. (1996). Influence of severe underlying pathology and hypovolemic shock on the development of acute pancreatitis in children, *J Pediatr Surg*, Vol.31, No.9, (September 1996), pp. 1256-1261

Berney, T.; Gasche, Y.; Robert, J.; Jenny, A.; Mensi, N.; Grau, G.; et al. (1999). Serum profile of interleukin-6, interleukin-8, and interleukin-10 in patients with severe and mild acute pancreatitis, *Pancreas*, Vol.18, No.4, (May 1999), pp. 371-377

Bollen, T.; Santvoort, H.; Besselink, M.; van Leeuwen, M.; Horvath, K.; Freeny, P. & Gooszen, H. (2007). The Atlanta classification of acute pancreatitis revisited. *Br J Surg*, Vol.95, No.1, (Jan 2008), pp. 6-21

Butler, K.; Venzon, D.; Henry, N.; Husson, R.; Mueller, B.; Balis, F.; Jacobsen, F.; Lewis, L. & Pizzo, P. (1993). Pancreatitis in human immunodeficiency virus-infected children receiving dideoxyinosine, *Pediatrics*, Vol.91, No.4, (April 1993), pp 747-751

Camp, J.; Polley, T. & Coran, A. (1994). Pancreatitis in children: diagnosis and etiology in 57 patients, *Pediatr Surg Int*, Vol. 9, No.7, (August 1994), pp 492-497

Canty, T. & Weinman, D. (2001). Treatment of pancreatic duct disruption in children by an endoscopically placed stent. *J Pediatr Surg*, Vol.36, No.2, (Feb 2001), pp. 345-348

Cay, A.; Imamoglu, M.; Bektas, O.; Ozdemir, O.; Arslan, M. & Sarihan, H. (2005). Nonoperative treatment of traumatic pancreatic duct disruption in children with an endoscopically placed stent, *J Pediatr Surg*, Vol.40, No.12, (2005), pp. e9-e12

Chang, Y.; Chao, H.; Kong, M.; Hsia, S.; Lai, M. & Yan, D. (2011). Acute pancreatitis in children, *Acta Paediatrica*, Vol.100, No.5, (May 2011), pp. 740–744

Clifton, M.; Pelayo, J.; Cortes, R.; Grethel, E.; Wagner, A.; Lee, H.; Harrison, M.; Farmer, D. & Nobuhara, K. (2007). Surgical treatment of childhood recurrent pancreatitis, *J Pediatr Surg*, Vol.42, No.7, (July 2007), pp. 1203-1207

Comfort, M. & Steinberg, A. (1952). Pedigree of family with hereditary chronic relapsing pancreatitis, *Gastroenterology*, No.21, pp 54-63

DeBanto, J.; Goday, P.; Pedroso, M.; et al. (2002). Acute pancreatitis in children. *Am J Gastoenterol*, Vol.97, No.7, (July 2002), pp. 1726-1731

DiMagno, M. & DiMagno, E. (2003). Chronic pancreatitis, *Current Opinion in Gastroenterology*, Vol.19, No.5, (September 2003), pp. 451-457

DuBay, D.; Sandler, A.; Kimura, K.; Bishop, W.; Eimen, M. & Soper, R. (2000). The modified Puestow procedure for complicated hereditary pancreatitis in children. *J Pediatr Surg*, Vol.35, No.2, (Feb 2000), pp. 343-348

Durie, P. (2010). Inherited pancreatic disorders of childhood. Cited 16/07/2011, available from www.pancreasfoundation.org/2010/04/inherited-pancreatic-disorders-of-childhood/

Garg, R.; Agarwala, S. & Bhatnagar, V. (2010). Acute pancreatitis induced by ifosfamide therapy, *J Pediatr Surg*, Vol.45, No.10, (October 2010), pp. 2071-2073

Goh, S.; Chui, C. & Jacobson, A. (2003). Childhood acute pancreatitis in a children's hospital, *Singapore Med J*, Vol.44, No.9, pp. 453-456

Haddock, G., Coupar, G., Youngson, G., MacKinlay G., & Raine P. (1994). Acute pancreatitis in children: A 15-year review, *J Pediatr Surg*, Vol. 29, No.6, pp. 719-722

Harb, R. & Naon, H. (2005). Idiopathic fibrosing pancreatitis in a 3-year-old girl: a case report and review of the literature, *J Pediatr Surg*, Vol.40, No.8, (August 2005), pp 1335-1340

Hebra, A.; Adams, S. & Thomas, P. (2009). Pediatric pancreatitis and pancreatic pseudocyst treatment and management. *Medscape Reference*. 21 Oct 2009. available from www.emedicine.medscape.com/article/933256-treatment

Hwang, S.; Paik, C.; Lee, K. Chung, W.; Jang, U. & Yang, J. (2010). Recurrent acute pancreatitis caused by an annual pancreas in a child, *Gastrointest Endosc*, Vol.72, No.4, (October 2010), pp. 848-849

Ibrahim, M.; Gabr, K.; Abdulrazik, M.; Fahmy, H. & El-Booq, Y. (2011). Acute pancreatitis in children: an experience with 50 cases, *Annals of Pediatric Surgery*, Vol.7, No.2, (April 2011), pp. 72–75

Jobst, M.; Canty, T. & Lynch, F. (1999). Management of pancreatic injury in pediatric blunt abdominal trauma, *J Pediatr Surg*, Vol.34, No.5, (May 1999), pp. 818-824

Kao, L.; Bulger, E.; Parks, D.; Byrd, G. & Jurkovich, G. (2003). Predictors of morbidity after traumatic pancreatic injury, *J Trauma*, Vol.55, No.5, pp 898-905

Keller, M.; Stafford, P. & Vane, D. (1997). Conservative management of pancreatic trauma in children, *Journal of Trauma-Injury Infection & Critical Care*, Vol.42, No.6, (June 1997), pp. 1097-1100

Kuhls, TL. (2004). Pancreatitis, in: *Textbook of pediatric infectious diseases*. Feigin RD. Cherry, Demmler, Kaplan (Eds). pp. 694-701, Saunders, ISBN 0-7216-9329-6, Philadelphia.

Lautz, T.; Chin, A. & Radhakrishnan, J. (2011). Acute pancreatitis in children: spectrum of disease and predictors of severity, *J Pediatr Surg*, Vol.46, No.6, (June 2011), pp. 1144-1149

Meehan, J. & Sawin, R. (2011). Robotic lateral pancreaticojejunostomy (Puestow), *J Pediatr Surg*, Vol.46, No.6, (June 2011), pp. e5-e8

Mehta, S. & Gittes G. (2005). Lesions of the pancreas and spleen. In: *Pediatric Surgery*, Ashcraft KW, Holcomb GW, Murphy JP, pp (639-645), Elsevier Saunders, ISBN 0721602223.

Miyano, T. (2006). The Pancreas, In: *Pediatric Surgery*, Grosfeld JL, O'Neil JA Jr, Fonkalsrud EW & Coran AG, pp (1671-1678), Mosby-Elsevier, ISBN 9780323028424, Philadelphia 2006.

Munoz, A. & Katerndahl, D. (2000). Diagnosis and management of acute pancreatitis. *Am Fam Physician*, No.62, pp. 164-174

Nydegger, A.; Couper, R. & Oliver, M. (2006). Childhood pancreatitis. *J Gastroenterology and Hepatology*, No.21, pp 499-509

Ohno, Y. & Kanematsu, T. (2008). Annular pancreas causing localized recurrent pancreatitis in a child: Report of a case, *Surgery Today*, Vol.38, No.11, pp. 1052-1055

Pfützer, R.; Myers, E.; Applebaum-Shapiro, S.; Finch, R.; Ellis, I.; Neoptolemos, J.; Kant, J. & Whitcomb, D. (2000). Novel cationic trypsinogen (PRSS1) N29T and R122C mutations cause autosomal dominant hereditary pancreatitis, *Gut*, Vol.50, No.2, (Feb 2002), pp. 271-272

Rabinovich, A.; Rescorla, F.; Howard, T.; Grosfeld, J. & Lillemoe, K. (2006) Pancreatic Disorders in Children: Relationship of Postoperative Morbidity and the Indication for Surgery, *The American Surgeon*, Vol.72, No.7, (July 2006), pp. 641-643

Raman, V.; Loar, R.; Renukuntia, V.; et al. Hyperglycemia and Diabetes Mellitus in Children With Pancreatitis. Journal of Pediatrics (04/01/2011) Vol. 158, No. 4, P. 612; March - 16 - 2011

Ridout, A. & Lakhoo, K. (2011). Pancreatitis, in: *Paediatric surgery: A comprehensive text for Africa*, Ameh EA, Bickler SW, Lakhoo K, Nwomeh BC, Poenaru D. Global Help. Pp. 507-511. ISBN 978-1-60189-091-7. www.global-help.org/publications/books/help_pedsurgeryafrica 00introductions.pdf

Saad, D.; Gow, K.; Cabbabe S.; Heiss, K. & Wulkan, M. (2005). Laparoscopic cystogastrostomy for the treatment of pancreatic pseudocysts in children. *J Pediatr Surg*, Vol.40, No.11, (November 2005), pp. e13-e17

Schmittenbecher, P.; Rapp, P. & Dietz, H. (1996). Traumatic and nontraumatic pancreatitis in pediatric surgery, *Eur J Pediatr Surg*, Vol.6, No.2, (April 1996), pp. 86-91

Segura, R. (2004). Useful clinical biological markers in diagnosis of pleural effusion in children, *Paediatr Respir Rev*, No.5 Suppl A:S205-12

Seitz, G.; Warmann, S.; Kirschner, H.; Haber, H.; Schaefer, J. & Fuchs, J. (2006). Laparoscopic cystojejunostomy as a treatment option for pancreatic pseudocysts in children—a case report. *J Pediatr Surg*, Vol.41, No.12, (December 2006), pp. e33-e35

Shah, R.; Chen, M.; Lobe, T.; Bufo, A.; Gross, E. & Whitington, G. (1997). Laparoscopic common duct exploration in a child with recurrent pancreatitis due to primary fungus ball in the terminal common bile duct, *J Laparoendosc Adv Surg Tech A*, Vol.7, No.1, pp. 63-67

Stringer, M.; Davison, S.; McClean, P.; Rajwal, S.; Puntis, J.; Sheridan, M.; Ramsden, W. & Woodley, H. (2005). Multidisciplinary Management of Surgical Disorders of the Pancreas in Childhood, *Journal of Pediatric Gastroenterology & Nutrition*, Vol.40, No.3, (March 2005), pp. 363-367 Teich, N.; Rosendahl, J.; Tóth, M.; Mössner, J. & Sahin-Tóth, M. (2006). Mutations of human cationic trypsinogen (PRSS1) and chronic pancreatitis. *Hum Mutat*, Vol.27, No.8, (Aug 2006), pp. 721-30

Uretsky, G.; Goldschmiedt, M. & James, K. (1999). Childhood Pancreatitis. American Family Physician. 1 May 1999. Available from www.aafp.org/afp/990501ap/2507.html

Weber, C. & Adler, G. (2003). Acute pancreatitis. *Current Opinion in Gastroenterology*, Vol.19, No.5, (September 2003), pp. 447-450

Werlin, S. (2003). Pancreatitis in children. *J Pediatr Gastroenterol Nutr*, Vol. 37, No.5, (November 2003), pp. 591-595

Whitcomb, D.; Gorry, M.; Preston, R.; Furey, W.; Sossenheimer, M.; Ulrich, C.; et al. (1996). Hereditary pancreatitis is caused by a mutation in the cationic trypsinogen gene, *Nat Genet*, No.14, pp. 141-145

Whitcomb, D. (1999). Hereditary pancreatitis: new insights into acute and chronic pancreatitis, *Gut*, No.45, pp. 317-22

Whitcomb, D. (2004). Value of genetic testing in the management of pancreatitis, *Gut*, No.53, pp. 1710-1717

Windsor, A.; Kanwar, S.; LI, A.; Barnes, E.; Guthrie, J.; Spark J.; Welsh, F.; Guillou, P.; Reynolds, J. (1998). Compared with parenteral nutrition, enteral feeding attenuates the acute phase response and improves disease severity in acute pancreatitis, *Gut*, No.42, pp. 431-435

Yoder, S.; Rothenberg, S.; Tsao, K.; Wulkan, M.; Ponsky, T.; Peter, S.; Ostlie D. & Kane, T. (2009). Laparoscopic Treatment of Pancreatic Pseudocysts in Children, *J Laparoendosc Adv Surg Tech A*. No.19 (April 2009) (Suppl 1) S37–S40

Zhu, Y.; Liu, F.; Zhou, X.; Gao, X.; Xu, Z. & Du, Y. (2011). Clinical and pathologic characteristics of pancreatic necrosis in critically ill children, *World J Emerg Med,* No.2, pp 111-116

Part 2

Pathogenesis

4

Coagulation Abnormalities in Acute Pancreatitis

Travis Gould*, Safiah Mai* and Patricia Liaw
McMaster University,
Canada

1. Introduction

Acute pancreatitis (AP) is a potentially lethal disorder with no specific medical treatment. AP is characterized by a spectrum of symptoms, ranging from a local inflammatory process to the more severe form (acute necrotizing pancreatitis) which is associated with a systemic inflammatory response and a mortality rate of 27-45%. A number of risk factors have been identified for AP including alcohol abuse, gallstones, abdominal surgery/injury, cigarette smoking, cystic fibrosis, endoscopic retrograde cholangiopancreatography, hypercalcemia, hyperparathyroidism, hypertriglyceridemia, infection, pancreatic cancer, and injury to the abdomen (Pandol et al., 2007). Alcohol abuse and the development of gallstones account for the majority of AP cases. In AP, inappropriate intracellular activation of digestive enzymes within the pancreas (e.g. trypsin, chymotrypsin, elastase) is the main initiating event. The development of acute necrotizing pancreatitis is usually associated with pancreatic glandular necrosis. Acinar cell apoptosis, the release of cytokines, activation of coagulation, tissue ischemia, and tissue necrosis are key factors in the progression of the condition, as well as in the development of associated extrapancreatic complications (Steinberg & Tenner, 1994; McKay & Buter, 2003; Pandol et al., 2007).

AP induces a strong inflammatory response in experimental animal models and in humans, and is independent of the initiating factor for acinar cell damage (Granger & Remick, 2005). The major inflammatory mediators in AP include tumor necrosis factor (TNF), interleukins 1, 6, and 8, chemokines, and platelet activation factor (Makhija & Kingsnorth, 2002). Release of proinflammatory mediators into the circulation results in a systemic inflammatory response syndrome (Granger & Remick, 2005).

Inflammatory mediators in turn can influence hemostasis. Indeed, the pathways of inflammation and coagulation are intimately linked. For example, pro-inflammatory cytokines (e.g. TNF, IL-1β) act in autocrine and paracrine loops to activate neutrophils and monocytes. These cytokines also activate endothelial cells by upregulating adhesion molecules (e.g. P- and E-selectins) and chemokines. This results in leukocyte recruitment to the site of injury. Activated monocytes and endothelial cells express tissue factor (TF), the "spark" that initiates the coagulation cascade. TF can also be expressed by cells in the injured pancreas. The TF/VIIa complex activates factor X to Xa (or factor XI to XIa), and the

* Denotes co-first Authors

factor Xa/factor Va complex converts prothrombin to thrombin. Thrombin not only forms the fibrin clot but is also a potent activator of protease activated receptor-1 (PAR-1). PAR-1 activation triggers pro-inflammatory responses including secretion of cytokines and growth factors, and upregulation of adhesion molecules.

In AP, coagulation abnormalities range from localized intravascular thrombosis to disseminated intravascular coagulation (DIC). Ultrastructural changes in the pancreas that accompany human AP include the infiltration of polymorphonuclear leukocytes into the stroma and parenchyma, intra- and extravascular accumulation of platelets, and microthrombi in blood vessels (Bockman et al., 1986). This chapter will provide an overview of the pathophysiology of acute pancreatitis with emphasis on coagulation abnormalities. The topics covered include dysregulation of coagulation and anticoagulant pathways, animal studies of AP, and the therapeutic potential of experimental interventions.

2. Overview of hemostasis

Hemostasis is a delicate balance between procoagulant (including platelets and clotting factors) and anticoagulant mechanisms (including blood flow and the production of anticoagulant proteins). It encompasses the vessel wall and endothelial cells, cellular constituents within the vessel (such as red blood cells, leukocytes, and platelets), soluble plasma proteins (coagulatory proteins and their moderators), as well as microparticles derived from leukocytes and platelets (Hoffman & Monroe, III, 2001). It is a physiologic process which modulates blood fluidity while also retaining the capacity to produce a hemostatic plug outside a damaged blood vessel. Thrombosis is a pathologic event inside the vessel lumen, consisting of platelet accumulation, adhesion, activation and aggregation, as well as tissue-factor-initiated thrombin generation and fibrin formation (Furie & Furie, 2007). The hemostatic process is tightly regulated in a healthy individual by a system of anticoagulant mechanisms (Dahlback, 2000; Esmon, 2000b; Esmon, 2009). Through these mechanisms, the transformation of blood from a liquid to a solid state (and vice versa) is tightly regulated by the multiple participants of the coagulation, anticoagulation, and fibrinolytic pathways. The following sections describe the key components of the hemostatic system and their relevance to AP. Biomarkers of hemostasis in acute human pancreatitis are summarized in Table 1.

3. Platelet activation in AP

Platelet adhesion at sites of vessel injury is a multistep process involving interactions between various platelet receptors and subendothelial adhesive ligands (Furie & Furie, 2007). The initial tethering of platelets to exposed subendothelial collagen is mediated by von Willebrand factor (VWF), a large multimeric protein secreted by endothelial cells and activated platelets (Furie & Furie, 2007; Lippi et al., 2009). Adherent platelets become activated and undergo a shape change, becoming spherical and extruding long filopodia that enhance platelet-platelet interactions. Activated platelets secrete ADP from their dense granules and synthesize and release thromboxane A_2. Released ADP and thromboxane A_2 bind to distinct receptors on nearby platelets and activate them, thereby recruiting additional platelets to the sites of injury. Activated platelets also secrete the contents of their alpha granules (e.g. VWF, platelet-derived growth factor, and coagulation cofactors V and

VIII) (Wagner & Burger, 2003). Finally, activated platelets promote blood coagulation via the expression of phosphatidylserine, a negatively charged phospholipid that is normally found on the inside of the platelet cell membrane. Assembly of coagulation factors on the activated platelet surface results in an explosive generation of thrombin (described in more detail below).

Evidence of increased platelet activation associated with pancreatitis has long been established in experimental animal models. In rabbits, administration of pancreatic fluid from patients with chronic pancreatitis induced platelet aggregation and activation (Prinz et al., 1984). In cases of acute pancreatitis, platelets have been shown to be activated, and their indices (mean platelet volume, platelet large cell ratio, and platelet distribution width) have also been shown to be elevated between onset and remission of AP (Mimidis et al., 2004). While a heightened platelet response is typical of patients with mild AP, a decreased platelet count (due to increased consumption of platelets) is observed in cases of severe AP. Low plasma levels of platelets in patients with AP are also associated with poor clinical outcome (Maeda et al., 2006).

4. Coagulation and fibrinolysis abnormalities in AP

Simultaneous to platelet activation, coagulation occurs in three overlapping stages: initiation, amplification, and propagation (Hoffman & Monroe, III, 2001). Tissue factor (TF) is the "spark" that initiates blood coagulation. Under normal conditions, TF is not expressed by cells that are in direct contact with blood (Butenas & Mann, 2004). After damage to the endothelial wall, however, TF is exposed to blood where it is free to bind plasma factor VIIa, forming TF-factor VIIa complex. TF is also expressed by macrophages and monocytes after stimulation by inflammatory mediators (Esmon, 1999; Nijziel et al., 2001; Bouchard & Tracy, 2003)

Tissue factor (TF) forms a complex with a small amount of circulating activated factor VII (FVIIa) and acts as a cofactor for increasing the ability of FVIIa to convert FX to FXa and FIX to FIXa at the cell surface (Osterud et al., 1978). FXa activates FV and together they convert a small amount of prothrombin to thrombin (Monroe et al., 1996). This is known as the initiation phase of coagulation. During the amplification phase, the small amount of thrombin generated initiates a positive feedback loop upon itself through further activation of FV, and thus, increased thrombin generation (Monroe et al., 1996). The initiation of large-scale thrombin generation begins with the formation of the tenase complex (which consists of FVIIIa and FIXa) and the prothrombinase complex (consisting of FVa and FXa) on an anionic surface such as activated endothelial cells or platelets (Hoffman & Monroe, III, 2001). This causes a thrombin burst, which further generates fibrin from fibrinogen. This rapid formation of thrombin also activates factor XIII and thrombin-activatable fibrinolysis inhibitor (TAFI). Factor XIIIa is then able to cross-link with fibrin strands to support and stabilize a fibrin meshwork, while TAFI protects the forming clot from plasmin-mediated fibrinolysis (Dahlback, 2000; Butenas & Mann, 2002).

Plasma levels of TF in AP patients have been shown to be higher than those of healthy volunteers, though there is no statistically significant difference in the TF levels between the severity groups of AP (Sawa et al., 2006). Plasma levels of TF in alcoholic severe AP with pancreatic necrosis was significantly higher than that in alcoholic severe AP without pancreatic necrosis or that in nonalcoholic severe AP with pancreatic necrosis. These findings suggest that an increase in plasma TF may be related to the development of pancreatic necrosis in alcoholic severe AP.

Other measurements of blood coagulation are the prothrombin time (PT) and the activated partial thromboplastin time (APTT) which measure the extrinsic and intrinsic coagulation pathways, respectively. Clinical studies have shown an elevated prothrombin time in patients with AP (Radenkovic et al., 2009). However, there have been no reports of significant deviations in partial thromboplastin time (APTT) or in F1+2 levels in patients with AP. While these measurements suggest early hemostatic disturbances of AP, their usefulness in predicting patient outcome is limited. Clinical studies which measure other parameters (most notably d-dimer and antithrombin) have demonstrated an improved specificity and sensitivity in predicting outcome for these parameters, when compared to the utility of either PT or APTT.

AP is also characterized by abnormalities in fibrinolysis. The fibrinolytic system counteracts fibrin deposition, thereby preventing excessive fibrin accumulation at sites of vascular injury and restoring blood flow. Plasmin, the enzyme that dissolves fibrin clots, is formed from plasminogen in the presence of tissue plasminogen activator (tPA) or urokinase plasminogen activator (uPA). Plasmin cleaves fibrin, resulting in the production of fibrin degradation products (e.g. D-dimer) (Adams & Bird, 2009).

The levels of DIC parameters (low levels of platelets and AT, and high levels of D-dimer) and thrombin-antithrombin complex upon admission have been found to be associated with increased severity and poor prognosis of AP (Maeda et al., 2006). A four-fold increase in D-dimer levels has been shown to be a marker of complicated AP (Salomone et al., 2003). In patients with severe AP, non-survivors have significantly higher levels of D-dimer and plasminogen activator inhibitor (PAI)-1 than survivors (Radenkovic et al., 2004). The high concentrations of D-dimer and PAI-1 in AP patients are indicative of a hypercoagulable state and microvascular coagulopathy which may lead to the formation of microthrombi and, ultimately, facilitate the progression of organ failure.

4.1 Anticoagulant abnormalities in AP

The potentially explosive nature of the coagulation cascade is tightly regulated by three natural anticoagulant systems: antithrombin (AT), the protein C (PC) pathway, and tissue factor pathway inhibitor (TFPI).

4.2 Antithrombin in AP

AT, a plasma serine protease inhibitor (serpin) synthesized and secreted by the liver, demonstrates broad inhibitory activity for enzymes of the coagulation cascade, particularly thrombin and factor Xa (Lippi et al., 2009). The rate of enzyme inhibition by AT is slow but is accelerated approximately 1000-fold in the presence of negatively charged polysaccharides such as pharmacologic heparin as well as heparan sulfate found on the endothelial cell surface (Bjork et al., 1992). The stimulatory effect of heparin and heparan sulfate is mediated by a unique pentasaccharide sequence which binds AT with high affinity. Binding of this pentasaccharide sequence evokes a conformational change in AT that facilitates its interaction with FXa but not with thrombin. To accelerate thrombin inhibition by AT, heparin must bind simultaneously to AT and thrombin, a process that bridges the enzyme and the inhibitor together in a ternary complex (Bjork et al., 1992). AT also demonstrates anti-inflammatory properties through the induction of prostacyclin release from endothelial cells, the inhibition of leukocyte-endothelium interactions (e.g. rolling and adhesion), the inhibition of procoagulant cellular signaling pathways, and the alteration of cellular receptor expression which modulate lysosomal proteinases, interleukin release, and soluble intercellular adhesion molecules (Mammen, 1998; Esmon, 2005).

In patients with AP, low levels of AT (< 69%) at admission were found to be associated with a poor prognosis (Maeda et al., 2006). In taurocholate-induced experimental pancreatitis in rats, high dose AT treatment was shown to improve survival (Bleeker et al, 1992). In cerulein-induced AP, AT supplementation inhibited the release of high mobility group box 1 protein (HMGB1) as well as other proinflammatory cytokines in rats (Hagiwara et al., 2009). However, in a systematic review of randomized trials, AT seems ineffective in improving overall mortality in critically ill patients (Afshari et al., 2007).

4.3 The protein C pathway in AP

The second natural anticoagulant is PC, a vitamin-K dependent glycoprotein synthesized by the liver. The PC pathway provides an "on site" and "on demand" anticoagulant response whenever thrombin is generated (Esmon, 2000c; Esmon, 2000a). Briefly, vascular injury initiates the coagulation cascade, ultimately resulting in thrombin generation and blood clot formation. Excess thrombin then binds to thrombomodulin (TM), a receptor found on the surface of vascular endothelial cells. The binding of thrombin to TM is critical for efficient protein C activation because this interaction induces a major specificity change in thrombin that increases its rate of protein C cleavage (ie. activation) by ~1000-fold. The conversion of PC to APC is augmented approximately 20-fold *in vivo* by the endothelial cell protein C receptor (EPCR). EPCR binds circulating protein C and presents it to the thrombin-TM complex. Activated protein C (APC), in conjunction with its cofactor protein S (PS), degrades coagulation cofactors Va and VIIIa on the surface of negatively-charged phospholipids (e.g. activated platelets).

Significant changes in protein C levels were observed in both experimental and clinical AP. In rabbits, a rapid decrease in PC levels was found after the induction of acute necrotizing pancreatitis (Ottesen et al., 1999). Serial measurements of PC in AP patients have shown a difference between surviving and non-surviving patients. Survivors exhibited a progressive normalization of PC levels in plasma, while patients who died exhibited no increase in PC levels (Radenkovic et al., 2004). Decreased PC levels may reflect an increased consumption of PC, vascular leakage, or impaired PC synthesis by the liver in the diseased state (Levi & ten Cate, 1999). Upregulated but insufficient generation of APC was shown to be associated with the development of multiorgan failure in severe AP (Lindstrom et al., 2006).

Plasma levels of soluble TM (important for PC activation) increase throughout the course of AP (Ida et al., 2009). Soluble TM levels were also significantly higher in non-surviving patient subgroups when compared with survivors. Exhibiting a specificity of 91% in predicting the prognosis of AP, sTM levels may be a useful prognostic marker for early mortality predictions.

4.4 Tissue Factor Pathway Inhibitor (TFPI) in AP

The third natural anticoagulant is tissue factor pathway inhibitor (TFPI), a Kunitz-type serine protease inhibitor that is produced by monocytes, macrophages, the liver, as well as endothelial cells (Lwaleed & Bass, 2006). It is stored mainly in three different regions of the body: in circulation, in the cytoplasm of platelets, and bound to the endothelium (DelGiudice & White, 2009). TFPI forms a quaternary complex with TF, factor FVIIa, and factor Xa, thereby preventing further production of factor Xa and factor IXa by the TF:VIIa complex and blocking additional generation of thrombin by factor Xa.

Yasuda et al. examined the levels of TFPI in patients with AP (Yasuda et al., 2009). Plasma TFPI levels in patients with AP were significantly higher than those in healthy volunteers, and plasma TFPI levels in severe AP were greater than those in mild AP. The elevation of TFPI appeared to be positively correlated with the severity, degree of necrosis, as well as incidence of organ dysfunction.

5. Therapeutic strategies in AP

Modulation of hemostasis may be an attractive strategy to treat AP. Experimental animal models include administration of activated protein C (APC) to improve microvascular coagulation and inflammation. Other strategies target procoagulant factors such as platelet activating factor (PAF), platelets, and factor VIIa.

5.1 Activated protein C in AP

Recombinant human APC (rAPC; Drotrecogin alpha activated; Xigris®) is the first biological agent to improve survival in patients with severe sepsis , a common co-morbidity associated with AP (Bernard et al., 2001; Bernard et al., 2004). Studies investigating the protective properties associated with APC treatment in vivo and in vitro have shown that APC functions not only as an anticoagulant, but also as a cytoprotective signaling molecule involved in inflammation, apoptosis, and vascular permeability. The protective effect of rAPC therapy in patients with severe sepsis likely reflects its ability to modulate the complex changes associated with sepsis pathophysiology.

The importance of the protein C anticoagulant pathway in AP was first studied in a rabbit model. Induction of severe AP caused a marked decrease in protein C activity compared to rabbits subjected to sham surgery (Ottesen et al., 1999), an effect that is also observed in non-surviving patients with AP. More recently, Chen et al. elucidated the effects of APC treatment on coagulation mechanisms in AP. In a 5% retrograde sodium taurocholate infusion rat model, pretreatment with 50 ug/kg of APC versus untreated rats with AP resulted in significant decreases in serum TNF, serum IL-8, and pancreatic matrix metalloproteinase 9 (MMP-9), an enzyme which degrades a wide range of extracellular matrix components (e.g. collagen, fibronectin, and gelatin). Moreover, APC-treated rats had significantly higher levels of pancreatic EPCR and TM, receptors critical for protein C activation. It has been shown that endotoxins increase shedding of membrane EPCR to produce soluble EPCR via MMP-9 (Gu et al., 2000) which respond to an increase in inflammatory cytokines (Wright & Friedland, 2004). It is proposed that APC treatment downregulates MMP-9 expression, thus reducing the shedding of EPCR to enhance endothelial EPCR cell expression in the pancreas. Following this study, the therapeutic effects of rAPC in AP have been demonstrated in various models of AP by different groups (Yamanel et al., 2005; Alsfasser et al., 2006; Chen et al., 2007) while others have shown no survival benefit attributed to treatment with APC (Akay et al., 2008).

The anti-inflammatory and protective functions of APC have been documented in severity-graded models of AP. In a 5% sodium taurocholate infusion model (via the common biliopancreatic duct) of acute necrotizing pancreatitis, it was found that treatment with recombinant human APC (bolus injection of 100 µg/kg) 6 hours following AP induction was associated with a decrease in pancreatic bacterial contamination as well as fewer mesenteric lymph nodes (Yamanel et al., 2005). APC-treated animals with AP also had significantly decreased amylase levels, plasma IL-6, and TNF-α by decreasing NF-κβ activation. Moreover, APC treatment resulted in improvements in pancreatic histology as reflected by the resolution of pancreatic edema, perivascular inflammation, acinar cell necrosis, and fat necrosis. This study found that APC neither worsened nor improved the hemorrhagic state of the pancreas in the experimental condition suggesting that the coagulation system remains intact despite significant pancreatic tissue injury in the early pathophysiology of acute necrotizing pancreatitis (Yamanel et al., 2005).

In a rat model of mild (cerulein injection) and severe AP (intravenous cerulein injection with intraductal glycodeoxycholic acid infusion), treatment with recombinant human APC at 100 ug/kg per hour for 6 hours significantly reduced inflammation in the lungs and pancreas and furthermore improved survival from 38%-86% ($p = 0.05$) (Alsfasser et al., 2006). Inflammation was characterized by the presence of myeloperoxidase (MPO) in the pancreas and lungs of rats with severe AP, which decreased significantly with APC treatment for 6 hours following induction of AP. MPO levels in the lungs were reduced to levels even lower than those in sham-operated rats, similar to levels observed in healthy mice, while MPO levels in the pancreas were reduced to those observed in sham-operated and healthy control animals, demonstrating the anti-inflammatory effect of APC (Alsfasser et al., 2006). In contrast, no significant changes in coagulopathy were observed in untreated rats with severe AP versus APC-treated rats. Coagulopathy associated with severe AP was characterized by significantly prolonged prothrombin and partial thromboplastin times, decreased fibrinogen, marked leukocytosis, and thrombocytopenia, which were not significant in untreated versus APC-treated rats. APC appears to offer a survival benefit by suppressing inflammation in the pancreas and lungs without concomitant reversal of the pancreatic tissue damage and coagulopathy observed in experimental severe AP (Satake et al., 1981; Alsfasser et al., 2006).

Further studies aimed at elucidating the mechanism by which APC treatment improves outcome in AP demonstrated the involvement of mitogen-activated protein kinases (MAPKs) (Chen et al., 2007). MAPKs are mammalian serine/threonine protein kinases known to amplify signals involved in differentiation, inflammation, and apoptosis (Robinson & Cobb, 1997). P38 MAPK and JNK/SAPK (c-Jun N-terminal kinase/stress-activated protein kinase) are stress-responding MAPKs which induce inflammatory pathways in the early pathogenesis of severe AP (Dabrowski et al., 2000; Samuel et al., 2003). In this study, severe AP was induced through retrograde infusion of a 5% sodium taurocholate solution via the pancreatic duct at 100 uL/min. Rats were pretreated before AP induction with a 50 ug/kg dose of APC, 10 ug/kg dose of APC, or CNI1493 (a synthetic molecule which significantly reduces AP severity by inhibiting MAPK phosphorylation thus attenuating inflammatory pathways (Lowenberg et al., 2004; Denham et al., 2000). In rats with severe AP, p38 MAPK and JNK2 proteins as well as inflammatory mediators TNF and IL-1β were significantly elevated. These effects were reversed in rats treated with the higher APC dose and CNI1493 (Chen et al., 2007). Decreases in the protein expression of MAPKs and cytokines in both treatments were comparable to levels in the healthy control group (Lowenberg et al., 2004; Wang et al., 2005; Chen et al., 2007). Moreover, APC treatment at 50 ug/kg and not CNI1493 significantly increased expression of ERK1/2 protein (Chen et al., 2007), the activation of which is known to protect against cell injury by promoting cellular regeneration (Sapieha et al., 2006).

These studies demonstrated that APC at a dose of 50 ug/kg inhibits p36 MAPK and JNK expression, thus reducing levels of proinflammatory cytokines like TNF and IL-1β in the pancreas. Additional protective effects of APC include the upregulation of ERK1/2 which promotes pancreatic cell regeneration and diminishes the severity of AP.

While some studies demonstrated the therapeutic potential of APC with high bolus APC injections (Yamanel et al., 2005; Chen et al., 2007) and hourly infusion (Alsfasser et al., 2006) treatments, others have suggested that APC offers no survival benefit in early phase AP (Akay et al., 2008). In a 5% sodium taurocholate rat AP model, APC was given hourly at the same dose given in the PROWESS study which tested the therapeutic effects of APC in sepsis patients (Bernard et al., 2001). Akay et al. found that APC treatment at 24 ug/kg per hour given 4 hours after AP induction resulted in significantly reduced serum IL-6 and amylase levels compared to untreated rats with AP (Akay et al., 2008). However, no significant improvements in pancreatic histology, pancreas oxidative stress, pancreas MPO, or renal function were observed. It is possible that that differences observed regarding the therapeutic benefit of APC may be due to dosage effects and differences in experimental design. The use of a lower dose of APC (24 ug/kg) may have been insufficient to offer any therapeutic benefit compared to the previous studies using 100 ug/kg of APC bolus or hourly (Yamanel et al, 2005; Alsfasser et al, 2006). Furthermore, the PROWESS trials used the 24 ug/kg per hour dose over 96 hours versus 5 hours in the experimental AP study (Akay et al., 2008). As such, studies testing the therapeutic effects of APC treatment in animal models of AP have yielded varying results.

5.2 Targeting Platelet Activating Factor (PAF) and platelets in AP

Modulation of platelet activating factor (PAF) has also been studied in experimental AP. PAF is a receptor-binding lipid and vasodilator that activates basophils, endothelial cells, platelets, and neutrophils. It is the most extensively studied experimental therapy in clinical trials of AP. In sodium taurodeoxycholate and trypsin injection models (via the biliopancreatic duct), PAF is released into the peritoneal fluid, bloodstream, and lung of rats (Kald et al., 1993). Furthermore, inhibition of PAF via an antagonist or an enzyme accelerating its degradation (acetylhydrolase) decreased inflammation characterized by marked reductions in pro-inflammatory cytokines (Lane et al., 2001; Hofbauer et al., 1998), pancreatic enzyme activation (Fujimura et al., 1992), and improved survival (Leonhardt et al., 1992; Dabrowski et al., 1995), hemodynamics (Ais et al., 1992), and histology (Dabrowski et al., 1995) in caerulein- (Fujimura et al., 1992; Lane et al., 2001; Hofbauer et al., 1998), deoxycholate- (Ais et al., 1992), taurocholate-infusion (Leonhardt et al., 1992; Dabrowski et al., 1995) and murine bile duct ligation models (Hofbauer et al., 1998).

The therapeutic effects of reducing pro-inflammatory platelet activity while maintaining its hemostatic abilities have also been studied. The inflammatory role of platelets was demonstrated in a study where platelet supernatant administered to platelet-depleted mice restored normal leukocyte recruitment (Tamagawa-Mineoka et al., 2007). In a cerulein model of AP, platelet depletion via an antibody (anti-GP1bα) reduced many markers of severe AP including serum amylase levels, acinar cell necrosis, interstitial pancreatic hemorrhage, inflammatory infiltration by neutrophils, pancreatic MPO, pancreatic macrophage inflammatory protein-2 (MIP-2), and circulating leukocytes and neutrophils (Abdulla et al., 2011a). This study along with others showed that platelets exert a pro-inflammatory response by invoking MIP-2 chemokine synthesis in pancreatic cells (macrophage and acinar cells) (Ramnath & Bhatia, 2006; Sun & Bhatia, 2007), a major signal for neutrophil infiltration and chemotaxis (Bhatia & Hegde, 2007; Li et al., 2004). Therefore targeting the inflammatory nature of platelets may have therapeutic potential in reducing pancreatic tissue injury and the severity of acute pancreatitis (Abdulla et al., 2011).

Measurement	Biomarker	Effect	Normal Value	AP Admission Value	References
Global Coagulation	PT (sec.)	Increased	9.8-12.7	13.46-13.92	1,2
	APTT (sec.)	NS†	21-39	32.99-33.22	1,2,3,4,5
	Platelet Count (10^4/μl)	NS†	9.2	Sur-vivor: 16.2 Non-Survivor: 6.8	1,6
	Fibrinogen (g/L)	Increased	1.8-3.5	3.7-5.39	1,2
Procoagulant Activity	D-dimer (ng/mL)	Increased	0-0.39	5.5-903.50	1,3,4,7,8
	TAT (μg/L)	Increased	1-16.1	11.8-25.3	3,4,6
	TF antigen (pg/ml)	Increased	120-140	363-721	7,9,10
	sP-selectin (ng/mL)	Increased	82-181	150-215	11,12,13
Fibrinolysis Pathway	Alpha-2-Antiplasmin (%)	Decreased	80-120	73.22-105.28	1,2
	PAI-1 (U/mL)	Increased	0.3-3.5	4.39-4.56	1,2,4
	Plasminogen (μg/mL)	Decreased	150 - 200	70.11-103.94	1,2,17
Anticoagulant Activity	AT (%)	Decreased	80-120	63.47- 81.47	1,2,4,5
	PC (%)	Decreased	81-173	52-84.75	1,2,4,5,8
	APC (%)	Decreased	100%	76-102	2
	Protein S (μg/mL)	Decreased	23.8-30.6	17.3-26.9	16
	sTM (ng/mL)	Increased	10.3-54	23.48-153.9	4,14,18
	TFPI (ng/mL)	Increased	26.4-28.6	34.6-40.4	15

[1]Radenkovic *et al.* 2009; [2]Radenkovic *et al.* 2004; [3]Mavrommatis *et al.* 2000; [4]Kinasewitz *et al.* 2004; [5]Collins *et al.* 2006; [6]Maeda *et al.* 2006; [7]Stief *et al.* 2007; [8]Lindstrom *et al.* 2006; [9]Sawa *et al.* 2006; [10]Gando *et al.* 1998; [11]Powell *et al.* 2001; [12]Ogura *et al.* 2001; [13]Osmanovic *et al.* 2000; [14]Lu *et al.* 2007; [15]Yasuda *et al.* 2009; [16]Uehara *et al.* 2009; [17]Vinazzer *et al.* 1988; [18]Ida *et al.* 2009;
†Denotes a non-significant value compared with normal controls.

Table 1. Biomarkers of hemostasis in human acute pancreatitis.

5.3 Inhibition of factor VIIa in AP

The effect of inhibiting FVIIa on experimental AP was investigated in an intraductal taurodeoxycholate infusion model of AP (Andersson et al., 2007). Administration of active-site inactivated FVII (FVIIai) and N-acetylcysteine (NAC, an anti-inflammatory antioxidant) 90 minutes prior to AP induction caused a significant reduction of MPO levels in distant organs like the lungs and ileum and reductions in plasma IL-6 and MIP-2 compared to saline controls 6 hours following AP induction (Andersson et al., 2007). This study suggests that coagulant mediators may potentially be therapeutic targets to decrease AP severity.

6. Conclusions

Coagulation abnormalities are a hallmark of AP and are related to disease severity. Results from experimental animal studies and human studies suggest that modulation of hemostasis may provide a therapeutic target for the treatment of AP. Inhibition of the coagulation cascade may prevent intravascular coagulation and inflammation in the pancreas and distant organs, thereby reducing systemic complications in patients with acute pancreatitis.

7. References

Abdulla, A., Awla, D., Hartman, H., Rahman, M., Jeppsson, B., Regner, S. et al. (2011). Role of platelets in experimental acute pancreatitis. *Br.J.Surg., 98,* 93-103.

Adams, R. L. & Bird, R. J. (2009). Review article: Coagulation cascade and therapeutics update: relevance to nephrology. Part 1: Overview of coagulation, thrombophilias and history of anticoagulants. *Nephrology.(Carlton.), 14,* 462-470.

Afshari, A., Wetterslev, J., Brok, J., & Moller, A. (2007). Antithrombin III in critically ill patients: systematic review with meta-analysis and trial sequential analysis. *BMJ, 335,* 1248-1251.

Ais, G., Lopez-Farre, A., Gomez-Garre, D. N., Novo, C., Romeo, J. M., Braquet, P. et al. (1992). Role of platelet-activating factor in hemodynamic derangements in an acute rodent pancreatic model. *Gastroenterology, 102,* 181-187.

Akay, S., Ozutemiz, O., Yenisey, C., Simsek, N. G., Yuce, G., & Batur, Y. (2008). Use of activated protein C has no avail in the early phase of acute pancreatitis. *HPB (Oxford), 10,* 459-463.

Alsfasser, G., Warshaw, A. L., Thayer, S. P., Antoniu, B., Laposata, M., Lewandrowski, K. B. et al. (2006). Decreased inflammation and improved survival with recombinant human activated protein C treatment in experimental acute pancreatitis. *Arch.Surg., 141,* 670-676.

Andersson, E., Axelsson, J., Pedersen, L. C., Elm, T., & Andersson, R. (2007). Treatment with anti-factor VIIa in acute pancreatitis in rats: blocking both coagulation and inflammation? *Scand.J.Gastroenterol., 42,* 765-770.

Bernard, G. R., Margolis, B. D., Shanies, H. M., Ely, E. W., Wheeler, A. P., Levy, H. et al. (2004). Extended evaluation of recombinant human activated protein C United States Trial (ENHANCE US): a single-arm, phase 3B, multicenter study of drotrecogin alfa (activated) in severe sepsis. *Chest, 125,* 2206-2216.

Bernard, G. R., Vincent, J. L., Laterre, P. F., LaRosa, S. P., Dhainaut, J. F., Lopez-Rodriguez, A. et al. (2001). Efficacy and safety of recombinant human activated protein C for severe sepsis. *New England Journal of Medicine, 344,* 699-709.

Bhatia, M. & Hegde, A. (2007). Treatment with antileukinate, a CXCR2 chemokine receptor antagonist, protects mice against acute pancreatitis and associated lung injury. *Regul.Pept., 138,* 40-48.

Bjork, I., Ylinenjarvi, K., Olson, S. T., & Bock, P. E. (1992). Conversion of antithrombin from an inhibitor of thrombin to a substrate with reduced heparin affinity and enhanced conformational stability by binding of a tetradecapeptide corresponding to the P1 to P14 region of the putative reactive bond loop of the inhibitor. *J.Biol.Chem., 267,* 1976-1982.

Bleeker, W. K., Agterberg, J., Rigter, G., Hack, C. E., & Gool, J. V. (1992). Protective effect of antithrombin III in acute experimental pancreatitis in rats. *Dig.Dis.Sci., 37,* 280-285.

Bockman, D. E., Buchler, M., & Beger, H. G. (1986). Ultrastructure of human acute pancreatitis. *International Journal of Pancreatology, 1,* 141-153.

Bouchard, B. A. & Tracy, P. B. (2003). The participation of leukocytes in coagulant reactions. *J.Thromb.Haemost., 1,* 464-469.

Butenas, S. & Mann, K. G. (2002). Blood coagulation. *Biochemistry (Mosc.), 67,* 3-12.

Butenas, S. & Mann, K. G. (2004). Active tissue factor in blood? *Nat.Med., 10,* 1155-1156.

Chen, P., Zhang, Y., Qiao, M., & Yuan, Y. (2007). Activated protein C, an anticoagulant polypeptide, ameliorates severe acute pancreatitis via regulation of mitogen-activated protein kinases. *J.Gastroenterol., 42,* 887-896.

Dabrowski, A., Boguslowicz, C., Dabrowska, M., Tribillo, I., & Gabryelewicz, A. (2000). Reactive oxygen species activate mitogen-activated protein kinases in pancreatic acinar cells. *Pancreas, 21,* 376-384.

Dabrowski, A., Gabryelewicz, A., & Chyczewski, L. (1995). The effect of platelet activating factor antagonist (BN 52021) on acute experimental pancreatitis with reference to multiorgan oxidative stress. *Int.J.Pancreatol., 17,* 173-180.

Dahlback, B. (2000). Blood coagulation. *Lancet, 355,* 1627-1632.

DelGiudice, L. A. & White, G. A. (2009). The role of tissue factor and tissue factor pathway inhibitor in health and disease states. *J.Vet.Emerg.Crit Care (San.Antonio.), 19,* 23-29.

Denham, W., Yang, J., Wang, H., Botchkina, G., Tracey, K. J., & Norman, J. (2000). Inhibition of p38 mitogen activate kinase attenuates the severity of pancreatitis-induced adult respiratory distress syndrome. *Crit Care Med., 28,* 2567-2572.

Esmon, C. (2000a). The protein C pathway. *Crit Care Med., 28,* S44-S48.

Esmon, C. T. (1999). Possible involvement of cytokines in diffuse intravascular coagulation and thrombosis. *Baillieres Best.Pract.Res.Clin.Haematol., 12,* 343-359.

Esmon, C. T. (2000b). Regulation of blood coagulation. *Biochim.Biophys.Acta, 1477,* 349-360.

Esmon, C. T. (2000c). The endothelial cell protein C receptor. *Thromb.Haemost., 83,* 639-643.

Esmon, C. T. (2005). The interactions between inflammation and coagulation. *Br.J.Haematol., 131,* 417-430.

Esmon, C. T. (2009). Basic mechanisms and pathogenesis of venous thrombosis. *Blood Rev., 23,* 225-229.

Fujimura, K., Kubota, Y., Ogura, M., Yamaguchi, T., Binnaka, T., Tani, K. et al. (1992). Role of endogenous platelet-activating factor in caerulein-induced acute pancreatitis in rats: protective effects of a PAF-antagonist. *J.Gastroenterol.Hepatol., 7,* 199-202.

Furie, B. & Furie, B. C. (2007). In vivo thrombus formation. *J.Thromb.Haemost., 5 Suppl 1,* 12-17.
Granger, J. & Remick, D. (2005). Acute pancreatitis: models, markers, and mediators. *Shock, 24 Suppl 1,* 45-51.
Gu, J. M., Katsuura, Y., Ferrell, G. L., Grammas, P., & Esmon, C. T. (2000). Endotoxin and thrombin elevate rodent endothelial cell protein C receptor mRNA levels and increase receptor shedding in vivo. *Blood, 95,* 1687-1693.
Hagiwara, S., Iwasaka, H., Shingu, C., Matsumoto, S., Uchida, T., & Noguchi, T. (2009). Antithrombin III prevents cerulein-induced acute pancreatitis in rats. *Pancreas, 38,* 746-751.
Hofbauer, B., Saluja, A. K., Bhatia, M., Frossard, J. L., Lee, H. S., Bhagat, L. et al. (1998). Effect of recombinant platelet-activating factor acetylhydrolase on two models of experimental acute pancreatitis. *Gastroenterology, 115,* 1238-1247.
Hoffman, M. & Monroe, D. M., III (2001). A cell-based model of hemostasis. *Thromb.Haemost., 85,* 958-965.
Ida, S., Fujimura, Y., Hirota, M., Imamura, Y., Ozaki, N., Suyama, K. et al. (2009). Significance of endothelial molecular markers in the evaluation of the severity of acute pancreatitis. *Surg.Today, 39,* 314-319.
Kald, B., Kald, A., Ihse, I., & Tagesson, C. (1993). Release of platelet-activating factor in acute experimental pancreatitis. *Pancreas, 8,* 440-442.
Lane, J. S., Todd, K. E., Gloor, B., Chandler, C. F., Kau, A. W., Ashley, S. W. et al. (2001). Platelet activating factor antagonism reduces the systemic inflammatory response in a murine model of acute pancreatitis. *J.Surg.Res., 99,* 365-370.
Leonhardt, U., Fayyazzi, A., Seidensticker, F., Stockmann, F., Soling, H. D., & Creutzfeldt, W. (1992). Influence of a platelet-activating factor antagonist on severe pancreatitis in two experimental models. *Int.J.Pancreatol., 12,* 161-166.
Levi, M. & ten Cate, H. (1999). Disseminated intravascular coagulation. *N.Engl.J.Med., 341,* 586-592.
Li, X., Klintman, D., Liu, Q., Sato, T., Jeppsson, B., & Thorlacius, H. (2004). Critical role of CXC chemokines in endotoxemic liver injury in mice. *J.Leukoc.Biol., 75,* 443-452.
Lindstrom, O., Kylanpaa, L., Mentula, P., Puolakkainen, P., Kemppainen, E., Haapiainen, R. et al. (2006). Upregulated but insufficient generation of activated protein C is associated with development of multiorgan failure in severe acute pancreatitis. *Crit Care, 10,* R16.
Lippi, G., Favaloro, E. J., Franchini, M., & Guidi, G. C. (2009). Milestones and perspectives in coagulation and hemostasis. *Semin.Thromb.Hemost., 35,* 9-22.
Lowenberg, M., Peppelenbosch, M. P., & Hommes, D. W. (2004). Therapeutic modulation of signal transduction pathways. *Inflamm.Bowel.Dis., 10 Suppl 1,* S52-S57.
Lwaleed, B. A. & Bass, P. S. (2006). Tissue factor pathway inhibitor: structure, biology and involvement in disease. *J.Pathol., 208,* 327-339.
Maeda, K., Hirota, M., Ichihara, A., Ohmuraya, M., Hashimoto, D., Sugita, H. et al. (2006). Applicability of disseminated intravascular coagulation parameters in the assessment of the severity of acute pancreatitis. *Pancreas, 32,* 87-92.
Makhija, R. & Kingsnorth, A. N. (2002). Cytokine storm in acute pancreatitis. *J.Hepatobiliary.Pancreat.Surg., 9,* 401-410.
Mammen, E. F. (1998). Antithrombin III and sepsis. *Intensive Care Med., 24,* 649-650.

McKay, C. J. & Buter, A. (2003). Natural history of organ failure in acute pancreatitis. *Pancreatology., 3,* 111-114.

Mimidis, K., Papadopoulos, V., Kotsianidis, J., Filippou, D., Spanoudakis, E., Bourikas, G. et al. (2004). Alterations of platelet function, number and indexes during acute pancreatitis. *Pancreatology., 4,* 22-27.

Monroe, D. M., Hoffman, M., & Roberts, H. R. (1996). Transmission of a procoagulant signal from tissue factor-bearing cell to platelets. *Blood Coagul.Fibrinolysis, 7,* 459-464.

Nijziel, M., van Oerle, R., van, '., V, van Pampus, E., Lindhout, T., & Hamulyak, K. (2001). Tissue factor activity in human monocytes is regulated by plasma: implications for the high and low responder phenomenon. *Br.J.Haematol., 112,* 98-104.

Osterud, B., Bouma, B. N., & Griffin, J. H. (1978). Human blood coagulation factor IX. Purification, properties, and mechanism of activation by activated factor XI. *J.Biol.Chem., 253,* 5946-5951.

Ottesen, L. H., Bladbjerg, E. M., Osman, M., Lausten, S. B., Jacobsen, N. O., Gram, J. et al. (1999). Protein C activation during the initial phase of experimental acute pancreatitis in the rabbit. *Dig.Surg., 16,* 486-495.

Pandol, S. J., Saluja, A. K., Imrie, C. W., & Banks, P. A. (2007). Acute pancreatitis: bench to the bedside. *Gastroenterology, 132,* 1127-1151.

Prinz, R. A., Fareed, J., Rock, A., Squillaci, G., & Wallenga, J. (1984). Platelet activation by human pancreatic fluid. *Journal of Surgical Research, 37,* 314-319.

Radenkovic, D., Bajec, D., Ivancevic, N., Milic, N., Bumbasirevic, V., Jeremic, V. et al. (2009). D-dimer in acute pancreatitis: a new approach for an early assessment of organ failure. *Pancreas, 38,* 655-660.

Radenkovic, D., Bajec, D., Karamarkovic, A., Stefanovic, B., Milic, N., Ignjatovic, S. et al. (2004). Disorders of hemostasis during the surgical management of severe necrotizing pancreatitis. *Pancreas, 29,* 152-156.

Ramnath, R. D. & Bhatia, M. (2006). Substance P treatment stimulates chemokine synthesis in pancreatic acinar cells via the activation of NF-kappaB. *Am.J.Physiol Gastrointest.Liver Physiol, 291,* G1113-G1119.

Robinson, M. J. & Cobb, M. H. (1997). Mitogen-activated protein kinase pathways. *Curr.Opin.Cell Biol., 9,* 180-186.

Salomone, T., Tosi, P., Palareti, G., Tomassetti, P., Migliori, M., Guariento, A. et al. (2003). Coagulative disorders in human acute pancreatitis: role for the D-dimer. *Pancreas, 26,* 111-116.

Samuel, I., Zaheer, S., Fisher, R. A., & Zaheer, A. (2003). Cholinergic receptor induction and JNK activation in acute pancreatitis. *Am.J.Surg., 186,* 569-574.

Sapieha, P. S., Hauswirth, W. W., & Di, P. A. (2006). Extracellular signal-regulated kinases 1/2 are required for adult retinal ganglion cell axon regeneration induced by fibroblast growth factor-2. *J.Neurosci.Res., 83,* 985-995.

Satake, K., Uchima, K., Umeyama, K., Appert, H. E., & Howard, J. M. (1981). The effects upon blood coagulation in dogs of experimentally induced pancreatitis and the infusion of pancreatic juice. *Surg.Gynecol.Obstet., 153,* 341-345.

Sawa, H., Ueda, T., Takeyama, Y., Yasuda, T., Matsumura, N., Nakajima, T. et al. (2006). Elevation of plasma tissue factor levels in patients with severe acute pancreatitis. *J.Gastroenterol., 41,* 575-581.

Steinberg, W. & Tenner, S. (1994). Acute pancreatitis. *New England Journal of Medicine, 330,* 1198-1210.

Sun, J. & Bhatia, M. (2007). Blockade of neurokinin-1 receptor attenuates CC and CXC chemokine production in experimental acute pancreatitis and associated lung injury. *Am.J.Physiol Gastrointest.Liver Physiol, 292,* G143-G153.

Tamagawa-Mineoka, R., Katoh, N., Ueda, E., Takenaka, H., Kita, M., & Kishimoto, S. (2007). The role of platelets in leukocyte recruitment in chronic contact hypersensitivity induced by repeated elicitation. *Am.J.Pathol., 170,* 2019-2029.

Wagner, D. D. & Burger, P. C. (2003). Platelets in inflammation and thrombosis. *Arterioscler.Thromb.Vasc.Biol., 23,* 2131-2137.

Wang, H., Zhang, Z. H., Yan, X. W., Li, W. Q., Ji, D. X., Quan, Z. F. et al. (2005). Amelioration of hemodynamics and oxygen metabolism by continuous venovenous hemofiltration in experimental porcine pancreatitis. *World J.Gastroenterol., 11,* 127-131.

Wright, K. M. & Friedland, J. S. (2004). Regulation of monocyte chemokine and MMP-9 secretion by proinflammatory cytokines in tuberculous osteomyelitis. *J.Leukoc.Biol., 75,* 1086-1092.

Yamanel, L., Mas, M. R., Comert, B., Isik, A. T., Aydin, S., Mas, N. et al. (2005). The effect of activated protein C on experimental acute necrotizing pancreatitis. *Crit Care, 9,* R184-R190.

Yasuda, T., Ueda, T., Kamei, K., Shinzaki, W., Sawa, H., Shinzeki, M. et al. (2009). Plasma tissue factor pathway inhibitor levels in patients with acute pancreatitis. *J.Gastroenterol., 44,* 1071-1079.

5

Prevention of Post-Endoscopic Retrograde Cholangiopancreatography Pancreatitis

Atsushi Sofuni and Takao Itoi
Department of Gastroenterology and Hepatology,
Tokyo Medical University Hospital,
Japan

1. Introduction

Endoscopic retrograde cholangiopancreatography (ERCP) is an essential modality for the diagnosis and therapy of pancreatobiliary disease. However, complications of ERCP-related procedures are also common. Post-ERCP pancreatitis (PEP), the most common and potentially serious complication of ERCP-related procedures, occurs in 1 - 9% of all procedures (1-16). Moreover, the PEP rate increases to 10 - 40% in cases with risk factors (1-16). In most cases, PEP is generally mild and requires only conservative treatment. However, substantial complications, occasionally fatal, can occur. Therefore, it is imperative to establish a strategy for preventing PEP based on medical, social, and economical circumstances. The prevention of PEP, according to various studies, is presently based on the elucidation of its underlying mechanisms, the identification of its risk factors, the administration of pharmacological drugs, and endoscopic procedures such as pancreatic stenting.

2. Mechanisms of post-ERCP pancreatitis

Various mechanisms of PEP have been suggested (1-25), which include obstruction of the outflow of pancreatic juice due to papillary edema or spasm of the sphincter of Oddi after ERCP procedures, chemical injury due to the injection of contrast material or leakage of intestinal juice to the pancreatic duct, mechanical injury of the pancreatic duct caused by the deep cannulation of a catheter and related devices including a guidewire, hydrostatic injury from the rise of pressure in the pancreatic duct due to repeated pancreatography with contrast agents, or the infusion of water or saline solution in manometry and pancreatic scope procedures, and thermal injury of the pancreas causing papillary edema due to radiofrequency ablation **(Table 1)**. One of the most likely mechanisms is impaired drainage from the pancreatic duct caused by papillary edema or spasm of the sphincter of Oddi after ERCP procedures (10-14,19,22,25). Another is local injury of the papilla and pancreatic duct as a result of ERCP procedures, or forceful and repetitive contrast injections causing local inflammation (1-20,26). This may lead to premature intracellular activation of proteolytic enzymes, consequently causing further damage and local inflammation as indicated by increased levels of cytokines, and possible initiation of a systemic inflammatory response with multi-organ involvement (1,10,11,13).

Papillary edema	Rise in pressure in the pancreatic duct due to retention of pancreatic juice accompanying papillary edema or spasm of the sphincter of Oddi after ERCP
Mechanical injury	Damage to the pancreatic duct due to deep cannulation with a catheter and related devices such as a guidewire
Hydrostatic injury	Rise in pressure in the pancreatic duct due to repeated pancreatography with a contrast agent or the infusion of water or saline solution in manometry and pancreatic scope procedures
Chemical injury	Injection of contrast agents and intestinal juice leakage to the pancreatic duct
Thermal injury	Inflammation of the pancreas causing papillary edema due to radiofrequency ablation

Table 1. Suggested mechanisms of post-ERCP pancreatitis

3. Risk factors of post-ERCP pancreatitis

PEP can be prevented by careful patient selection with full consideration of the risk factors for PEP. Previous researchers have reported several factors which may increase the risk of PEP (1-27). A meta-analysis of 15 prospective cohort studies and 52 retrospective cohort studies previously evaluated and elucidated the risk factors of PEP.

Freeman et al. (1,2) reported that the high risks of PEP were associated with both patient-related risk factors and procedure-related risk factors on multivariate analysis of prospective studies and meta-analyses (Table 2). In their review, they advocated special caution in performing ERCP-related procedures in patients with specific patient-related risk factors (e.g., young age, female gender, suspected sphincter of Oddi dysfunction (SOD), prior PEP, recurrent pancreatitis, and absence of chronic pancreatitis) and procedure-related risk factors (e.g., pancreatic duct injection, pancreatic sphincterotomy, balloon dilation of an intact biliary sphincter, difficult or failed cannulation, and pre-cut (access) sphincterotomy).

Young age
Female gender
Suspected sphincter of Oddi dysfunction (SOD)
Prior post-ERCP pancreatitis
Recurrent pancreatitis
Absence of chronic pancreatitis
Pancreatic duct injection
Initial pancreatography
Two or more pancreatic duct injections
Pancreatic sphincterotomy
Minor papilla sphincterotomy
Balloon dilation of intact biliary sphincter
Difficult or failed cannulation
Pre-cut (access) sphincterotomy
Procedure time $\geqq$ 30 min
Pancreatic tissue sampling by any method
IDUS (pancreatic duct)
Trainee involvement
Non-placement of pancreatic stent after ERCP procedures

Table 2. Risk factotrs of post-ERCP pancreatitis on multivariate analysis

Cheng et al. (3) also reported the risk factors of PEP in a large prospective multivariate analysis as patient-related risk factors (e.g., suspected SOD, a history of PEP, and young age (< 60 yrs)) and procedure-related risk factors (e.g., previous minor papilla sphincterotomy, pancreatic duct injections of 2 or more, and trainee involvement).

We previously (28) identified the risk factors of PEP on multivariate analysis as procedure-related risk factors such as initial pancreatography, non-placement of a pancreatic stent (PS) after ERCP procedures, procedure time of 30 min or more, pancreatic-tissue sampling by any method, pancreatic-intraductal ultrasonography (IDUS), and difficulty of cannulation (≥ 15 min). Moreover, we evaluated the correlation between the number of risk factors and PEP. We found a statistically significant association between PEP and the number of risk factors ($P = 0.011$), and the frequency of PEP was statistically significant when there were more than 3 risk factors ($P = 0.001$).

Special consideration should be taken for risk factors, as indicated by multivariate analysis and meta-analysis, in performing ERCP-related procedures, although these procedures also involve comparatively wide-ranging variables such as the experience of the endoscopist.

4. Prevention attempts

To date, there have been several attempts to prevent PEP in terms of patient selection considering the risk factors of PEP, pharmacological drug administration and endoscopic procedures.

4.1 Pharmacological prophylaxis

Chemoprophylaxis to reduce the synthesis and secretion of proteolytic enzymes (octreotide or somatostatin), protease inhibitors (gabexate mesilate, ulinastatin, nafamostat, or aprotinin), antibiotics, and nonsteroidal anti-inflammatory drugs (NSAIDs) have been used to prevent PEP (1,29-42) (Table 3). Numerous randomized controlled trials (RCTs) and several meta-analyses have been performed to evaluate the efficacy of pharmacological drugs for preventing PEP. Freeman et al. evaluated and reviewed the results of previous studies (1), and found that most of these studies failed to show clearly the efficacy of pharmacological drugs, although some promising drugs for preventing PEP were indicated. However, their results should be interpreted in consideration of a lack of unified study design, for example, the selection of high-risk cases, mixed high-risk and non-high-risk cases, and a variety of criteria to define PEP. The outcomes varied and there is as yet no consensus on whether or not chemoprophylaxis is useful for preventing PEP.

4.1.1 Gabexate mesilate

Andriulli et al. (29) demonstrated that gabexate mesilate was effective for PEP evaluation. However, they found that the prophylactic use of gabexate mesilate did not prevent ERCP-related pancreatic damage, even in patients at high risk for PEP in an additional study of the same subject group. Four other meta-analyses (29-32) of RCTs clearly showed that gabexate mesilate was ineffective in preventing PEP, (odds ratio [OR], 0.67; 95% confidence interval [CI], 0.31 - 1.47) and that it was not useful in preventing severe pancreatitis, death, hyperamylasemia, or abdominal pain (30). On the other hand, another meta-analysis which considered the administration schedule (31) showed that the incidence of PEP after long-term infusion (12 h) of gabexate mesilate was significantly decreased by 5.2% (95% CI, 1.1 - 9.4, P = 0.01), although an examination of short-term infusion (within 12 h) failed to show its usefulness in PEP.

Medication	Assessment	Meta-analyses	RCTs
Gabexate mesilate (long-term infusion)	Effective		
Nitroglycerin	Possibly effective		
Antibiotics	Possibly effective		
NSAIDs	Possibly effective	Effective	
Somatostatin (long-term infusion)	Possibly effective	Possibly effective	
Somatostatin (bolus injection)		Effective	
Gabexate mesilate (short-term infusion)	Ineffective	Ineffective	Effective
Ulinastatin			Possibly effective
Semapimod			Possibly effective
Octreotide	Ineffective	Ineffective	
Somatostatin (short-term infusion)	Ineffective	Ineffective	
Calcium inhibitors	Ineffective		
Lidocaine (local administration)	Ineffective		
Nonionic contrast medium	Ineffective		
Steroids	Ineffective	Ineffective	
PAF inhibitors	Ineffective		
IL-10	Ineffective		
Heparin	Ineffective		
Allopurinol	Ineffective	Ineffective	
N-acetylcysteine			Ineffective

RCT, randomized controlled trial; PAF, platelet activating factor; IL, interleukin; NSAIDs, nonsteroidal anti-inflammatory drugs

Refs. (1,42) with alterations

Table 3. Pharmacologocal interventions to reduce risk of post-ERCP pancreatitis

4.1.2 Ulinastatin

Tsujino et al. (33) in their multicenter RCT showed that ulinastatin significantly lowered the incidence of PEP in the ulinastatin-administered group compared with the control group (2.9% vs. 7.4%, P = 0.041). Another RCT, which compared a group given a high dosage of ulinastatin (450,000 U) with a group given a low dosage of ulinastatin (150,000 U) and a group administered gabexate mesilate (900 mg) showed PEP rates of 6.5%, 8.5%, and 4.3%, respectively, indicating no significant differences among the groups (34). Ueki et al. conducted a RCT which compared a group given ulinastatin (150,000 units) and a group given gabexate mesilate (600 mg) and demonstrated a similar PEP rate in both groups, indicating no difference between the 2 groups (35). Chen at al. in their meta-analysis (36) showed that the incidence of PEP was significantly reduced by ulinastatin (OR, 0.53; 95% CI, 0.31 - 0.89; P = 0.02), as well as the incidence of hyperamylasemia (OR, 0.42; 95% CI, 0.30 - 0.59; P < 0.00001); however, subsequent sensitivity and subgroup analyses produced conflicting results. The authors concluded that ulinastatin had value in preventing PEP in average-risk patients when administered intravenously at a dose of at least 150,000 U, given immediately before ERCP.

4.1.3 Somatostatin and octreotide

A meta-analysis (32) of 9 RCTs showed a PEP rate of 7.3% in control groups and 5.3% in the groups administered somatostatin and octreotide (OR, 0.73, 95% CI, 0.54 - 1.006; relative risk [RR], 0.734, 95% CI, 0.535 - 1.006), indicating no significant difference between the 2 groups. In contrast, a different meta-analysis (31) showed that in terms of the administration schedule of somatostatin, long-term infusion (12 h) was associated with a decrease in PEP rate by 7.7% (95% CI, 3.4 - 12.0; P < 0.0001). Short-term infusion (within 12 h) of somatostatin failed to show usefulness in preventing PEP. A study with bolus injections revealed that a bolus injection of somatostatin significantly reduced the PEP rate by 8.2% (95% CI, 4.4 - 12.0; P < 0.0001). A meta-analysis of the bolus injection groups in 3 other RCTs showed that a bolus injection of somatostatin was useful in preventing PEP (OR, 0.271, 95% CI, 0.138 - 0.536; difference in incidence 8.2%, 95% CI, 4.4 - 12.0; number needed to treat [NNT] = 12, 95% CI, 8 - 23).

A meta-analysis of 15 RCTs involving octreotide demonstrated that the overall examination of 2,621 cases failed to show the usefulness of octreotide in preventing PEP (OR, 0.78; 95% CI, 0.57 - 1.08) (38). However, when the analysis was limited to a total of 1,714 cases including the cases in 5 RCTs in which more than 200 cases were studied, it was shown that the PEP rate was significantly decreased by octreotide (OR, 0.50; 95% CI, 0.32 - 0.79; P = 0.003; NNT, 31).

4.1.4 Nonsteroidal anti-inflammatory drugs

A meta-analysis of 6 RCTs involving the administration of NSAIDs showed that the PEP rate was significantly lower in the NSAID-administered group (8.9% vs. 16.8%; OR, 0.46; 95% CI, 0.32 - 0.65; P < 0.0001) (39). Of these 6 RCTs, a meta-analysis of 4 RCTs evaluating a rectally administered drug showed that the single use of NSAIDs just before or after ERCP was useful in preventing PEP (4.4% vs. 12.5%; RR, 0.36; 95% CI, 0.22 - 0.60; NNT, 15) (40). A subgroup analysis of the same 4 RCTs demonstrated that in the NSAID-administered group, there was a significant decrease in the PEP rate in both the low-risk group (RR, 0.29; 95% CI, 0.12 - 0.71; P = 0.006) and the high-risk group (RR, 0.40; 95% CI, 0.23 - 0.72; P = 0.002) (41).

Allopurinol, steroids, N-acetylcysteine, and mitogen-activated protein kinase inhibitors all failed to show a significant preventative effect in PEP (42).

4.1.5 Endoscopic procedures

Careful pancreatic duct injection and avoiding cannulation trauma are essential in performing ERCP-related procedures. Moreover, the placement of a PS with internal and external flanges, or a nasopancreatic drainage tube (9,10) has been performed. To prevent PEP, some endoscopists have inserted a naso-pancreatic drainage tube into the pancreatic duct (9,10) or employed a flanged PS, apparently not considering the possible advantages of spontaneous dislodgement (10-14,19,20). A temporary PS has recently become commercially available and has been reported to be effective in preventing PEP (1,15,17-20,25). PSs are classified into those with and without flanges on the pancreatic ductal side. The former is unlikely to naturally dislodge, and endoscopic removal is often necessary. As for the latter unflanged PS, the rate of natural dislodgement within a short period is high (1,17,25), and re-insertion of an endoscope for removal is generally unnecessary.

Several, mainly non-prospective, randomized studies (9-12,14,18-21) have evaluated endoscopic drainage using a PS with flanges on both sides, unlike our pancreatic duct spontaneous dislodgement stent (PSDS), for preventing PEP in high-risk patients (Table 4). The results suggested that the frequency of PEP decreased, and the PS provided a maintained drainage route when the papilla was blocked as a result of edema, or spasm of the sphincter of Oddi, or both, after the procedure.

Recently, Freeman et al. (17) found that the insertion of a PS in high-risk patients reduced the frequency of PEP by 4 - 23%. In contrast, Smithline et al. (12) reported that PS insertion did not confer a significant beneficial effect in patients with previous biliary sphincterotomy.

Sofuni et al. conducted 3 RCTs (15,28,43) to prospectively evaluate the usefulness of PSDS for PEP prophylaxis. In a preliminary single-center RCT (15), they evaluated PEP prophylaxis using the same unflanged 5-Fr PSDS in 80 consecutive patients, including those who underwent simple ERCP and those who received additional manipulation of the papilla through several stressful examinations including manometry, IDUS, and aspiration of pure pancreatic juice (PPJ). The trial revealed that a temporary unflanged 5-Fr PS reduced the frequency of PEP.

Study (yr)	Study design	No. of patients	Procedures	Pancreatitis rate		
				Non-PD stent	PD stent	P
Smithline, 1993	RCT*	93	Precut biliary ES, SOD, small ducts	18%	14%	0.299
Sherman, 1996	RCT (abstract)	93	Precut biliary ES	21%	2%	0.036
Vandervoort, 1996	(abstract)	127	Pancreatic duct manipulation	18%	8.3%	>0.05
Tarnasky, 1998	RCT	80	Biliary ES for SOD	26%	7%	0.03
Elton, 1998	Retrospective, c.c.[#]	194	Pancreatic ES for all indications	12.5%	0.7%	<0.003
Patel, 1999	RCT (abstract)	36	Pancreatic ES for SOD	33%	11%	>0.05
Vandervoort, 1999	Prospective, c.c.	42	Pancreatic brush cytology	28.1%	0%	0.08
Aizawa, 2001	Retrospective, c.c.	40	EPBD for stone removal	6%	0%	0.11
Fogel, 2002	Retrospective, c.c.	436	Biliary +/ - pancreatic ES for SOD	28.2%	13.5%	<0.05
Norton, 2002	Retrospective, c.c.	28	Endoscopic ampullectomy	11.1%	20%	>0.05
Fazel, 2003	RCT	76	Difficult cannulation, ES, SOD	28%	5%	<0.05
Freeman, 2004	Prospective, c.c.	225	Pancreatic stent in high risk therapeutic ERCP	66.7%	14.4%	0.06
Catalano, 2004	Retrospective, c.c.	103	Endoscopic ampullectomy	16.7%	3.3%	0.10
Rashdan, 2004	Retrospective, c.c.	2283	SOD, divisum therapy, precut ES	N.A.	7.6-14.6**	N.A.
Tsuchiya, 2007	RCT*	64	All patients needed ERCP procedures	28.1%	6.2%	0.02
Sofuni, 2007	RCT*	201	All patients needed ERCP procedures	13.6%	3.2%	0.019
Sofuni, 2011	RCT*	426	15 risk factors for post-ERCP pancreatitis	15.2%	7.9%	0.021

*Randomized controlled trial, [#] case control; SOD, sphincter of Oddi dysfunction; ES, endoscopic sphincterotomy; EPBD, endoscopic balloon dilation; PD, pancreatic duct; N.A., not available; **, evaluation of stent characteristics on the rate of post-ERCP pancreatitis

Ref. (1) with alterations

Table 4. Studies of pancreatic atent for prevention of post-ERCP pancreatitis

A multi-center RCT (43) of 6 endoscopy units based on a previous study (15) demonstrated that the insertion of PSDS significantly reduced the frequency of PEP (3.2% vs. 13.6%, P =0.019). In particular, in cases of hyperamylasemia, the placement of a PSDS significantly reduced the mean serum amylase level (767 vs. 1364 IU/l). This previous study clearly showed the efficacy of PSDS in preventing PEP.

Finally, another RCT (28) conducted in 37 large endoscopic units evaluated whether or not the placement of a PSDS would prevent pancreatitis after ERCP-related procedures in patients with any of the risk factors for PEP, as well as identified risk factors for PEP. The results demonstrated that the placement of a PSDS significantly reduced the frequency of PEP in the analysis, excluding invalid cases (7.9% vs. 15.2%, P = 0.021). A total of 6 risk factors for PEP were identified.

Four meta-analyses (13,44-46) for prophylactic PS placement and PEP indicated that prophylactic temporary stent placement significantly reduces the risk of PEP.

A meta-analysis by Andriulli et al. (44) showed that PEP developed in 16.5% of controls, and in 5.1% or 9.6% of the stent group on per-protocol (PP) or intention-to-treat (ITT) analyses. Analysis of 4 RCTs showed that PEP developed in 24.1% of controls, and in 6.1% or 12.0% of the stented patients on PP or ITT analyses. The risk was significantly lower in the stent group than in the controls (OR, 0.44; 95% CI, 0.24 - 0.81). The ORs for mild to moderate PEP were reduced in the stent group (OR, 0.537; 95% CI, 0.283 - 1.021), as well as those for severe PEP (OR, 0.123; 95% CI, 0.021 - 0.726). These trials indicated the benefits of pancreatic stenting in the prophylaxis of PEP; however, further randomized studies are needed before endorsing the routine use of this endoscopic procedure.

Choudhary et al. (45) have recently found that PS placement decreases the risk of PEP and hyperamylasemia in high-risk patients. They concluded in a meta-analysis of RCTs that prophylactic PS placement decreased the odds of PEP (OR, 0.22; 95% CI, 0.12 - 0.38; P < 0.01). Stents also decreased the level of hyperamylasemia (weighted mean difference, -309.22; 95% CI, -350.95 to -267.49; P ≤ 0.01). Similar findings were also noted in other non-randomized studies.

Mazaki et al. (46) in their meta-analysis showed that PS placement after ERCP reduces the risk of PEP. They concluded that PS placement was associated with a statistically significant reduction in PEP (RR, 0.32; 95% CI, 0.19 - 0.52; P < 0.001). Subgroup analysis with stratification according to PEP severity showed that pancreatic stenting was beneficial in patients with mild to moderate PEP (RR, 0.36; 95% CI, 0.22 - 0.60; p < 0.001) and in patients with severe PEP (RR, 0.23; 95 % CI, 0.06 - 0.91; P = 0.04). Subgroup analysis according to patient selection demonstrated that pancreatic stenting was effective for both high-risk and mixed-case groups.

Freeman et al. (1,20) also reported that unsuccessful cases of stent placement were at higher risk of PEP. Therefore, the PS insertion method for such risk factor cases, and for those in which cannulation is difficult should involve only the insertion of a guidewire before the main procedure. Moreover, it is occasionally difficult to place a stent in anatomic deformity cases. In such cases, the careful use of the Radifocus R (Termo, Tokyo, Japan) guidewire or a 0.025-inch guidewire will enable successful stent placement. Taken together, PS placement is a strategy for preventing PEP which has been shown to be the most effective procedure related to prevention of PEP.

Recently, to increase the success rate of primary deep biliary cannulation and reduce the risk of PEP, a wire-guided cannulation method has been proposed. However, several prospective studies (50-52) provided conflicting results as to whether the wire-guided cannulation technique reduces PEP risk compared with the standard method. Further RCTs are needed to confirm the effectiveness of this method.

4.1.6 Type of stent

Stents with various diameters (3 - 7-Fr), lengths (2.0 - 12 cm), and with or without flanges have been used in previous studies of PEP. However, the optimal stent has not been determined (25,53).

An internal flange is likely to make spontaneous PS dislodgment difficult, and in such cases, generally, the PS has to be removed 7 - 14 days after placement by additional endoscopy, which may not only injure the pancreatic duct, but also be an economic burden. An unflanged stent designed to pass spontaneously from the pancreatic duct may obviate the need for a second endoscopic procedure for stent retrieval. It may also reduce the overall cost of treatment and procedures, and the pancreatic duct is less likely to be injured by an internal flange when the PS dislodges spontaneously. It has been reported that 86% of 3-Fr stents spontaneously dislodged (25).

Unflanged duodenal pigtail- and straight-type stents may spontaneously dislodge into the duodenum owing to pancreatic juice flow or friction with passing food. According to previous RCTs (15,43), unflanged duodenal pigtail- and straight-type stents spontaneously dislodge at a higher rate. The spontaneous dislodgement rates were 93.8% and 95.7%, and the durations until dislodgement were 2.7 and 2 days on average, respectively. The straight type of PS shape on the duodenal side is an important feature facilitating stent placement. Although the unflanged pigtail-type stent may be spontaneously dislodged at a higher rate due to friction with passing food and duodenal peristalsis, the handling of the short duodenal pigtail-type stent is slightly complicated, for example, the possible sudden forward movement of the stent on release, thus it requires close attention and experience. The straight-type PS with a flange on the duodenal side is easier to place than the pigtail-type PS.

Long-term PS retention is a significant risk factor with respect to chronic pancreatitis (1,25-28). Rashdan et al. (25) reported that 3 - 4-Fr stents are more effective than traditionally used stents for preventing PEP, and that 5 - 6-Fr stents cause more significant stent-induced pancreatic duct changes than 3 - 4-Fr stents. However, 3 - 4-Fr stents require a small-caliber guidewire (0.018 - 0.025 inches), and the use of a small-caliber guidewire is difficult and requires a high level of experience (1,25-27). In contrast, the 0.035-inch guidewire used with the 5-Fr PS is relatively easy to use for stent placement.

5. Conclusion

PEP is the most common and potentially serious complication of ERCP-related procedures. The current optimal strategy for preventing PEP is considered to include the elucidation of its underlying mechanisms, identification of risk factors, administration of pharmacological drugs, and endoscopic procedures such as pancreatic stenting. The placement of a PS currently remains the most effective strategy for preventing PEP.

6. Acknowledgements

The authors are indebted to Mr. Roderick J. Turner, Assistant Professor Edward F. Barroga and Professor J. Patrick Barron, Chairman of the Department of International Medical Communications of Tokyo Medical University for their review of this manuscript. We also thank the members of The Japan Pancreatic Stent-Study Group (JPS-SG). No external financial support for this study was provided. Both authors report that they have no conflicts of interest associated with this study.

7. References

[1] Freeman ML, Nalini M, Guda M. Prevention of post-ERCP pancreatitis: a comprehensive review. Gastrointest Endosc 2004; 59:845-64.

[2] Freeman ML, DiSario JA, Nelson DB, et al. Risk factors for post-ERCP pancreatitis: a prospective, multicenter study. Gastrointest Endosc 2001; 54:425-34.

[3] Cheng CL, Sherman S, Watkins JL, et al. Risk factors for post-ERCP pancreatitis: A prospective multicenter study. Am J Gastroenterol 2006;101:139-47.

[4] Freeman ML, Nelson DB, Sherman S, et al. Complications of endoscopic biliary sphincterotomy. N Engl J Med 1996; 335:909-18.

[5] Masci E, Toti G, Mariani A, et al. Complications of diagnostic and therapeutic ERCP: a prospective multicenter study. Am J Gastroenterol 2001;96:417-23.

[6] Mehta SN, Pavone E, Barkun JS, et al. Predictors of post-ERCP complications in patients with suspected choledocholithiasis. Endoscopy 1998;30:457-63.

[7] Sherman S, Ruffolo TA, Hawes RH, et al. A prospective series with emphasis on the increased risk associates with sphincter of Oddi dysfunction and nondilated bile ducts. Gastroenterology 1991;101:778-82.

[8] Vandervoort J, Soetikno RM, Tham TC, et al. Risk factors for complications after performance of ERCP. Gastrointest Endosc 2002;56:652-6.

[9] Elton E, Howell DA, Parsons WG, et al. Endoscopic pancreatic sphincterotomy: indications, outcome, and a safe stentless technique. Gastrointest Endosc 1998;47:240-9.

[10] Fazel A, Quadri A, Catalano MF, et al. Does a pancreatic duct stent prevent post-ERCP pancreatitis? A prospective randomized study. Gastrointest Endosc 2003;57:291-4.

[11] Tarnasky PR, Palesch YY, Cunningham JT, et al. Pancreatic stenting prevents pancreatitis after biliary sphincterotomy in patients with sphincter of Oddi dysfunction. Gastroenterology 1998;115:1518-24.

[12] Smithline A, Silverman W, Rogers D, et al. Effect of prophylactic main pancreatic duct stenting on the incidence of biliary endoscopic sphincterotomy-induced pancreatitis in high-risk patients. Gastrointest Endosc. 1993;39:652-7.

[13] Singh P, Das A, Isenberg G, et al. Does prophylactic pancreatic stent placement reduce the risk of post-ERCP acute pancreatitis? A meta-analysis of controlled trials. Gastrointest Endosc 2004;60:544-50.

[14] Catalano MF, Linder JD, Chak A, et al. Endoscopic management of adenoma of the major duodenal papilla. Gastrointest Endosc.2004;59:225-32.

[15] Tsuchiya T, Itoi T, Sofuni A, et al. A temporary inner unflanged 5Fr pancreatic duct stent to prevent post-ERCP pancreatitis. A preliminary and single center randomized controlled trial study. J Hepatobiliary Pancreat Surg. 2007;14:302-7.

[16] Sherman S, Lehman G, Freeman M, et al. Risk factors for post-ERCP pancreatitis: A prospective multicenter study. Am J Gastroenterol 1997;92(suppl 9):1639

[17] Freeman ML. Role of pancreatic stents in prevention of post-ERCP pancreatitis. J Pancreas 2004;5:322-7.

[18] Fogel EL. Eversman D, Jamidar P, et al. Sphincter of Oddi dysfunction: Pancreaticobiliary sphincterotomy with pancreatic stent placement has a lower rate of pancreatitis than biliary sphincterotomy alone. Endoscopy 2002;34:280-5.
[19] Aizawa T, Ueno N. Stent placement in the pancreatic duct prevents pancreatitis after endoscopic sphincter dilation for removal of bile duct stones. Gastrointest Endosc 2001;54:209-13.
[20] Freeman ML, Overby C, Qi D. Pancreatic stent insertion: Consequence of failure and results of a modified technique to maximize success. Gastrointest Endosc 2004;59:8-14.
[21] Vandervoort J, Soetikno RM, Montes H, et al. Accuracy and complication rate of brush cytology from bile duct versus pancreatic duct. Gastrointest Endosc 1999;49:322-7.
[22] Cotton PB, Lehman G, Vennes J, et al. Endoscopic sphincterotomy complications and their management: an attempt at consensus. Gastrointest Endosc 1991;37:383-93.
[23] Tarnasky P, Cunningham J, Cotton P, et al. Pancreatic sphincter hypertension increases the risk of post-ERCP pancreatitis. Endoscopy 1997;29:252-7.
[24] Sherman S, Troiano FP, Hawes RH, et al. Sphincter of Oddi manometry: decreased risk of clinical pancreatitis with use of a modified aspirating catheter. Gastrointest Endosc 1990;36:462-6.
[25] Rashdan A, Fogel EL, Mchenry Jr. L, et al. Improved stent characteristics for prophylaxis of post-ERCP pancreatitis. Clin Gastroenterol Hepatol 2004;2:322-9.
[26] Johnson GK, Geenen JE, Johanson JF, et al. Evaluation of post-ERCP pancreatitis: potential causes noted during controlled study of differing contrast media. Gastrointest Endosc 1997;46:217-22.
[27] Testoni PA, et al. Risk factors for post-ERCP pancreatitis in high- and low-volume centers and among expert and non-expert operators: a prospective multicenter study. Am J Gastroenterol. 2010;105:1753-61.
[28] Sofuni A, Maguchi H, Itoi T et al. Endoscopic pancreatic duct stents reduce the incidence of post-endoscopic retrograde cholangiopancreatography pancreatitis in high risk patients. Clin Gastroenterol Hepatol. 2011 Jul 9. Clin Gastroenterol Hepatol. 2011 Oct;9(10):851-8.
[29] Andriulli A, Leandro G, Niro G, et al. Pharmacologic treatment can prevent pancreatic injury after ERCP: a meta-analysis. Gastrointest Endosc. 2000;51:1-7.
[30] Zheng M, Chen Y, Yang X, et al. Gabexate in the prophylaxis of post-ERCP pancreatitis: a meta-analysis of randomized controlled trials. BMC Gastroenterol. 2007;7:6–13.
[31] Rudin D, Kiss A, Wetz RV, et al. Somatostatin and gabexate for post-endoscopic retrograde cholangiopancreatography pancreatitis prevention: meta-analysis of randomized placebo-controlled trials. J Gastroenterol Hepatol. 2007;22:977–83.
[32] Andriulli A, Leandro G, Federici T, et al. Prophylactic administration of somatostatin or gabexate does not prevent pancreatitis after ERCP: an updated meta-analysis. Gastrointest Endosc. 2007;65:624–32.
[33] Tsujino T, Komatsu Y, Isayama H, et al. Ulinastatin for pancreatitis after endoscopic retrograde cholangiopancreatography: a randomized, controlled trial. Clin Gastroenterol Hepatol. 2005;3:376–83. 55
[34] Fujishiro H, Adachi K, Imaoka T, et al. Ulinastatin shows preventive effect on post-endoscopic retrograde cholangiopancreatography pancreatitis in a multicenter prospective randomized study. J Gastroenterol Hepatol. 2006;21:1065–9.

[35] Ueki T, Otani K, Kawamoto K, et al. Comparison between ulinastatin and gabexate mesylate for the prevention of post-endoscopic retrograde cholangiopancreatography pancreatitis: a prospective, randomized trial. J Gastroenterol. 2007; 42:161–7. 44.
[36] Chen S, Shi H, Zou X et al. Role of ulinastatin in preventing post-endoscopic retrograde cholangiopancreatography pancreatitis: the Emperor's New Clothes or Aladdin's Magic Lamp? Pancreas. 2010;39(8):1231-7.
[37] Andriulli A, Leandro G, Federici T, et al. Prophylactic administration of somatostatin or gabexate does not prevent pancreatitis after ERCP: an updated meta-analysis. Gastrointest Endosc. 2007;65:624–32.
[38] Bai Y, Gao J, Zou DW, et al. Prophylactic octreotide administration does not prevent post-endoscopic retrograde cholangiopancreatography pancreatitis: a meta-analysis of randomized controlled trials. Pancreas. 2008;37:241–6.
[39] Dai HF, Wang XW, Zhao K. Role of nonsteroidal anti-inflammatory drugs in the prevention of post-ERCP pancreatitis: a meta-analysis. Hepatobiliary Pancreat Dis Int. 2009;8:11–6.
[40] Elmunzer BJ, Waljee AK, Elta GH, et al. A meta-analysis of rectal NSAIDs in the prevention of post-ERCP pancreatitis. Gut. 2008;57:1262–7.
[41] Zheng MH, Xia HH, Chen YP. Rectal administration of NSAIDs in the prevention of post-ERCP pancreatitis: a complementary meta-analysis. Gut. 2008;57:1632–3.
[42] Arata S, Takada T, Hirata K, et al. Post-ERCP pancreatitis. J Hepatobiliary Pancreat Sci. 2010;17:70-8.
[43] Sofuni A, Maguchi H, Itoi T, et al. Prophylaxis of post-endoscopic retrograde cholangiopancreatography pancreatitis by an endoscopic pancreatic spontaneous dislodgement stent. Clin Gastroenterol Hepatol. 2007;5:1339-46.
[44] Andriulli A, Forlano R, Napolitano G et al. Pancreatic duct stents in the prophylaxis of pancreatic damage after endoscopic retrograde cholangiopancreatography: a systematic analysis of benefits and associated risks. Digestion. 2007;75:156-63.
[45] Choudhary A, Bechtold ML, Arif M. et al. Pancreatic stents for prophylaxis against post-ERCP pancreatitis: a meta-analysis and systematic review. Gastrointest Endosc. 2011 ;73:275-82.
[46] Mazaki T, Masuda H, Takayama T. Prophylactic pancreatic stent placement and post-ERCP pancreatitis: a systematic review and meta-analysis. Endoscopy. 2010;42:842-53.
[47] Sherman S, Hawes RH, Savides TJ, et al. Stent-induced pancreatic ductal and parenchymal changes: correlation of endoscopic ultrasound with ERCP. Gastrointest Endosc 1996;44:276-82.
[48] Smith MT, Sherman S, Ikenberry SO, et al. Alterations in pancreatic ductal morphology following polyethylene pancreatic stent therapy. Gastrointest Endosc 1996;44:268-75.
[49] Raju GS, Gomez G, Xiao SY, et al. Effect of a novel pancreatic stent design on short-term pancreatic injury in a canine model. Endoscopy 2006;38:260-5.
[50] Lella F, Bagnolo F, Colombo E et al. A simple way of avoiding post-ERCP pancreatitis. Gastrointest Endosc 2004;59:830–4.

[51] Bailey AA, Bourke MJ, Williams SJ et al. A prospective randomized trial of cannulation technique in ERCP: effects on technical success and post- ERCP pancreatitis. Endoscopy 2008;40:296–01.
[52] Cennamo V, Fuccio L, Zagari RM et al. Can a wire-guided cannulation technique increase bile duct cannulation rate and prevent post-ERCP pancreatitis?: A meta-analysis of randomized controlled trials. Am J Gastroenterol. 2009;104:2343-50.
[53] Chahal P, Tarnasky PR, Petersen BT, et al. Short 5Fr vs long 3Fr pancreatic stents in patients at risk for post-endoscopic retrograde cholangiopancreatography pancreatitis. Clin Gastroenterol Hepatol. 2009;7:834-9.

6

Recurrent Pancreatitis

Vincenzo Neri
University of Foggia,
Italy

1. Introduction

The nosological definition of inflammatory pancreatic diseases appears rather difficult and uncertain, as proved by the great number of classifications which have been proposed in the last few decades, showing that the definition and classification of this disease is still under critical review. The reason is the reduced availability or, in the majority of the cases, the absence of histological findings which can be connected to a clinical picture that moreover is often subject to evolutions. A not negligible role in generating uncertainties is played by the very diversified territorial distribution of the various forms of pancreatitis: this provides to the different observers different and often hardly reconcilable experiences. Therefore, the succeeding classifications are based exclusively on clinical or laboratory data or on imaging exams. We can consider as stable references the basic anatomo-clinical correspondences. It is preliminarily acquired that the parenchymal phlogistic process recognizes its origin in the self-digestive effect of the same pancreatic proteolytic enzymes. Self-limiting parenchymal inflammation characterizes mild and moderate acute pancreatitis. Self-digestive processes of serious entity with parenchymal necrosis and peripancreatic fluid collections manifest themselves as severe acute pancreatitis (SAP). Finally, chronic pancreatitis is histologically characterized by fibrosis, sclerosis and calcifications. Historically, the rigorous and well-defined distinction between acute and chronic pancreatitis has represented for a long time the basis of classifications in which acute and chronic pancreatitis were substantially considered two different diseases but, in the course of time, important modifications have taken place. In fact, currently this distinction is in discussion due to the imaging of the main bile duct and of the duct of Wirsung and above all due to the more comprehensive, prolonged and detailed clinical observations which allow to estimate the sometimes long evolution of pancreatitis. These observations show that acute and chronic forms overlap (Bassi & Butturini , 2007). The onset and/or the acute manifestations of chronic pancreatitis are considered and also the acute pancreatitis which, because of the repeated acute episodes, evolve anatomo-clinically towards chronicity. Recurrent acute pancreatitis is characterized by several acute episodes which follow the first attack. On the whole, the risk of recurrence for pancreatitis with different etiology is contained (20-30%). On the contrary the patients who present a second attack have a much higher risk of further recurrences and therefore require a rigorous diagnostic investigation. Biliary lithiasis and excessive alcohol consumption are the more frequent causes of pancreatitis, reaching as a whole the total incidence of 80% (Barthet, 2001; Gullo et al, 2002). However, the frequency rate between biliary and alcoholic etiology is subject to great variations in relation to geographic distribution. Moreover, even if with much contained frequency, numerous other causes of pancreatitis are recognized which may manifest as recurrent and which, on the whole, represent 20% of the total (Ferec & Maire, 2005; Hastier, 2005) : hereditary, metabolic pancreatitis (hyperlipidemia, hypercalcaemia, steroids), from neoplastic ductal obstruction (intraductal papillary mucinous neoplasms (IPMN), periampullary tumors,etc), from congenital anomalies (pancreas divisum, annular pancreas, anomalies of the biliopancreatic junction), from dysfunction of the sphincter of Oddi, from drugs and toxic substances, trauma and infections and finally post-endoscopic retrograde cholangiopancreatography (ERCP) pancreatitis. Among all the various forms of recurrent pancreatitis, the conditions based on the obstruction of the flow of pancreatic secretions amenable to endoscopic treatment (ERCP-Endoscopic Sphincterotomy (ES)) are in evidence: biliary pancreatitis, dysfunction of the sphincter of Oddi, pancreas divisum. The object of our interest is the anatomo-clinical condition of recurrent pancreatitis. Pancreatic inflammatory diseases may evolve towards chronicity because of either the episodic increase of the phlogistic response and/or the recurrence of acute attacks. In pancreatitis with different etiopathogenesis it is useful to examine which are the possible different pathogenetic modalities of pancreatitis recurrence and its possible evolution. On the basis of the clinical presentation, acute pancreatitis, in particular those of biliary etiology, can be subdivided in mild, moderate and severe: the former, which include clinical forms of different relevance and extension, represent the majority of acute pancreatitis (75%). Severe forms constitute the remaining 25%. Among these an ulterior 20% is represented by forms of particular and sudden severity (early severe acute pancreatitis (ESAP)) (Beger & Rau , 2007). Pancreatitis incidence increases stably with the increase of the average age of population and with the increased incidence of biliary lithiasis and alcohol consumption. Unlike in chronic pancreatitis in which fibrosis does not revert and there is no total recovery with restoration of the original condition, patients with an attack of acute pancreatitis, particularly in mild/moderate forms, show an almost complete anatomical and functional recovery. However, there remains still the possibility of other recurrent attacks. The reason of this possible evolution can be recognized in at least two circumstances: either the initial and effective cause persists or it is not completely removed by the therapeutic intervention: biliary lithiasis or biliary sludge, cholelithiasis, inflammatory papillary stenosis, invariated alcohol consumption, tumors obstructing the main pancreatic duct. Also severe pancreatitis with extended necrotic parenchymal areas can evolve into chronic pancreatitis for successive stenosis of the main pancreatic duct. The possibility of the evolution of an acute inflammatory process into a chronic phlogistic condition returns therefore in evidence. The distinction between acute and chronic pancreatitis is based on the natural history, the characteristics of the clinical picture and the anatomo-pathological alterations. Acute pancreatitis starts out in patients with no history of related illness and with the possibility of a complete resolution especially in mild/moderate forms. On the contrary, the anatomical and functional recovery in severe forms can be compromised. Moreover in SAP with severe impairment of the general clinical conditions and important structural alterations, the prognosis is serious. In chronic pancreatitis the organ impairment and the persistence of painful symptomatology of moderate severity characterize the intervals between the acute attacks. However, the acute attack, both in acute and chronic pancreatitis, is characterized by acute onset and by very similar symptoms. Therefore, in the absence of an histological exam and of prolonged observation, the distinction between the two forms may be difficult. Regarding this point, SAP and ESAP often with biliary etiopathogenesis and with impairment of clinical conditions, must be considered with attention. In fact, the acute onset in chronic pancreatitis and severe acute pancreatitis may be distinguished for the presence in the latter of a severe impairment of clinical conditions which impairs the prognosis. All these considerations contribute to establish a connection between acute and chronic forms. The inflammatory process underlying acute pancreatitis can resolve if the recurrence of acute episodes is interrupted in the early stages. But, if the conditions which determine the recurrence of the acute attacks persist, like for example papillary sclerosis or obstruction with reflux in the duct of Wirsung, then inflammation will be able to evolve into fibrosis and acute pancreatitis will evolve anatomically and clinically into chronic pancreatitis. Therefore, recurrent pancreatitis may be considered the clinical condition which constitutes the bridge between acute and chronic pancreatitis. In fact, pancreatic inflammation may show a chronic evolution through the recurrence of acute episodes. Thus it is important to establish through which anatomical alterations and how in the pancreatitis of various etiologies this evolution is determined.

2. Biliary pancreatitis

Pathogenetic modalities of recurrent pancreatitis are well evident in biliary pancreatitis. Recurrent acute biliary pancreatitis is caused by obstacle in the papillary patency with abnormal biliopancreatic flow. Papillary obstacle, caused by gallstones, biliary sludge, cholesterol cristals, sclerosis or edema, determines biliopancreatic reflux in the pancreatic duct with consequent pancreatitis. Therefore, restoring the normal transpapillary flow and cleaning the common bile duct (CBD) can prevent pancreatitis recurrences. This pathogenetic pattern of acute biliary pancreatitis (ABP) is by now widely documented (Frossard et al.,2008; Lee et al, 1992; Opie, 1901; Pandol SJ, 2006; Wang et al, 2009). The incidence of recurrent biliary pancreatitis is reported to widely vary between 30% and 60% in patients who did not undergo cholecystectomy and ES, often with a short interval between the first and the second attack: 4-6 weeks (Heider et al, 2006; Van Geenen et al, 2009). Our purpose is to evaluate the possibility and the means to prevent recurrent acute biliary pancreatitis. Detailed examination of an homogeneous series contributes to clarify the anatomo-clinical details. The study evaluated the patients with ABP admitted to our hospital in the period September 1997 - December 2010. We collected a total of 261 cases, mean age 49 (20-86), M 112 - F 149, including 203 (77,7%) mild/moderate and 58 (22,3%) severe pancreatitis (Tab 1). Among moderate pancreatitis, we recognized 31 (15,7%) moderate/severe pancreatitis, characterized by extensive pancreatic and peripancreatic inflammation with fluid collections and mild necrosis, without however impairment of the general clinical conditions (Heider et al, 2006; Nealon et al, 2004). We selected, through the medical records, the patients who had a first attack of ABP, distinguishing them from the ones who had previously suffered from one or more episodes of ABP. The patients with a first attack of onset were on the whole 188 (72,3%), while those with previous repeated episodes were 73 (28%). Among the 73 recurrent pancreatitis, 12 (16,4%) were severe and 61 (83,6%) moderate/mild (Tab. 2).

MEAN AGE	SEX	Dir. BIL. < 2 mg/dl	Dir. Bil. 2-5 mg/dl	AST/ALT x3 iU/l	gamma-GT >200 iU/l	ALP >150 iU/l	CBD size (US)> 8 mm	Cholecystic Lithiasis
49 (20-86)	F 149 M 112	60.4%	39.6%	26.8%	59.9%	53.6%	40.7%	100%
EDEMATOUS				187			71.64%	
NECROTIZING				74			28.36%	
PERIPANCREATIC FLUID COLLECTION				95/261			36.39%	

Table 1. Demographic data, percentage incidence of biliary lithiasis and cholestasis tests, pancreatitis morphology (US/CT) in 261 acute biliary pancreatitis at the admission in our Hospital.

MEAN AGE	SEX	Dir. Bil. < 2 mg/dl	Dir. Bil. 2-5 mg/dl	AST/ALT x3 iU/l	gamma-GT >200 iU/l	ALP >150 iU/l	CBD size (US)>8mm	Cholecystic Lithiasis
54 (28-76)	F 44 M 29	47.2%	52.8%	31.2%	64.3%	59.4%	48.2%	100%
EDEMATOUS				54		73.97%		
NECROTIZING				19		26.03%		
PERIPANCREATIC FLUID COLLECTION				33/73		45.20%		

Table 2. Demographic data, percentage incidence of biliary lithiasis and cholestasis tests, pancreatitis morphology (US/CT) in 73 recurrent acute pancreatitis at the admission in our Hospital.

The acute episode of pancreatitis was defined by the presence of abdominal epi-mesogastric pain radiating through to the back and by increased serum amylase and lipase levels. To establish the gallstone etiology of pancreatitis, we searched, in all patients, on ultrasonography, gallbladder lithiasis and/or gallstones, sludge, microlithiasis etc. in the CBD or also a dilatation of the CBD (>8 mm). Laboratory cholestasis tests were on average positive in 40% of patients: direct bilirubin between 2 and 5 mg/l, alkaline phosphatase >150 U/l and gamma-GT >200 U/l. Alcohol consumption in these patients had also been excluded. The severity of pancreatic involvement was assessed with abdominal ultrasound (US) at the admission and with computed tomography (CT) (Balthazar criteria)(Balthazar et al, 1990) after 48-72-hours. The patients with previous attacks of recurrent acute pancreatitis have not been submitted, during the previous hospitalizations, to any specific therapy for pancreatitis (ERCP/ES, cholecystectomy), but only to simple supportive therapy. In this group, with recurrent pancreatitis, control of gallstone etiology, laboratory cholestasis tests and the CT pancreatic involvement were not dissimilar compared to all patients. All patients underwent the complete treatment for ABP, adjusted according to the degree of severity of the disease: intensive therapy, clinical and instrumental monitoring of papillary patency,

ERCP/ES (209/261=80%) within 72 hours from the onset in all severe pancreatitis (58) (in 3 cases this procedure was unsuccessful and in 7 cases it was delayed for 10 days), in all recurrent pancreatitis (73), in all moderate/severe pancreatitis (31) with extensive inflammatory pancreatic and peripancreatic involvement, fluid collection and mild pancreatic necrosis (as shown by CT), but without organ failure and finally in moderate/mild pancreatitis with laboratory cholestasis tests and instrumental (US/MRCP) confirmation of papillary obstacle (lithiasis, microlithiasis, sludge in CBD, papillary edema, stenosis, etc.) (59/203, 29%). The treatment was completed with laparoscopic cholecystectomy: 254 video-laparocholecystectomies (VLC) and 7 open cholecystectomies. The timing of cholecystectomy varied according to the severity of pancreatitis; generally, we waited for the stabilization of the pancreatic and peripancreatic phlogosis/necrosis and of the patient's clinical conditions. After the treatment and the discharge, all the patients were introduced in a follow-up program (clinical and instrumental control after 90 and 180 days). The 73 patients with recurrent pancreatitis, after the standard therapeutic program and the discharge, entered a follow-up program with clinical and instrumental controls at 90 and 180 days. Forty-two (57,5%) patients were monitored (31 patients could not be reached): the results of the follow-up showed, beside the absence of critical episodes, the stable normalization of laboratory and instrumental cholestasis tests at the first (90 days) and at the second control (180 days) (Tab 3). A further recurrence has occurred only in 2 patients (2/42 = 2,7%) with a moderate/mild pancreatitis at the 145th day from the discharge. Once the persistence of the papillary obstacle for incomplete sphincterotomy had been assessed, the resolution was obtained with medical therapy and a new ES.

Tot. Bil.	ALP	AST/ALT	Amylase	Lipase	gamma-GT	CBD size (US)	Recurrence
0.80 mg/dl	115 iU/l	24/50 iU/l	220 iU/l	110 iU/l	38 iU/l	6 mm	2 (2.7%)

Table 3. Recurrent acute biliary pancreatitis 42/73 (57.5%) : follow-up (180 days)
Cholestasis tests were on average normal.

The same controls in 88 patients (88/188 = 46,8%) with a first attack of acute pancreatitis, at 90 and 180 days from the discharge resulted normal, in the absence of new acute episodes (Tab 4).

Tot. Bil.	ALP	AST/ALT	Amylase	Lipase	gamma-GT	CBD size (US)	Recurrence
0.90 mg/dl	112 iU/l	28/40 iU/l	95 iU/l	158 iU/l	54 iU/l	5 mm	–

Table 4. Acute biliary pancreatitis 88/188 (46,4%) : follow-up (180 days)
Cholestasis tests were on average normal.

We believe that ES has a control role in the therapy of ABP. Biliary pancreatitis presents clinical findings of different severity. Signs and symptoms of reference, always present, consist in epigastric pain with acute onset and characteristic radiation to the back and evident increase of serum amylase and lipase levels. Moderate/mild pancreatitis, with pancreatic or peripancreatic edema, is not accompanied by impairment of the patient's general clinical conditions, requires only supportive therapy and generally evolves towards a spontaneous recovery. In these patients cholecystectomy is indicated and is performed, as a general rule, while the patient is still hospitalized. In moderate/mild pancreatitis ES is not generally indicated because the papillary obstacle is transient and probably incomplete. In the cases showing clinical and laboratory signs or ultrasound evidence of cholestasis, instrumental control of the bile duct with magnetic resonance cholangiopancreatography (MRCP) is proposed. ERCP/ES is used as therapy only in case of lithiasic obstacles or biliary sludge in the CBD or papillary stenosis. Moreover the advisability of an instrumental control of the bile duct with MRCP is discussed in patients with mild acute pancreatitis who do not show any clinical or instrumental sign of cholestasis, as an additional exam beside the routine abdominal ultrasonography before cholecystectomy. The incidence of gallstones in the population of western countries is about 15% and among these patients about 10-15% have choledocholithiasis (Tazuma, 2006). The literature data show that a very variable range (45-75%) of patients with acute biliary pancreatitis has stones in the CBD (Barro et al,2005; Young et al,2003). The cases with acute biliary pancreatitis include mild/moderate self-limiting forms with transient papillary obstacle, which are not accompanied by clinical, laboratory or instrumental signs of cholestasis. For these mild/moderate forms of acute pancreatitis the use of invasive procedures to explore the CBD is not advisable, while it is necessary to demonstrate the absence of stones in the CBD. For these reasons in patients with mild/moderate acute biliary pancreatitis without increase of cholestasis indexes and in the absence of dilatation of intra and extra-hepatic biliary ducts, it is useful to know if obstacles are present in the CBD. These patients should undergo a MRCP to determine the conditions of the CBD before cholecystectomy. In these cases, in fact, the extensive use of MRCP can be useful for a significant reduction of the number of non-therapeutic ERCP/ES and their associated complications. The clinical scenario is, in 20-30% of cases, a severe pancreatitis characterized by extensive pancreatic and peripancreatic necrosis, fluid collections at risk of infection, possible systemic inflammatory response syndrome (SIRS) with impairment of the patient's clinical conditions which always requires starting immediately intensive therapy. Besides, 20% of SAP show an early severity - ESAP - with development within 72 hours of multiple organ failure and within 2 weeks of infection of the pancreatic and peripancreatic necrotic collections with high mortality (40-60%). Thus, in all severe pancreatitis it is necessary a prolonged control of the pancreatic and peripancreatic necrotic collections which are exposed to infectious complications. Early (within 72 hours) ES has proved to be successful to maintain and to control the evolution of the inflammatory process and also safe to prevent close inflammatory-necrotic recurrences, which are caused by the persistence of the papillary obstacle and of the biliary reflux in the pancreatic duct (Folsch et al, 1997; Heider et al, 2006; Hernandez et al, 2004; Kimura et al, 2006; Neoptolemos et al, 1988; Sungler et al, 2007 ; Van Geenen et al, 2009). Cholecystectomy is definitely indicated, but should be programmed once the patient's clinical conditions are stable. Another clinical manifestation of biliary pancreatitis is the moderate form. Its nosological definition is rather difficult and uncertain, placed between the much better identifiable mild and severe forms. Among the moderate forms it is significant, to therapeutic goals, to identify the moderate/severe forms (Heider et al,2006) which are characterized by pancreatic necrosis, not exceeding 30% of the parenchyma at the CT control, edema and phlogosis of the retroperitoneal peripancreatic lodge with possible fluid collections. In these forms impairment of the patient's clinical conditions with multi-organ dysfunction is absent. Also, infection of the fluid collections occurs rarely. The resolution of symptoms occurs in a relatively short time, 10 days on average; return to normality of serum amylase and lipase levels is slower and so is the resolution of the pancreatic and peripancreatic phlogosis/necrosis and the fluid collections reabsorption. Also in these cases early (within 72 hours) ES is effective to reduce the risk of an often even earlier recurrence of pancreatitis. Cholecystectomy can be performed when the patient's clinical conditions are restored, almost always during the same hospitalization. The pathogenesis of acute biliary pancreatitis is based on the alteration of transpapillary flow caused by edema and/or mechanical obstacle which determines the pancreatic intra-ductal reflux. Thus ES by normalizing the biliopancreatic transpapillary flow removes the morphofunctional alteration and reduces the risk of pancreatitis recurrences, which present themselves sometimes with acute close episodes. Besides, ERCP/ES allow at the same time to clean the CBD in case of sludge, microlithiasis or stones. Once the initial pathogenesis has been defined, it remains to establish which patients with acute biliary pancreatitis should undergo ES. ES is indicated in severe and in moderate/severe pancreatitis, and, of course, in acute recurrent pancreatitis, irrespective of the presence of laboratory, clinical and instrumental signs of cholestasis or of a lithiasic obstacle in the CBD which, if present, constitute further motive for ES. On the contrary, moderate/mild pancreatitis does not require endoscopic treatment unless cholestasis is present. In patients with recurrent pancreatitis, according to the pathogenetic sequence papillary obstacle / biliopancreatic reflux, the necessity to restore the papillary patency with ES is assumed. In our experience recurrent pancreatitis is present in 30% of acute biliary pancreatitis treated. Recurrent pancreatitis occupies a nosographic place which presents a special interest because it can represent the connection between acute pancreatitis and chronic pancreatitis. A relevant contribution to the definition of the therapeutic choice and of the possible nosological organization which may clarify the possible evolutions of acute pancreatitis (ex: recurrent acute pancreatitis evolving to chronification of the phlogistic lesions) may come from the careful and extended clinical observation integrated with repeated instrumental verifications: US-CT-MRCP. In fact, ever since its onset, we can consider pancreatitis as a difficult disease to classify, whose possibilities of evolution can be influenced by numerous etiopathogenetic factors and which should be subject to a dynamic follow- up. Acute pancreatitis can evolve into the chronic form as the result of recurrences of repeated episodes of papillary obstruction secondary to edema and to sclerotic evolution of the inflammatory reaction of the sphincter of Oddi. Biliary lithiasis, with passage of stones, biliary sludge, microstones or with persistent lithiasic obstacle of the papilla, plays a considerable role in the genesis of the sclerosis of the sphincter of Oddi. In this light, ES in the treatment of recurrent acute biliary pancreatitis may have a role of prevention against an hypothesized papillary fibrotic evolution of the phlogosis with consequent chronification. The process that brings to pancreatic fibrotic alterations corresponds clinically to repeated episodes of typical abdominal pains and increased levels of serum amylase and lipase which are caused by recurrences of acute pancreatitis. The episodes of parenchymal inflammation evolve towards the self-limitation of the phlogosis without sequels, as an alternative to the evolution towards chronification. The recurrent pancreatitis presents itself with the anatomopathological substrate of an acute inflammatory focus during the course of chronic pancreatitis. In a general picture, the possible evolutions of the pancreatic inflammations are self-limitation, progression with self-digestion and extensive necrosis of the parenchyma and of the surrounding tissues, or an evolution with predominance of fibrosis and calcifications which characterize chronic phogosis. Finally, ES plays a double preventive role, interrupting the recurrence of acute attacks and the possible chronification of the phlogistic process. Recurrent acute biliary pancreatitis has been caused, in patients discharged from the hospital without additional treatment, by persistent papillary obstacle (small stones, sludge, microlithiasis, cholesterol crystals). Therefore we confirm the therapeutic validity of instrumental control (US/MRCP) and the possible treatment (ERCP/ES) of papillary or biliary lithiasic obstacle for the prevention of recurrent acute biliary pancreatitis. ES plays an important role in the treatment of ABP and a most important role in recurrent pancreatitis because of the persistent papillary obstacle. In severe, moderate/severe and recurrent pancreatitis, instrumental confirmation of papillary obstacle is not necessary because this is persistent. On the contrary, in mild/moderate pancreatitis laboratory, US and MRCP confirmation of papillary or CBD lithiasic obstacle is useful prior to ERCP/ES because the papillary obstacle is transient. Patients with mild/moderate pancreatitis without cholestasis indexes should undergo instrumental control with MRCP for lithiasic obstacles in the CBD prior VLC because in a very variable range (45-75%) of acute biliary pancreatitis stones are present in the CBD. The results of these evaluations show the efficacy of the therapeutic program with ERCP/ES in the prevention of recurrent acute biliary pancreatitis with mini-invasive approach. The pathogenetic modalities of recurrent pancreatitis are well defined and obvious in the forms with biliary aetiology. However there are recurrent pancreatitis also among pancreatitis with different aetiology: these are less frequent pancreatitis for which a smaller number of observations is available and therefore with a somewhat uncertain characterization.

3. Alcoholic pancreatitis

The diagnosis of alcoholic pancreatitis is based on the definition of alcohol consumption and on the presence of anatomopatological alterations assessed with morphological examinations (X-rays, CT, EUS, wirsungraphy): parenchymal anomalies and of the excretory ducts with or without calcifications. In the course of alcoholic pancreatitis, recurrent episodes of acute pancreatitis can evolve into chronic pancreatitis and the effective and determining way of the recurrence of acute attacks can be evidenced (Gorelick, 2003; Spanier et al,2008; Whitcomb, 2005). In fact, most observers currently believe that chronic pancreatitis which follows prolonged ethanol abuse reflects repeated but subclinical, episodes of acute pancreatic injury. These repeated episodes of pancreatic injury with necrosis lead to fibrosis which characterizes chronic pancreatitis (Kloppel,1999). There are numerous theories since long presented in literature which propose an explanation of the lesive action of alcohol on pancreatic parenchyma but none of them is completely acquired. Alcohol would cause hypertriglyceridemia, fat acid and ethyl esters formation, that is formation of oxygen free radicals, causing pancreatic phlogistic damage. According to another hypothesis, alcohol alters the composition of pancreatic secretions with reduction of inhibiting enzymes and proteins precipitation forming intraductal plugs. Ductal obstruction causes increase in endoluminal pressure and consequent phlogosis with multiple foci of pancreatitis. Also the spasm of the sphincter of Oddi has been attributed to the action of alcohol.

4. Processes obstructing the flow of pancreatic juice, pancreas divisum

Obstructions of various nature of the main pancreatic excretory duct can cause pancreatitis too, in the parenchymal territory proximal to the obstruction. The obstacle can be a ductal neoplasia (IPMN) (Fazel et al ,2005) or a papillary alteration (periampullary diverticula, duodenal ulcer, duodenal Crohn, post-traumatic stenosis of the duct of Wirsung), or pancreas divisum (Arya et al, 2006; Gelrud et al, 2004). Pancreas divisum can cause acute pancreatitis for the small-caliber of the minor papilla which represents an obstacle to pancreatic flow. The endoscopic control of pressure in the pancreatic duct shows values more elevated than in normal patients. This hypothesis is at the basis of the therapeutic procedure of sphincterotomy of the pancreatic minor papilla. Therapeutic success reaches 80% (Bradley & Stephan,1996). The pancreatitis from ductal obstruction can present itself with an acute attack, orienting clinically to an acute form involving all the gland, but the histological characteristics are attributable to a chronic phlogosis which is limited to the portion of gland proximal to the obstruction. Also in this case, the evolution of the anatomo-pathological lesion is characterized by the sequence phlogosis-proteolisis-necrosis-fibrosis. In advanced stages of chronic pancreatitis ductal stenoses and gallstones can be the base of acute attacks of pancreatitis. However, recurrent acute attacks are documented also in the early stages of alcoholic chronic pancreatitis (Garg et al,2007). In summary, it is not well established whether initial chronic pancreatitis is the cause of recurrent acute pancreatitis or whether, on the contrary, acute recurrent attacks of pancreatitis evolve into chronic pancreatitis. In general, for pancreatitis caused by an obstacle to the flow of pancreatic secretions, the treatment consists in the removal of the obstacle. However, the specific treatment is deeply diversified according to the nature of the obstacle: ampullary and periampullary tumors and intraductal neoplastic stenoses must be removed surgically; small pancreatic stones or phlogistic stenosis can be treated with endoscopical procedures.

5. Hereditary pancreatitis

In hereditary pancreatitis (Ferec & Maire,2005; Whitcomb, 1999), the intraparenchymal activated trypsinogen is not inhibited by the antienzymes which are inactive for genetic causes, that is because it is present trypsin rendered genetically resistant to antitrypsin. The effect is a series of recurrent episodes of pancreatitis which induce parenchymal chronic alterations with fibrosis, calcifications and sclerosis.

6. Autoimmunitary pancreatitis

The autoimmunitary phlogistic process in pancreatitis is characterized by a sclerotic effect (Hamano et al, 2001) with conspicuous lymphoplasmacellular infiltrates. In these cases, phlogosis is delimited sometimes in a mass which, if in the pancreatic head, can cause biliopancreatic ductal obstruction, simulating a neoplastic lesion (autoimmune lymphoplasmacellular pancreatitis or eosinophilic pancreatitis).

7. Metabolic pancreatitis

Possible recurrences of acute attacks with phlogosis which evolve into fibrosis and chronic sclerosis occur for hypercalcaemia and hyperlipidemia. Hypercalcaemia (in hyperparathyroidism) causes pancreatitis for the increased activation of proteolytic digestive enzymes. Hyperlipidemia causes pancreatitis because chylomicrons and free fat acids in excess interfere with pancreatic microcirculation. The circulatory alteration is the base of ductal obstructions of fibrous origin (obstructive mechanism).

8. Pancreatitis in celiac disease

Celiac disease (CD) is an immune mediated enteropathy caused by permanent insensivity to gluten in genetically susceptible individuals. Some recent reports have shown an association between acute pancreatitis and CD. A recent epidemiological study has shown that patients with CD have a higher risk than the general population for development of acute pancreatitis with epigastric pain and biochemical and radiographic confirmation (Ludvigsson et al, 2007). There are in the literature many pathogenetic mechanisms to explain the development of pancreatitis in patients with CD. T helper cell class 1 (TH1) cytokine up-regulation in CD may be predisposing factor for acute pancreatitis (Ludvigsson et al,2007). Another hyphotesis suggests that malnutrition can cause pancreatitis (Ludvigsson et al, 2007). However there is no evidence to show improvement of pancreatitis after correction for malnutrition. The mechanism for recurrent pancreatitis in CD may be papillary stenosis resulting from localized duodenal inflammation (Patel et al, 1999; Sood et al, 2007). The ES is the possible treatment. On the other hand it is also postulated that the improvement of recurrent episody of pancreatitis is a result of gluten restriction (Patel et al, 1999)).

9. Idiopathic pancreatitis

Idiopathic pancreatitis, that is with undefined etiology, represent approximately 20% of all cases. Among them, however, an important number can be ascribed to biliary forms with microstones or biliary sand of which there is no sure confirmation, that is they are caused by dysfunction of the sphincter of Oddi , generally of difficult demonstration.

10. Sphincter of Oddi dysfunction

Sphincter of Oddi dysfunction (SOD) can be due to stenosis or dyskinesia. Stenosis is a structural alteration due to inflammation and consequent stenosis (ex. passage of stones). Dyskinesia, instead, is a functional disorder with hypertonia. Stenosis or dyskinesia can involve the biliary sphincter, the pancreatic sphincter or the common sphincter. The clinical pictures may be slightly different if the alteration involves the biliary sphincter (pain of biliary type, biliary enzymes increase) or the pancreatic sphincter (pain of pancreatic type, recurrent attacks of pancreatitis). In summary, the phlogistic process is due to the obstruction and to the increased pressure in the pancreatic excretory system. The therapeutic indication in SOD is endoscopic sphincterotomy. Criteria for this diagnosis are represented by dilatation (> 8 milimeter) of the common bile duct, delayed emptying (more than 45 ') after ERCP, increased levels of alkaline phosphatase and gamma-GT during the episodes of pain. Certainty of diagnosis is based on finding, on manometry during ERCP, elevated pressure in the sphincter of Oddi (> 40 mmHG). Tc-99m iminodiacetic acid (IDA) cholescintigraphy is helpful for the diagnosis. It is moreover possible that the dysfunction of the sphincter of Oddi be present also in patients who did not undergo cholecistectomy. Three levels of diagnostic certainty are distinguished. In type 1 SOD the three clinical criteria above mentioned are present and manometry of the sphincter is superfluous. In type 2 SOD two clinical criteria are present or or only one but this one must not be pain. In this case manometry of the sphincter of Oddi is necessary and is pathological in half of the cases. Lastly in type 3 SOD only pain is present in the right hypochondriac region. Manometry of the sphincter is necessary. Moreover, in these cases of uncertain assessment the answer to the sphincterotomy is not sure (Vassiliou & Laycock,2008). In fact endoscopic sphincterotomy, in particular of pancreatic sphincter, can prevent the recurrence of dysfunction of the sphincter of Oddi in 60% of cases (Elta, 2008).

In conclusion, the sequence of physiopathologic events which underlies pancreatic parenchymal phlogosis has overlapping characteristics in acute and chronic pancreatitis. The inflammatory process, caused by ductal obstruction or for cleansing, by the biliary reflux, of the mucosa of the main pancreatic duct, is determined by the action, in the acinar cells of pancreas, of the same proteolytic enzymes produced there. Chronic pancreatitis is caused by repeated episodes of subclinic acute pancreatitis with parenchymal necrosis evolving into fibrosis. Therefore, the hypotheses to consider are the activation of proteolytic enzymes and of trypsinogen in the same acinar cells or the reduced inhibitory action of antienzymes that is, in the end, the activated intraparenchymal diffusion of the pancreatic secretions activated in the lumen of the excretory duct for the alteration of its mucous barrier. Recurrent, also subclinical, episodes of acute pancreatitis with phlogosis and necrosis evolve into the fibrosis and the sclerosis of chronic pancreatitis. It must still be explained how the obstruction of the main pancreatic duct or of smaller ducts can induce the intracellular activation of proteolytic enzymes. Steer (Steer,1998) has advanced the hypothesis of the colocalization. According to this hypothesis, based on experimental data, enzymes like trypsinogen and lyisosomial hydrolase as catepsin B are localized together in the cytoplasmic vacuoli. In these conditions catepsin B can activate trypsinogen into trypsin which with its proteolytic action causes self-digestion and intraparenchymal phlogosis. The intensity of the inflammatory response can regulate the severity of pancreatitis.

11. References

Arya S, Rana SS, Sinha SK et al (2007) Coexistence of chronic calcific pancreatitis and celiac disease. *Gastrointest Endosc* vol. 63 pp 1080-1081

Balthazar EJ, Robinson DL, Megibow AJ et al. (1990) : Acute pancreatitis : value of CT in establishing prognosis. *Radiology* vol. 174 , pp. 331-336.

Barro J, Soetikno RM, Carr-Locke DL, (2005) : Early endoscopic sphincterotomy in acute pancreatitis : is it indicated advisable , not indicated, or contraindicated? A proposal for clinical practise. In *Clinical Pancreaotology for practising Gastroenterologists and Surgeons*. Dominguez-Numoz JE , Ed. 1st ed. Oxford : Blackwell , pp. 113-124

Barthet M. (2001) : Comment poser le diagnostic positif et etiologique de pancreatite aigue? *Gastroenterol Clin Biol* vol. 25 , pp. 1S 12-1S 17

Bassi C, Butturini G (2007) : Definition and classification of pancreatitis. In *Surgery of Liver, Biliary tract and pancreas.* Blumgart LH Ed. Saunders-Philadelphia, pp. 685-690

Beger HG, Rau BM (2007) : Severe acute pancreatitis: Clinical course and management. *World J Gastroenterol* ; vol. 13 , pp. 5043-51.

Bradley EL, Stephan RN. (1996) : Accessory duct sphincterotomy is preferred for long term prevention of recurrent acute pancreatitis in patients with pancreas divisum. *J Am Coll Surg* vol. 183 , pp. 65 - 70

Elta GH. (2008) Sphincter of Oddi dysfunction and bile duct microlithiasis in acute idiopathic pancreatitis. *World J Gastroenterol* vol. 14, pp. 1023-26

Fazel A, Geenen JE, MoezArdalan K et al (2005) Intrapancreatic ductal pressure in sphincter of Oddi dysfunction. *Pancreas* vol. 30 pp 359-362

Ferec C, Maire F (2005) : Pancreatites d'origine genetique. In *Traitè de Pancreatologie clinique.* Levy P, Ruszniewski P., Sauvanet A. Edts. Flammarion Ed. Paris, pp. 50-56

Folsch UR, Nitsche R, Ludtke R et al (1997) : Early ERCP and papillotomy compared with conservative treatment for acute biliary pancreatitis. The German Study Group on Acute Biliary Pancreatitis. *N Engl J Med* vol. 336, pp. 237-242

Frossard JL, Steer ML, Pastor CM (2008) Acute pancreatitis. *Lancet* vol. 371 pp. 143-152

Garg PK, Tandan RK, Madan K. (2007) Is biliary microlithiasis a significant cause of idiopathic recurrent acute pancreatitis? A long-tem follow-up study. *Clin Gastroenterol Hepatol* vol. 5 , pp. 75-79

Gelrud A, Sheth S, Banerjee S et al (2004). Analysis of cystic fibrosis gener product (CFTR) function in patients with pancreas divisum and recurrent acute pancreatitis. *Am J Gastroenterol* vol. 99 pp 1557-1562

Gorelick FS (2003) Alcohol and zymogen activation in the pancreatic acinar cell. *Pancreas* vol. 27 pp 305-310

Gullo L, Migliori M, Olah A et al (2002) Acute pancreatitis in five european countries : etiology and mortality. *Pancreas* vol. 24 , pp. 223-227

Hamano H, Kawa S, Horinchi A et al (2001) High serum IgG4 concentrations in patients with sclerosing pancreatitis. *N Engl J Med* vol. 344 pp 732-738

Hastier P (2005) : Pancreatites metaboliques. In *Traitè de Pancreatologie clinique,* Levy P, Ruszniewski P, Sauvanet A, Edts Flammarion Ed. Paris , pp. 56-58

Heider TR, Brown AB, Grimm IS, et al. (2006) : Endoscopic Sphyncterotomy permits internal laparoscopic cholecystectomy in patients with moderately severe gallstone pancreatitis. *J. Gastro Surg* vol. 10 , pp. 1-5.

Hernandez V, Pascual I, Almela P et al (2004) Recurrence of acute gallstone pancreatitis and relationship with cholecystectomy or endoscopic sphincterotomy. *Am J Gastroenterol* vol. 99 pp 2417-2423

Kimura Y, Takada T, Kawarada Y et al (2006) JPN guidelines for the management of acute pancreatitis : treatment of gallstone-induced acute pancreatitis. *J Hepatobiliary Pancreat Surg* vol. 13 pp 56-60

Kloppel G (1999) Progression from acute to chronic pancreatitis: a pathologist's view. *Surg Clinic. North Am.* vol. 79, pp. 801 - 814

Lee SP, Nicholls JF, Park HZ (1992) : Biliary sludge as a cause of acute pancreatitis. *N Engl J. Med* vol. 326 , pp. 529-593

Ludvigsson JF, Montgomery SM, Ekbom A. (2007) : Risk of pancreatitis in 14.000 individuals with celiac disease. *Clin Gastroenterol Hepatol* vol. 5, pp. 1347-1353

Nealon WH, Bawdamiak J, Walser EM. (2004) : Appropriate timing of cholecystectomy in patients who present with moderate to severe gallstone pancreatitis associated acute pancreatitis with peripancreatic fluid collections. *Ann. Surg.* no. 239 , vol. 741-751.

Neoptolemos JP, Carr-Locke DL, London NJ et al (1988) : Controlled trial of urgent endoscopic retrograde cholangiopancreatography and endoscopic sphincterotomy versus conservative treatment for acute pancreatitis due to gallstones. *Lancet* vol. 332, pp. 979-983

Opie EL (1901) : The aetiology of acute hemorrhagic pancreatitis. *Bull. Johns Hopkins Hosp.* vol. 12, pp. 182-188

Pandol SJ (2006) : Acute pancreatitis. *Curr Opin Gastroenterol* vol. 22 pp :481-486

Patel RS, Johlin JFC, Murray JA (1999) : Celiac disease and recurrent pancreatitis. *Gastrointest Endosc* vol. 50, pp. 823-827

Sood A, Midha V, Sood N, et al. (2007) : Coexistence of chronic calcific pancreatitis and celiac disease. *Ind J Gastroenterol* vol. 26, pp. 1080-1081

Spanier BW, Dijkgraaf MG, Bruno MJ (2008) Epidemiology, aetiology and outcome of acute and chronic pancreatitis : An update. *Best Pract Res Clin Gastroenterol* vol. 22 pp. 45-63

Steer ML (1998) : The early intra-acinar cell events which occur during acute pancreatitis. The Frank Brooks Memorial Lecture. *Pancreas* vol. 17, pp. 31-37

Sungler P, Holzinger J, Waclawiczek HW et al (2007) Novel concepts in biology and therapy : biliary pancreatitis: urgent ERCP and early elective laparoscopic cholecystectomy. *Blackwell Science*, Oxford pp 373-376

Tazuma S. (2006) : Gallstone disease : epidemiology pathogenesis and classification of biliary stones (CBD and intra-hepatic) *Best Res Clin. Gastroenterol* vol.20 , pp. 1075-83

Van Geenen EJM, Van der Peet DL, Mulder CJJ et al (2009) Recurrent acute biliary pancreatitis : the protective role of cholecystectomy and endoscopic sphincterotomy. *Surg Endosc* vol. 23 pp 950-956

Vassiliou MC, Laycock WS. (2008) Biliary Dyskinesia. In *Biliary tract surgery*. Munson JL Ed. Surgical Clinics of North America. Saunders vol. 88 , pp. 1260-1267

Wang GJ, Gao CF, Wei D et al (2009) Acute pancreatitis: Etiology and common pathogenesis. *World J Gastroenterol* vol. 15 pp 1427-1430

Whitcomb DC (1999) Conference report. The first international Symposium on hereditary pancreatitis. *Pancreas* vol. 18 , pp. 1-12

Whitcomb DC (2005) Genetic polymorphisms in alcoholic pancreatitis. *Dig Dis* vol. 23 pp 247-254

Young YP, Lo SF, Yip AW. (2003) : Role of ERCP in the management of predicted mild acute biliary pancreatitis. *Asian J Surg* vol. 26 , pp. 197-201.

Part 3

Diagnosis

7

Acute Pancreatitis: Presentation and Risk Assessment

Ashok Venkataraman and Preston B. Rich
The University of North Carolina at Chapel Hill, North Carolina, USA

1. Introduction

Acute pancreatitis is the third most common gastrointestinal disease diagnosis at hospital discharge. (Browse 2003) Although many etiologies exist, the most common causes worldwide are gallstone disease and excessive alcohol consumption. However, one-third of pancreatitis cases have no association with alcohol, no associated biliary tract disease, and no pancreatic duct obstruction, and are thus labelled idiopathic. Despite a documented increase in the overall incidence of acute pancreatitis in several countries, disease related mortality has progressively declined over the years. This improvement is in part due to advances in disease management, including better diagnostics and treatment modalities. (Baron 2001)

Acute pancreatitis is a pathological condition in which activated pancreatic enzymes leak into the substance of the pancreas and initiate auto-digestion of the gland. Most episodes of acute pancreatitis are mild and self-limiting and do not require aggressive intervention. In marked contrast, approximately one fifth of patients develop severe acute pancreatitis which is associated with a mortality rate that can exceed 30%. (Bradley and Dexter 2010).

Pancreatitis occurs with equal frequency in men and women, despite the common association of gallstones with female gender. Although the peak incidence of pancreatitis is in the fourth and fifth decades of life, it can occur at any age.

2. Signs and symptoms

The most common presenting symptom of acute pancreatitis is pain. Typically the discomfort begins suddenly, high in the epigastrium, and steadily increases in severity until movement is intentionally limited and respiratory excursion is reduced. It is often unrelenting and may radiate through to the back, classically just to left of mid-line. Frequently, a complex of nausea, vomiting and retching accompanies the abdominal pain. Although many acute abdominal conditions can cause nausea, and vomiting, pancreatitis is often associated with a specific pattern of persistent nausea between cyclical bouts of emesis without nausea prior to initiation of the pain. (Mergener and Baillie 1998)

Many patients report having eaten an unusually large meal or drunk alcohol an hour or so before the pain began (Mergener and Baillie 1998). When the pain is severe, any movement of the lower chest wall and abdomen exacerbates the discomfort, often resulting in rapid shallow breathing and a sensation of dyspnea. In advanced cases, patients may develop tetanic muscle twitches, cramps and spasms related to associated hypocalcemia associated with the development of intra-abdominal fat necrosis. (Browse 2003)

As the condition progresses, retroperitoneal inflammation and trans-capillary leak reduce intravascular volume resulting in tachycardia with peripheral vasoconstriction generating a pale skin tone and diaphoresis. A paralytic intestinal ileus may develop, resulting in abdominal distension, a quiet abdomen to auscultation, and aggravation of nausea. Advanced cases may be associated with retroperitoneal haemorrhage, causing bruising and discoloration in the left flank (Grey Turner's sign) and around the umbilicus (Cullen's sign); both are late signs of extensive inflammatory destruction of the pancreas and peri-pancreatic tissues. (Dickson et al 1984)

Physical findings often consist of tenderness to palpation in the upper abdomen and abdominal distension, with severe cases producing diffuse abdominal guarding with discrete epigastric fullness secondary inflammatory exudate present in the lesser sac. Over time, this collection can organize, resulting in the formation of a pancreatic pseudocyst or lesser sac abscess. (Browse 2003)

3. Laboratory assessment, risk assessment and prognostic systems

Multiple risk assessment and classification systems have been developed over the years to assist in the clinical assessment of patients presenting with acute pancreatitis. These systems have been formulated in an attempt to predict the severity of a given episode of pancreatitis, and therefore aid in directing disease- appropriate management plans. Notable tools include the Atlanta Classification, Ranson's Criteria, the Acute Physiology and Chronic Health Evaluation (APACHE) II systems, and the Balthazar CT Severity Index (CTSI). (Brisinda, Vanella et al. 2011)

3.1 Biochemical values used for prognostication

Biochemical markers, including serum amylase and lipase, have been traditionally utilized in the diagnosis of acute pancreatitis. Newer indices have been reported to yield higher correlations with the presence of pancreatitis and have demonstrated improved prognostic value. (Gates 1999)

3.1.1 Serum amylase and lipase

Serum amylase and lipase levels are the most commonly obtained biochemical markers of pancreatic disease, particularly for evaluation of the presence of acute pancreatitis. However, the utility of these enzyme markers is complicated by significant limitations, including low sensitivity and specificity (Young 1989). In aggregate, there are many causes of elevated serum amylase levels, and amylase levels may only be moderately elevated or even normal in proven cases of acute pancreatitis of all degrees of severity (Clavien et al. 1989).

While an amylase level of three times the upper limit of normal is often recommended to support a clinical diagnosis of acute pancreatitis, the magnitude of the observed hyperamylasemia has limited direct correlation with disease severity (Clavien et al. 1989). Furthermore, after reaching a peak serum concentration, the subsequent return of amylase levels to previously normal levels does not necessarily correlate with resolution of clinical illness, limiting the value of serial measurements (Young 1989). If hyperamylasemia temporally persists in conjunction with clinical symptoms, consideration should be given to the presence of a pseudocyst or peri-pancreatic abscess. Clinical studies have demonstrated that serum amylase levels can be normal in one-fifth of diseased patients, elevated in one-quarter of well patients, and that the magnitude of serum elevation has poor statistical correlation with disease severity or ultimate prognosis. (Vissers, Abu-Laban et al. 1999)

Serum lipase is the acinar enzyme most often recommended to replace or supplement amylase levels for the diagnosis of acute pancreatitis. At a cut-off of five times the upper limit of normal, an elevated lipase is virtually diagnostic for pancreatitis, approaching 100% specificity; however, its sensitivity is limited to 60% (Kazmierczak et al. 1993). Given these considerations, using a multiple of twice the upper limit of normal may offer high specificity without significantly compromising sensitivity. Although few studies have examined the prognostic value of elevated lipase levels in acute pancreatitis, most suggest poor correlation with disease severity, similar to amylase. (Vissers, Abu-Laban et al. 1999)

Simultaneous measurements of both serum lipase and amylase have not been shown to improve diagnostic accuracy, and no advantage has been demonstrated over assaying lipase alone (Viel et al. 1990). While serum lipase measurements are comparable to amylase in terms of speed, cost, and availability, evidence suggests that lipase is the more accurate assay for acute pancreatitis (Clave et al. 1995). As a result, in institutions where both tests are available, it is recommended that lipase replace amylase as the initial enzymatic test for acute pancreatitis. Regardless of the marker employed, it is important to appreciate that the absolute levels of neither amylase nor lipase have prognostic value in established disease. (Vissers, Abu-Laban et al. 1999)

3.1.2 Blood Urea Nitrogen (BUN)

Some studies have demonstrated that an elevated Blood Urea Nitrogen (BUN) level at admission and subsequent temporal increases in BUN levels during the initial 24 hours of hospitalization are independent risk factors for mortality in acute pancreatitis (Wu et al. 2009). Serial BUN measurements have also been shown to provide prognostic accuracy comparable to the more complex APACHE II score for early prediction of in-hospital mortality (Papachristou et al. 2010). Among patients with an elevated BUN value at admission (>20 mg/dL), a decrease of at least 5 mg/dL at 24 hours is associated with a reduced risk of in-hospital death. In contrast, among patients with a normal BUN value at admission, even modest increases in the BUN level (≥ 2mg/dL) are associated with an increased risk of mortality (Wu, Bakker et al. 2011). Due to its correlation with outcome, an algorithm based on early changes in BUN level has been developed to aid clinicians in evaluating patient responses to early resuscitation efforts in pancreatitis. (Wu, Bakker et al. 2011)

3.1.3 Coagulation parameters: D-dimer and tissue factor

Coagulation disorders are known to occur in the early phase of severe acute pancreatitis and the D-dimer of fibrinogen is a commonly used clinical parameter to assess the hemostatic system (Salomone et al. 2003). Studies have demonstrated that serum D-dimer levels significantly differ between pancreatitis patients with and without key clinical differentiators such as the progression to multiple organ dysfunction syndromes, the eventual need for surgical intervention, and the development of both pancreatic and secondary infection (Radenkovic et al. 2009). Furthermore, serum D-dimer levels have been demonstrated to correlate well with two traditional markers of severity in acute pancreatitis, namely the APACHE II score and C-reactive protein serum levels (Papachristou, Whitcomb 2004). As such, the D-dimer assay may be a useful, easy, and inexpensive early prognostic marker of the evolution and complications of acute pancreatitis. (Ke, Ni et al. 2011) Several studies have demonstrated elevated levels of circulating Tissue factor (TF) to be present in patients presenting with acute pancreatitis (Yasuda et al. 2009). Furthermore, a weak statistical correlation between assayed serum TF levels and disease severity has been observed (Yasuda et al. 2009). Further studies will be required to characterize this relationship. (Andersson, Axelsson et al. 2010)

3.1.4 C-reactive protein (CRP)

C-reactive protein (CRP) is an acute phase reactant that is elevated in several inflammatory conditions and serves as a non-specific marker for inflammation (Wilson et al 1989). In acute pancreatitis, CRP levels commonly peak on the 3rd or 4th day after symptom onset, with 48-hour values of 150 mg/dL often accepted as a predictor of subsequent disease severity (Dervenis et al. 1999). It has been demonstrated that peak CRP levels of ≥210 mg/dL can differentiate severe acute pancreatitis from milder forms with a sensitivity of 83-84% and a specificity of 74-85%. (Wilson et al. 1989) Similar studies have shown that high CRP levels have an overall accuracy of 93% in detecting pancreatic necrosis. CRP levels are easy to measure, widely available, and relatively inexpensive to perform. One disadvantage of CRP is its delayed serum peak (48-72 hours), although this delay is also inherent in other methods used for severity assessment in acute pancreatitis such as the Ranson criteria. (Yadav, Agarwal et al. 2002)

3.1.5 Hemoconcentration

Recently, hemoconcentration has been identified as a strong risk factor and an early marker for the develpment of necrotizing pancreatitis and organ failure (Baillargeon, Ramagopal et al. 1998). Admission hematocrit (Hct) ≥ 47 and failure of admission Hct to decrease by 24 h represent strong risk factors for the development of severe pancreatitis. (Yadav, Agarwal et al. 2002). The sensitivity of hematocrit as a marker for necrotizing pancreatitis is 72% at admission and increases to 94% at 24 hours; specificity is 83 and 69%, respectively. (Baillargeon, Ramagopal et al. 1998)

The relationship between hemoconcentration and the development of pancreatic necrosis has been studied extensively in experimental animal models (Hotz et al. 1995). These studies have shown that early hemoconcentration in acute pancreatitis contributes significantly to the impairment of the pancreatic microcirculation and to the subsequent progression to pancreatic necrosis (Hotz et al. 1995). Patients presenting with an elevated admission hematocrit or those demonstrating an admission hematocrit that does not decrease by 24 hours are at high risk for complications (Brown, Orav et al. 2000). Consideration in this patient cohort should be given to early intensive care unit admission for vigorous fluid resuscitation, supportive care, and continous hemodynamic monitorring. In contrast, patients who do not exhibit these criteria may have a lower likelihood of developing severe pancreatitis and could represent a group that requires less intensive care. (Brown, Orav et al. 2000)

3.1.6 Interleukins and procalcitonin

Interleukins, particularly IL-6 and IL-8, have been identified as serum markers of disease severity in acute pancreatitis (Heath et al. 1993 and Rau et al 1997). Although predictive accuracies have varied in several clinical studies, meta-analyses performed to assess their utility in predicting severe acute pancreatitis have demonstrated promising correlations. (Gregoric, Sijacki et al. 2010)

IL-6 is a cytokine produced by a wide variety of cell types, including macrophages (Xing et al 1994). It drives the hepatic acute phase response and as such may be one biochemical step closer than CRP to the underlying inflammatory process in acute pancreatitis. Serum levels of IL-6 in patents with severe pancreatitis can be elevated as early as five hours after admission; pooled sensitivities range between 81.0% and 83.6%, specificities between 75.6 and 85.3%, and odds ratios of between 3. 43 and 4.90 in predicting disease severity (Aoun, Chen et al. 2009). IL-8 serum levels also have been found to correlate with pancreatitis, with pooled sensitivities identified between 65.8 and 70.9% and specificities of 66.5% and 91.3% for days 1 and 2 of disease presentation. (Aoun, Chen et al. 2009)

Procalcitonin (PCT) is the inactive propeptide of the hormone calcitonin, which is involved in calcium homeostasis (Assicot et al. 1993). In patients with acute pancreatitis, PCT has been shown to predict the subsequent development of infected pancreatic necrosis and has been demonstrated to be a predictor of severity and organ failure in patients with acute pancreatitis (Riche et al. 2003). Sensitivity analyses performed on multiple studies have demonstrated that a serum PCT value greater than 0.5 ng/mL is an accurate predictor of severe acute pancreatitis (Mofidi, Suttie et al. 2009). In studies where daily serum PCT levels were measured, it was noted that patients who subsequently developed infected pancreatic necrosis had a sustained increase in serum PCT levels and that the degree of PCT increase reflected the severity of systemic inflammation and progresion to multiorgan dysfunction (Rau et al. 1997). Furthermore, it has been observed that serum PCT levels tend to decrease with clinical improvment (Rau et al. 1997).

The identification of pancreatic necrosis is clinically important because patients with sterile pancreatic necrosis are often treated with supportive care only, whereas infected pancreatic necrosis generally requires surgical or radiologic intervention (Büchler et al. 2000). Infected pancreatic necrosis is classically diagnosed by microbial culture of material obtained using image-guided FNA of pancreatic tissue. Unlike FNA, the measurement of PCT is non-invasive and is not hindered by the potential for image-directed sampling error. Furthermore, PCT levels are not affected by antifungal and antimicrobial systemic coverage, and remain elevated in infected pancreatic necrosis (Rau et al. 1997). However, it is important to note that PCT is a nonspecific marker of infectious complications in critically ill patients, and as a result other infective foci need to be excluded carefully when interpreting PCT measurements in pancreatitis.. (Mofidi, Suttie et al. 2009)

3.2 Systems based risk models

3.2.1 Atlanta classification

Most recent attempt to standardize severity criteria in acute pancreatitis The 1992 Atlanta Symposium was convened to standardize severity criteria and nomenclature in acute pancreatitis (Bradley 1993). A major step forward at the time was the establishment of a universal definition of severe pancreatitis. Objective criteria of severity and outcome were defined by both local and systemic parameters (Table 1.) In addition, universal standards to define "predicted severe" pancreatitis were adopted based on the two most popular scoring systems, namely the Ranson criteria and the Acute Physiology and Chronic Health Evaluation II (APACHE II) criteria. "Predicted severe" pancreatitis was defined as either a score of three or more in Ranson criteria, or eight or more in APACHE-II criteria. (Gates 1999)

Severity Criteria	**Definitions**
Organ Failure	
Cardiovascular	Systolic blood pressure < 90 mm Hg (after resuscitation)
Respiratory	PaO_2 < 60mmHg (8 kPa)
Renal	Serum creatinine > 177 µmol/l (2mg/dl) after resuscitation
Gastrointestinal Haemorrhage	>500 ml/ 24h
Systemic Complications	
Coagulation System	Platelet count < 100 × 109/l
	Fibrinogen level < 1g/l
	Fibrin split products >80µg/mL
Metabolic	Corrected serum calcium < 1.85 mmol/l (7.5 mg/dl) serum lactate levels > 5mmol/l
Local Complications	
Acute fluid collections	Occur early in the natural history of acute pancreatitis and lack a fibrous capsule
Pseudocyst	Occurs at least 4 weeks after the onset of symptoms and has a fibrous capsule
Pancreatic abscess	A localised collection of pus containing little or no necrotic pancreatic material
Pancreatic necrosis	Pathological features : diffuse or focal area of nonviable pancreas that maybe associated with peripancreatic fat necrosis CT features : an area of non-enhancing pancreas measuring > 3 cm in diameter or 30% of pancreatic tissue

Table 1. Atlanta Classification for Severe Pancreatitis

Threshold scores for assignment of "predicted severe" pancreatitis

≥ 3 Ranson criteria
≥ 8 APACHE II criteria

Although the Atlanta Classification has proven useful, a more thorough classification system could incorporate assessment of clinical severity with more objective measurements of anatomic pathology in and around the pancreas. In addition, the Atlanta Classification fails to differentiate between the two discrete peaks in mortality (early and late) observed with pancreatitis. (Brisinda, Vanella et al. 2011)

3.2.2 Ranson criteria

Ranson proposed the first numerical grading system for acute pancreatitis in 1974, focusing on several commonly observed clinical and hematochemical variables (Ranson et al. 1974). With an increased number of risk factors present, there is a corresponding increase in mortality rate (Ranson et al. 1974). In patients with less than three positive signs no significant associated mortality is observed, whereas in patients with at least six signs the mortality rate is over 50% (Ranson 1995). Furthermore, individuals with a score greater than six often develop necrotising pancreatitis (Ranson 1995). This system is particularly useful at the two extremes of the scale, with less discriminating power between; correlation with severity of disease or the eventual development of necrosis in patients with a score of 3-5 is deficient. (Brisinda, Vanella et al. 2011)

At admission	**During initial 48 hours**
Age > 55 years	Hematocrit decrease > 10%
White blood cell count > 16000/µl	Blood urea nitrogen increase >5mg/dl (>1.8 mmol/l)
Serum glucose level > 200 mg/dl (>11.1 mmol/l)	Calcium < 8 mg/dl (<2 mmol/l)
Serum lactate dehydrogenase > 350 IU/l	PaO2 < 60 mmHg
Aspartate Aminotransferase > 250 IU/l	Base deficit > 4 mEq/l
	Fluid sequestration > 6 l

Table 2. Ranson criteria for non- gallstone pancreatitis

At admission	**During initial 48 hours**
Age > 70 years	Hematocrit decrease > 10%
White blood cell count > 18000/µl	Blood urea nitrogen increase >5mg/dl (>1.8 mmol/l)
Serum glucose level > 220 mg/dl (>12.2 mmol/l)	Calcium < 8 mg/dl (<2 mmol/l)
Serum lactate dehydrogenase > 400 IU/l	PaO2 < 60 mmHg
Aspartate Aminotransferase > 250 IU/l	Base deficit > 5 mEq/l
	Fluid sequestration > 4 l

Table 3. Ranson criteria for gallstone pancreatitis

The Ranson scoring system was derived from statistical analysis of multiple clinical and laboratory parameters from consecutive patients who were tested for significant correlation with disease outcome (Ranson et al. 1974). The result was an 11-point conglomerate of predictive factors, five of which were to be obtained on admission and the remaining six within 48 hours of presentation. Because the first group of patients analysed had a preponderance of alcohol-associated disease, a second analysis was later performed with patients manifesting gallstone pancreatitis. (Ranson et al. 1974) Thus, two separate Ranson criteria currently exist for gallstone and non-gallstone pancreatitis, as illustrated above.

The Ranson scoring system has important merits, along with some deficits. Clear benefits include its ease of use and its clinical correlation, with an estimated sensitivity of 72%, specificity of 76%, positive predictive value of 51%, and negative predictive value of 89. (Gates 1999)

However, many physicians inappropriately apply the non-gallstone criteria to patients with gallstone pancreatitis, which accounts for a third of all cases of acute pancreatitis. Furthermore, patients are often incorrectly classified as having "predicted mild" pancreatitis before 48 hours; using the Ranson criteria, patients may only be classified as "predicted severe" or "pending" pancreatitis before the 48 hour mark. Importantly, the Ranson criteria have not been validated for continued temporal monitoring of the patient's condition. A repeat assessment with the criteria at say, 72 hours, cannot be accurately interpreted with the tool. It is also important to note that the Ranson criteria have not been validated for used in children. (Gates 1999)

3.2.3 Glasgow criteria

The Glasgow criteria (Imrie) were originally introduced in the late 1970's and early 1980'sand have since been modified three times. (Imrie et al. 1978). The original Glasgow, or modified system, has been used for the prediction of mortality, and like the Ranson, performs well. It yields an estimated sensitivity of 63%, specificity of 84%, positive predictive value of 52%, and negative predictive value of 89% (Steinberg 1990). When

Variables for the Glasgow Scoring System
Age > 55 years
White blood cell count > 15000 / μl
PaO2 < 60 mmHg (8 kPa)
Serum lactate dehydrogenase > 600 units/l
Serum aspartate aminotransferase > 200 units/l[a]
Serum albumin < 32g/l
Serum calcium < 2 mmol/l
Serum glucose > 10 mmol/l
Serum urea > 16 mmol/l

[a] Removed from revised Glasgow outcome score.
Each variable has a binary score of 0 or 1. The outcome score is derived from the sum of all variables at 48 hours after presentation.

Table 4. Glasgow (Imrie) severity scoring system for acute pancreatitis

Physiologic Variable	High Abnormal Range								Low Abnormal Range	
	+4	+3	+2	+1	0	+1	+2	+3	+4	**Points**
Temperature (rectal °C)	>41	39-40.9		38.538.9	36-38.4	34-35.9	32-33.9	30-31.9	≤29.9	
Mean Arterial Pressure (mmHg)	≥160	130-159	110-129		70-109		50-69		≤49	
Heart Rate	≥180	140-179	110-139		70-109		55-69	40-54	≤39	
Respiratory Rate	≥50	35-49		24-34	12-24	10-11	6-9		≤5	
Oxygenation: A-a DO_2 <u>or</u> P_aO_2 (mmHg) FiO_2 > 0.5 record A-a DO_2 FiO_2 < 0.5 record P_aO_2	≥500	350-499	200-349		< 200 P_aO_2 > 70	P_aO_2 61-70		P_aO_2 55-60	P_aO_2 < 55	
Arterial pH (preferred) Serum HCO_3 (venous mEq/l) **(not preferred, may use if no ABGs)**	≥7.7 ≥52	7.6-7.69 41-51.9		7.5-7.59 32-40.9	7.33-7.49 22-31.9		7.25-7.32 18-21.9	7.15-7.24 15-17.9	<7.15 <15	
Serum Sodium (mEq/l)	≥180	160-171	155-159	150-154	130-149		120-129	111-119	≤110	
Serum Potassium (mEq/l)	≥7	6-6.9		5.5-5.9	3.5-5.4	3-3.4	2.5-2.9		<2.5	
Serum Creatinine (mg/dl) Double point score for acute renal failure	≥3.5	2-3.4	1.4-1.9		0.6-1.4		<0.6			

Table 5. Continued

Physiologic Variable	High Abnormal Range								Low Abnormal Range	
Hematocrit (%)	≥60		50-59.9	46-49.9	30-45.9		20-29.9		<20	
White Blood Count (total/mm³) (in 100s)	≥40		20-39.9	15-19.9	3-14.9		1-2.9		<1	
Glasgow Coma Score (GCS) Score = 15 minus actual GCS										
Total Acute Physiology Score (sum of above 12 points)										
Age points (years) ≤44= 0; 45 – 54 = 2; 55 – 64 = 3; 65 – 74 = 5; ≥75 = 6										
Chronic Health Points (see below)										
Total APACHE II Score (Add together points from A + B + C)										

Chronic Health Points: If the patient has a history of severe organ system insuffiency or is immunocompromised as defined below, assign points as follows:
2 points for nonoperative or emergency postoperative patients
2 points for elective postoperative patients
Liver insufficiency: Biopsy proven cirrhosis; Documented portal hypertension; Episodes of past upper GI bleeding attributed to portal hypertension; Prior episodes of hepatic failure / encephalopathy / coma. ***Cardiovascular***: New York Heart Association Class IV Heart Failure. ***Respiratory***: Chronic restrictive, obstructive or vascular disease resulting in severe exercise restriction, i.e. unable to climb stairs or perform household duties; Documented chronic hypoxia, hypercapnia, secondary polycythemia, severe pulmonary hypertension (> 40 mmHg), or respirator dependency. ***Renal***: Receiving chronic dialysis. *Immunosuppression*: The patient has received therapy that suppresses resistance to infection e.g. immunosuppression, chemotherapy, radiation, long term or recent high dose steroids, or has a disease that is sufficiently advanced to suppress resistance to infection, e.g. leukemia, lymphoma, AIDS.

Table 5. Acute Physiology and Chronic Health Evaluation II (APACHE-II) Worksheet Adapted from *Crit Care Med* 13(10): 818-829. (Knaus, Draper et al. 1985) compared to Ranson, it may be less sensitive while adding increased specificity. Any Glasgow data point may be scored at any time during the first 48 hours of presentation, but like Ranson, the Glasgow system is not valid for repeat measurements beyond 48 hours and cannot be applied to children (Gates 199). During the initial 48 hours, a patient may be classified only as having "severe" or "pending" pancreatitis. (Gates 1999)

3.2.4 Acute Physiology and Chronic Health Evaluation II (APACHE-II)

The Acute Physiology and Chronic Health Evaluation II (APACHE-II) assessment has become popular more recently. The system is comparatively complex and more difficult to perform because 12 different physiologic measurements are used (Larvin 1989). The higher the total score, the more severe the episode of acute pancreatitis, which corresponds to an increase in predicted morbidity and mortality (Wilson et al. 1990). One major advantage of the APACHE-II numeric system compared with other systems is that it can be used throughout the patient's hospital course, aiding evaluation and monitoring of response to therapy. (Knaus, Draper et al. 1985)

The APACHE-II system was developed as a general measure of disease severity and not specifically as a tool for describing acute pancreatitis. Each physiologic parameter is weighted from 0 to 4, and an aggregate score is tabulated (Knaus, Draper et al. 1985). Unlike the Ranson and Glasgow criteria, APACHE-II can provide a valid prediction of mild pancreatitis on admission. The APACHE-II is valid for repeated measures throughout hospitalization and it represents a universal measurement of disease severity, obviating the need for a separate score for acute pancreatitis. The APACHE II performs very well as a prognostic tool, with sensitivity and specificity rates of 75% and 92% respectively (Wilson et al. 1990).

3.2.5 Bedside Index for Severity in Acute Pancreatitis (BISAP)

A newer prognostic scoring system, the Bedside Index for Severity in Acute Pancreatitis (BISAP) has been proposed as an accurate method for early identification of patients at risk for in-hospital mortality (Wu, Johannes et al. 2008). The BISAP combines findings of physical examination, vital signs, routine laboratory data, and imaging studies to derive a five-point score (Wu, Johannes et al. 2008).

Individual Components of the BISAP Scoring System
BUN > 25mg/dl
Impaired mental status (Glasgow Coma Scale Score < 15)
Age > 60 years
Pleural effusion detected on imaging
SIRS, ≥ 2 or more of the following: Temperature <36°C or >38°C Respiratory Rate >20 breaths/min or $PaCO_2$ <32 mmHg Pulse > 90 beats/min WBC count > 12,000 or <4,000 cells/mm^3 or >10% immature neutrophils (bands

Adapted from *Gut* 57(12): 1698-1703 (Wu, Johannes et al. 2008)

Table 6. BISAP Scoring System

The BISAP uses five ordinal points: urea nitrogen (BUN) >25 mg/dl, impaired mental status as defined by evidence of disorientation or alteration in mental status, presence of Systemic Inflammatory Response Syndrome (SIRS), age > 60 years, and the presence or absence of pleural effusions (Singh, Wu et al. 2009).

SIRS is defined by the presence of ≥ 2 of the following criteria:

Pulse >90 beats/min, respirations >20/min or $PaCO_2$ <32 mmHg, temperature >38°C of <36°C, WBC count > 12,000 or <4,000 cells/mm^3 or >10% immature neutrophils (bands).

The presence of each variable contributes one point to a total 5-point score, and is obtained within 24 hours of admission; there is no requirement for additional computation, and the assessment of mental status is the only subjective parameter involved. It should be noted, however, that the SIRS criterion is a composite parameter that involves four separate but related criteria. Essentially, the BISAP is an eight-variable system cumulatively applied to calculate five points. (Wu, Johannes et al. 2008)

Studies have demonstrated that the BISAP score can predict mortality risk (Wu, Johannes et al. 2008). Studies have demonstrated that a BISAP score ≥ 3 is associated with higher mortality when compared to scores < 3; high specificity and negative predictive values were observed using these ordinal values (Wu, Johannes et al. 2008). Furthermore, it has been shown that BISAP scores ≥ 3 predict the development of organ failure, persistent organ failure, and the evolution of pancreatic necrosis. (Singh, Wu et al. 2009)

The key advantages of the BISAP include its relative ease of use and application of parameters that are commonly obtained either at presentation or within 24 hours of presentation (Wu, Johannes et al. 2008). The score appears generalizable, having been initially formulated and validated using a large number of patients across 389 hospitals, reflecting a broad spectrum of health-care delivery. (Singh, Wu et al. 2009)

The BISAP score cannot readily distinguish transient organ dysfunction from more persistent organ dysfunction at 24 hours (sensitivity of 38%, specificity 92%, PPV 58%, and NPV 84%), an important clinical distinction since the latter group suffers the majority of morbidity and mortality in acute pancreatitis (Zimmerman et al. 1994). The BISAP score may prove more useful in the triage of patients to levels of care intensity on initial evaluation rather than being used to predict the development of persistent organ failure and its consequences. (Papachristou, Muddana et al. 2010)

In summary, the BISAP score is a reliable prognostic tool enabling classification of patients with acute pancreatitis into mild or severe groups, and its components are clinically relevant and easy to obtain. It is important to recognize that an inherent limitation of all such scoring systems is their conversion of continuous variables into binary values of equal weight and thus fail to capture synergistic or multiplicative effects based on interactions of interdependent systems.

3.3 Imaging based risk models

3.3.1 Ultrasonography

Ultrasonography (US) may be useful in the early assessment of acute pancreatitis to evaluate the biliary system for the presence of gallstones or common bile ductal stones. However, US use is often technically limited to applications in the early staging of acute pancreatitis due to the presence of overlying bowel gas secondary to paralytic intestinal ileus. In aggregate, abnormal US findings are seen in 33-90% of patients with acute pancreatitis; a diffusely enlarged and hypoechoic gland is consistent with interstitial edema, while extrapancreatic fluid collections (e.g., lesser sac, anterior pararenal space) can be detected in patients with severe disease. (Balthazar 2002)

3.3.2 Computed Tomography (CT)

Most of the clinical and laboratory parameters discussed thus far are applied to evaluate the systemic effects of pancreatitis, and only indirectly infer the presence and degree of pancreatic damage. The use of Computed Tomography (CT) in acute pancreatitis has increased in the last decade as it offers improved anatomic visualization, direct assessment of the extent of parenchymal injury, and identification of local complications (Dervenis et al. 1999). The CT Severity Index (CTSI) derived by Balthazar et al. has become the standard objective assessment for the description of CT findings in acute pancreatitis. (Balthazar 2002)

The first described CT grading index was based on radiographic images obtained without the addition of intravenous (IV) contrast (Hill et al. 1982). Using the scoring system, it was demonstrated that patients with high grade pancreatic damage (grades D or E) had a mortality rate of 14% and a morbidity rate of 54%, as compared with no mortality and a morbidity rate of only 4% in lesser affected patients (groups A, B or C.) Due to the lack of IV contrast, its main drawback was an inability to reliably depict pancreatic necrosis (Balthazar, Robinson et al. 1990).

A major significant improvement has been achieved in early CT grading systems with the introduction of an incremental contrast bolus CT technique (Kivisaari et al. 1983). Contrast-enhanced CT has been used effectively to directly characterize and quantify pancreatic parenchymal injury. Investigators have shown that the attenuation values of pancreatic parenchyma during an intravenous contrast bolus study can be used as an indicator of pancreatic necrosis and as a predictor of disease severity (Dervenis et al. 1999).

Patients with mild interstitial pancreatitis have an intact but vasodilated capillary network and therefore exhibit uniform enhancement of the pancreatic gland (Balthazar 2002). To the contrary, areas of diminished or no enhancement are indicative of decreased blood flow and reveal pancreatic zones of ischemia or necrosis (Balthazar 2002). An excellent correlation has been documented between necrosis, length of hospitalization, development of complications, and death. Furthermore, the extent of pancreatic necrosis has also been proven to be of clinical importance with prognostic and therapeutic implications (Vitellas et al. 1999). Studies have shown that patients with less than 30% necrosis exhibited no mortality and a 48% morbidity rate, while larger areas of necrosis (30-50% and >50%) were associated with morbidity rates of 75-100% and mortality rates of 11-25% (Balthazar, Robinson et al. 1990).

The CT Severity Index (CTSI) was designed to improve the early prognostic value of CT in cases of acute pancreatitis and is based on IV contrast-enhanced imaging (Balthazar, Robinson et al. 1990). The grading and allocation of points takes into consideration the CT grade as well as the extent of necrosis and is illustrated in the table below. It has been demonstrated that a statistically significant correlation exists between morbidity and mortality and the CTSI score (Balthazar, Robinson et al. 1990). Studies have shown that patients with a severity index of 0 or 1 exhibit a 0% mortality rate and no morbidity, while patients with a severity index of 2 had no mortality and a 4% morbidity rate (Balthazar, Robinson et al. 1990). In contrast, a severity index of 7-10 yields a 17% mortality rate and a 92% complication rate. (Balthazar, Robinson et al. 1990) In a clinical study comparing BISAP, Ranson criteria, APACHE-II, and CTSI, CTSI was the most accurate in predicting pancreatic necrosis. (Papachristou, Muddana et al. 2010)

CT grade	Grade Points	Necrosis (in percentage)	Necrosis Points	CT severity index[b]
Normal (A)	0	0	0	0
Focal, diffuse enlargement, contour irregularity, inhomogenous attenuation (B)	1	0	0	1
B + peripancreatic haziness/strand densities (C)	2	< 30	2	4
B + C + one ill-defined peripancreatic fluid collection (D)	3	30 - 50	4	7
B + C + two ill-defined peripancreatic fluid collections (E)	4	< 50	6	10

[a] Balthazar
[b] Grade points are added to points assigned for percentage of necrosis.

Table 7. Computed Tomography Severity Index[a]

Adapted from Eur J Gastroenterol Hepatol 23(7): 541-551 (Brisinda, Vanella et al. 2011) of presentation may show only equivocal findings of pancreatitis, and that CT scans obtained 3 days after clinical onset yield higher accuracy in the depiction of pancreatic necrosis (Vitellas et al. 1999). Thus, it is recommended that when the clinical diagnosis of pancreatitis is in doubt, an initial early CT be used to confirm the clinical suspicion or to help detect alternative acute abdominal conditions that mimic acute pancreatitis. For staging, however, more reliable results are obtained with the use of intravenous bolus contrast-enhanced CT performed 48-72 hours after the onset of an acute attack of pancreatitis. (Balthazar 2002)

It appears that the CTSI is an anatomically oriented scoring system that aids in identifying local complications from pancreatitis, while clinical scores, such as the APACHE-II, may be superior for predicting associated organ failure and systemic complications (Lankisch et al. 2000). In patients with predicted severe disease or those manifesting a severe clinical course within the first 48 hours of presentation, the CTSI appears superior to other scoring systems in predicting overall pancreatitis severity and pancreatic necrosis. (Chatzicostas, Roussomoustakaki et al. 2003) At present, it appears that clinical scores are the best way to stratify the immediate management of acute pancreatitis, particularly the requirement for intensive care, and that the value of CT is greater in evaluating intermediate term management. (Alhajeri and Erwin 2008)

3.3.3 Magnetic Resonance Imaging (MRI)

The development of high field strength magnetic resonance imaging (MRI), rapid gradient-echo breath hold techniques, and fat suppression methodologies has made MR imaging an excellent alternative imaging modality to aid in the evaluation of patients with acute pancreatitis (Lecesne et al. 1999). It is particularly useful in patients who cannot receive iodinated contrast material due to allergic reactions or renal insufficiency. Gadolinium-enhanced T1 weighted gradient-echo MR images can depict pancreatic necrosis as areas of non-enhanced parenchyma (Fulcher, Turner 1999). Fat-suppression images are also helpful in defining subtle, diffuse, or focal parenchymal abnormalities. T2 weighted images can accurately depict fluid collections, pseudocysts, and areas of haemorrhage. (Balthazar 2002)

4. Conclusion

Acute pancreatitis is a dynamic entity with varying degrees of severity. Most episodes of acute pancreatitis are generally mild, but up to a third of cases may progress to severe pancreatitis. This is associated with a significant increase in associated mortality and complications. The key to effectively managing the patient with an episode of acute pancreatitis is early identification and diagnosis, followed by an appropriate assessment of severity. Appropriate evaluation of severity and prognosis is of great help in aiding the clinician in administering appropriate care. The clinician needs to be able to determine which patients will benefit from invasive intervention or transfer to a critical care unit, with the availability of its attendant intensive laboratory and cardiorespiratory monitoring.

A variety of prognostication systems for acute pancreatitis have been developed over the years to better categorize disease severity and predict clinical outcomes. There are three commonly employed types of predictors of the severity of acute pancreatitis: individual biological markers, multi-parameter scorings systems, and imaging-based systems. Within each category there are several individual systems, each with unique advantages and disadvantages. Given the currently available tools, the majority of patients presenting with acute pancreatitis will benefit from a rational and informed combination of these complimentary but distinct systems. In an era where intensive and invasive techniques are available to manage the local and systemic complications of pancreatitis, the ability to appropriately identify patients who will benefit from these interventions in a timely fashion is an important adjunct to their care.

5. References

Alhajeri A and Erwin S. (2008) "Acute pancreatitis: value and impact of CT severity index." Abdom Imaging 33(1): 18-20.

Andersson E, Axelsson J, et al. (2010) "Tissue factor in predicted severe acute pancreatitis." World J Gastroenterol 16(48): 6128-6134.

Aoun E, Chen J, et al. (2009). "Diagnostic accuracy of interleukin-6 and interleukin- 8 in predicting severe acute pancreatitis: a meta-analysis." Pancreatology 9(6): 777-785.

Assicot M, Gendrel D, Carsin H, Raymond J, et al. (1993) "High serum procalcitonin concentrations in patients with sepsis and infection." Lancet 341: 515–518.

Baillargeon JD, Ramagopal V, Tenner SM, et al. (1998) "Hemoconcentration as an early risk factor for necrotizing pancreatitis." Am J Gastroenterol 93:2130–2134.

Balthazar EJ(2002) "Acute pancreatitis: assessment of severity with clinical and CT evaluation." Radiology 223(3): 603-613.

Balthazar EJ, Robinson DL, et al. (1990) "Acute pancreatitis: value of CT in establishing prognosis." Radiology 174(2): 331-336.

Balthazar EJ, Ranson JHC, Naidich DP, et al. (1985) "Acute pancreatitis: prognostic value of CT." Radiology 156:767–772.

Baron TH. (2001) "Predicting the severity of acute pancreatitis: is it time to concentrate on the hematocrit?" Am J Gastroenterol 96(7): 1960-1961.

Bradley EL. (1993) "A clinically based classification system for acute pancreatitis: summary of the Atlanta International Symposium." (1993). Arch Surg 128:586–5909

Bradley EL and Dexter ND. (2010) "Management of severe acute pancreatitis: a surgical odyssey." Ann Surg 251(1): 6-17.

Brisinda G, Vanella S, et al. (2011) "Severe acute pancreatitis: advances and insights in assessment of severity and management." Eur J Gastroenterol Hepatol 23(7): 541-551.

Brown A, Orav J, et al. (2000) "Hemoconcentration is an early marker for organ failure and necrotizing pancreatitis." Pancreas 20(4): 367-372.

Browse NL. (2003) An Introduction to the Symptoms and Signs of Surgical Disease. London, Great Britain, Arnold, Hodder Headline Group.

Büchler MW, Gloor B, Müller CA, Friess H, Seiler CA, Uhl W. (2000) "Acute necrotizing pancreatitis: treatment strategy according to the status of infection." Ann Surg 232: 619–626.

Chatzicostas C, Roussomoustakaki M, et al. (2003) "Balthazar computed tomography severity index is superior to Ranson criteria and APACHE II and III scoring systems in predicting acute pancreatitis outcome." J Clin Gastroenterol 36(3): 253-260.

Clave P, Guillaumes S, Blanco I et al. (1995) "Amylase, lipase, pancreatic isoamylase, and phospholipase A in diagnosis of acute pancreatitis." Clin Chem 41: 1129–1134.

Clavien PA , Burgan S, Moossa AR. (1989) "Serum enzymes and other laboratory tests in acute pancreatitis." Br J Surg 76: 1234–1243.

Dervenis C, JohnsonCD, Bassi C, et al. (1999) "Diagnosis, objective assessment of severity, and management of acute pancreatitis." Int J Pancreatol (25):195–210.

Dickson AP, Imrie CW. (1984) "The incidence and prognosis of body wall ecchymosis in acute pancreatitis." Surg Gynecol Obstet 159(4):343-7

Fulcher AS, Turner MA. (1999) "MR pancreatography: a useful tool for evaluating pancreatic disorders." RadioGraphics 19:5-24.

Gates LK, Jr. (1999) "Severity scoring for acute pancreatitis: where do we stand in 1999?" Curr Gastroenterol Rep 1(2): 134-138.

Gregoric P, Sijacki A, et al. (2010) "SIRS score on admission and initial concentration of IL-6 as severe acute pancreatitis outcome predictors." Hepatogastroenterology 57(98): 349-353.

Heath D, Cruickshank A, Gudgeon M, Jehanli A, et al. (1993) "Role of interleukin-6 in mediating the acute phase protein response and potential as an early means of severity assessment in acute pancreatitis." Gut 34:41-5.

Hill MC, Barkin J, Isikoff MB, et al. (1982) "Acute pancreatitis: clinical vs. CT findings." AJR Am J Roentgenol 139:263-269.

Hotz HG, Schmidt J, Ryschich EW, et al. (1995) "Isovolemic hemodilution with dextran prevents contrast medium induced impairment of pancreatic microcirculation in necrotizing pancreatitis of the rat." Am J Surg 169:161–6.

Imrie CW, Benjamin IS, Ferguson JL, et al. (1978) "A single-center double-blind trial of Trasylol therapy in primary acute pancreatitis." Br J Surg 65:337–341.

Kazmierczak S, Catrou P, VanLente F. (1993) "Diagnostic accuracy of pancreatic enzymes evaluated by use of multivariate data analysis." Clin Chem 39: 1960–1965.

Ke L, Ni HB, et al. (2011) "D: -dimer as a marker of severity in patients with severe acutepancreatitis." J Hepatobiliary Pancreat Sci.

Kivisaari L, Somer K, Standertskjold-Nordenstam CG, et al. (1983) "Early detection of acute fulminant pancreatitis by contrast enhanced computed tomography." Scand J Gastroenterol 18:39-41.

Knaus WA, Draper EA, et al. (1985) "APACHE II: a severity of disease classification system." Crit Care Med 13(10): 818-829.

Larvin M, McMahon MJ. (1989) "APACHE II score for assessment and monitoring of acute pancreatitis." Lancet 2:201–204.

Lankisch PG, Wamecke B, Bruns D, et al. (2000) "The APACHE II score on admission to hospital is unreliable to diagnose necrotizing and thus severe pancreatitis" Int J Pancreatol 28:130-131.

Lecesne R, Taourel P, Bret PM, et al. (1999) "Acute pancreatitis: interobserver agreement and correlation of CT and MR cholangiopancreatography with outcome." Radiology 211:727-735.

Mergener K, Baillie J. (1998) "Acute pancreatitis" Brit Med Journal 316:44-48.

Mofidi R, Suttie SA, et al. (2009) "The value of procalcitonin at predicting the severity of acute pancreatitis and development of infected pancreatic necrosis: systematic review." Surgery 146(1): 72-81.

Papachristou GI, Muddana V, et al. (2010) "Comparison of BISAP, Ranson's, APACHE-II, and CTSI scores in predicting organ failure, complications, and mortality in acute pancreatitis." Am J Gastroenterol 105(2): 435-441; quiz 442.

Papachristou GI, Whitcomb DC. (2004) " Predictors of severity and necrosis in acute pancreatitis." Gastroenterol Clin North Am. 33:871-890.

Radenkovic D, Bajec D, Ivancevic N et al. (2009) "D-dimer in acute pancreatitis: a new approach for an early assessment of organ failure." Pancreas 38:655–660.

Ranson JH, Rifkind KM, et al. (1974) "Prognostic signs and the role of operative management in acute pancreatitis". Surgery, Gynecology & Obstetrics 139 (1): 69–81.

Ranson JH. (1995) "The current management of acute pancreatitis." Adv Surg. 28:93–112

Rau B, Steinbach G, Gansauge F, Mayer JM, et al. (1997) "The potential role of pro calcitonin and interleukin 8 in the prediction of infected necrosis in acute pancreatitis." Gut 41:832-40.

Riche FC, Cholley BP, Laisne MJ, Vicaut E. (2003) "Inflammatory cytokines, C reactive protein, and procalcitonin as early predictors of necrosis infection in acute necrotizing pancreatitis." Surgery 133: 257–262 et al. (2003) "Coagulative disorders in human acute pancreatitis: role for the D-dimer." Pancreas (26):111–116

Singh VK, Wu BU, et al. (2009) "A prospective evaluation of the bedside index for severity in acute pancreatitis score in assessing mortality and intermediate markers of severity in acute pancreatitis." Am J Gastroenterol 104(4): 966-971.
Steinberg WM. (1990) "Predictors of severity of acute pancreatitis." Gastroenterol Clin North Am 19:849–861.
Viel J, Foucault P, Bureau F, et al. (1990) "Combined diagnostic value of biochemical markers in acute pancreatitis." Clin Chim Acta 189:191–198
Visser RJ, Abu-Laban RB, et al. (1999) "Amylase and lipase in the emergency department evaluation of acute pancreatitis." J Emerg Med 17(6): 1027-1037.
Vitellas KM, Paulson EK, Enns RA, et al. (1999) "Pancreatitis complicated by gland necrosis: evolution of findings on contrast-enhanced CT." J Comput Assist Tomogr 23:898-905.
Wilson C, Heads A, Shenkin A, et al. (1989) C-reactive protein, antiproteases, and complement factors as objective markers of severity in acute pancreatitis." Br J Surg 76:177–181.
Wilson C, Heath DI, Imrie CW. (1990) "Prediction of outcome in acute pancreatitis: a comparative study of APACHE II, clinical assessment and multiple factor scoring systems." Br J Surg 77:1260–1264.
Wu BU, Bakker OJ, et al. (2011) "Blood urea nitrogen in the early assessment of acute pancreatitis: an international validation study." Arch Intern Med 171(7): 669-676.
Wu BU, Johannes RS, et al. (2008) "The early prediction of mortality in acute pancreatitis: a large population-based study." Gut 57(12): 1698-1703.
Wu BU, Johannes RS, et al. (2009) " Early changes in blood urea nitrogen predict mortality in acute pancreatitis." Gastroenterology 137(1):129-135.
Xing Z, Jordana M, Kirpalani H, Driscoll KE, et al. (1994) "Cytokine expression by neutrophils and macrophages in vivo: endotoxin induces tumor necrosis factor-alpha, macrophage inflammatory protein-2, interleukin-1 beta, and interleukin-6 but not RANTES or tranforming growth factor -beta 1 mRNA expression in acute lung inflammation." Am J Resp Cell Mol Bio 10(2):148-53
Yadav D, Agarwal N, et al. (2002) "A critical evaluation of laboratory tests in acute pancreatitis." Am J Gastroenterol 97(6): 1309-1318.
Yasuda T, Ueda T, Kamei K, Shinzaki W, et al. (2009) "Plasma tissue factor pathway inhibitor levels in patients with acute pancreatitis." J Gastroenterol. 44:1071-1079
Young M. (1989) "Acute diseases of the pancreas and biliary tract." (1989) Emerg Med Clin North Am 7: 555–573.
Zimmerman JE, Rousseau DM, Duffy J et al. (1994). "Intensive care at two teaching hospitals: an organizational case study." Am J Crit Care 3:129–138.

8

Imaging Appearances of Autoimmune Pancreatitis

Koji Takeshita
Teikyo University School of Medicine, Japan

1. Introduction

Autoimmune pancreatitis (AIP) is a rare disorder of presumed autoimmune etiology with specific pathologic features, and is an increasingly recognized clinical condition. AIP is characterized histologically by fibrosis with dense infiltration of T lymphocytes and IgG4-positive plasma cells in the peripancreatic and interlobular area of the pancreas (1-4). Patients with AIP usually have serum markers of autoimmune disorders, such as increased IgG4 and antinuclear antibodies. Although clinical features and symptoms are nonspecific, association with many other autoimmune disorders have also been reported (5-10). Therefore AIP should be considered in differential diagnosis when a patient with another autoimmune condition presents with symptoms related to the pancreas and biliary tract.

AIP has been described in literature to respond well to steroid therapy. Also, imaging appearances of AIP improve with steroid therapy, so imaging can be used in evaluation of treatment (11-16). Correct diagnosis is essential for appropriate treatment planning and to avoid unnecessary surgery. In particular, differentiation of AIP from pancreatic malignancies is very important, and several characteristic imaging features have been reported (16-18).

This article presents imaging appearances of AIP described in several radiological publications.

2. Imaging findings of AIP

AIP is mainly indicated by an imaging procedure such as contrast enhanced computed tomography (CT) or magnetic resonance imaging (MRI) (16, 18-22).

The classic finding of contrast enhanced CT that is diagnostic or highly suggestive of AIP is the diffuse sausage shaped enlargement of the entire pancreas with homogeneous attenuation, moderate enhancement and featureless, pencil sharp borders, absent of the normal pancreatic clefts (Figure1-4). The pancreas is covered with a thin capsular-like low density rim that possibly represents inflammatory exudates (Fig 1ab). Usually there is no calcification, peripancreatic fluid collection or vascular involvement. Though the diffuse form is most commonly reported in literature, focal forms have been reported, and the involved segment may mimic a pancreatic tumor, consequently most patients with focal forms of AIP underwent surgery, because of preoperative diagnoses of pancreatic carcinoma (Figure 4)(16-18, 23, 24).

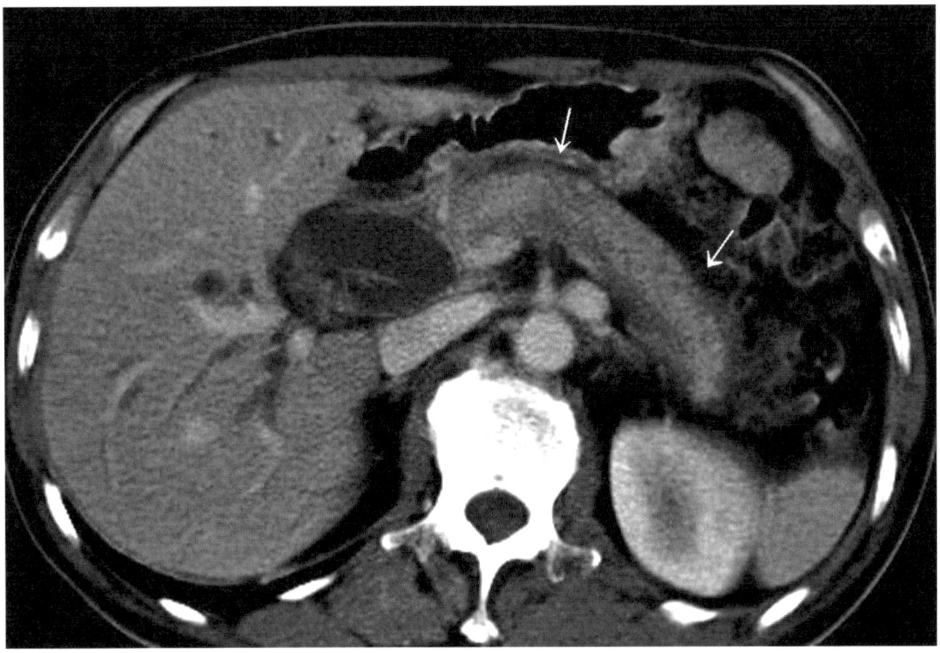

A

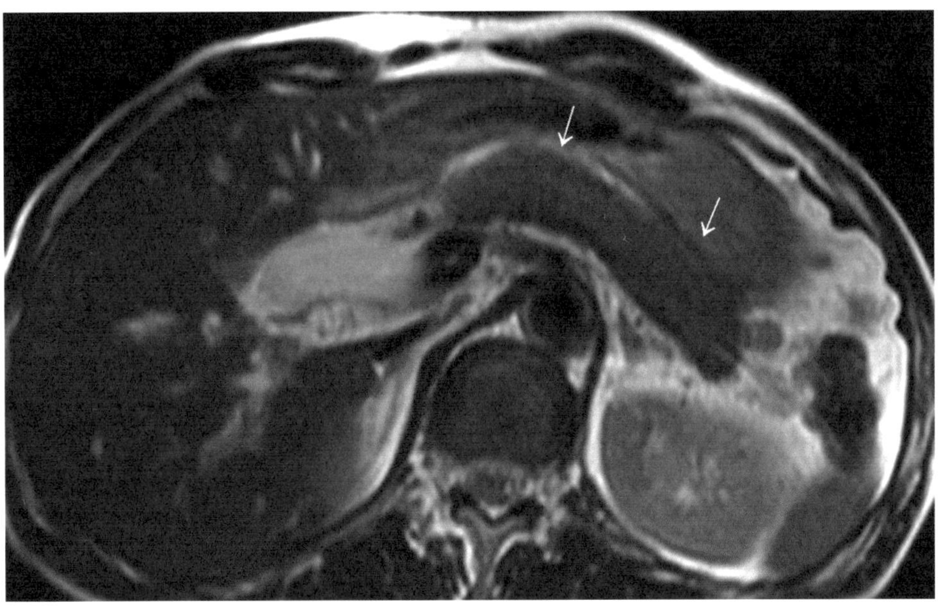

B

A, Contrast enhanced axial CT scan shows diffuse enlargement of the pancreas with sharp borders and minimal peripancreatic stranding (arrow), B, MRI shows diffuse pancreatic enlargement with minimal high signal intensity on T2-weighted MR images.

Fig. 1. (A,B) Images obtained in 58-year-old man with diffuse form of AIP who had jaundice and abdominal pain at presentation.

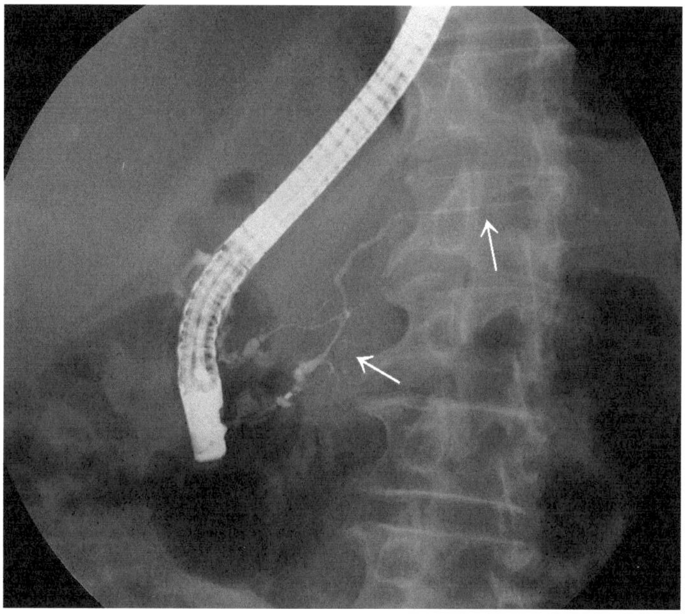

C

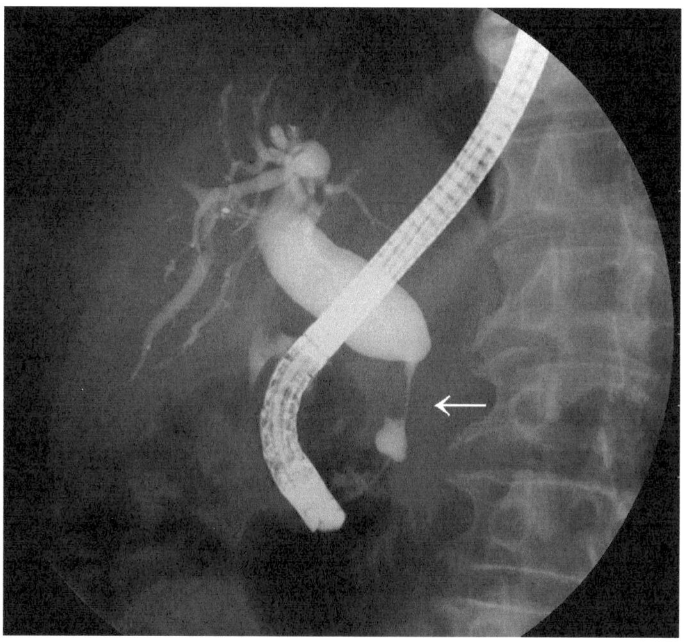

D

Endoscopic retrograde cholangiopancreatographic (ERCP) image shows diffuse narrowing of pancreatic duct with irregular walls (C; arrrows), and focal stricture in distal common bile duct (D; arrrow).

Fig. 1. (C,D) Images obtained in 58-year-old man with diffuse form of AIP who had jaundice and abdominal pain at presentation.

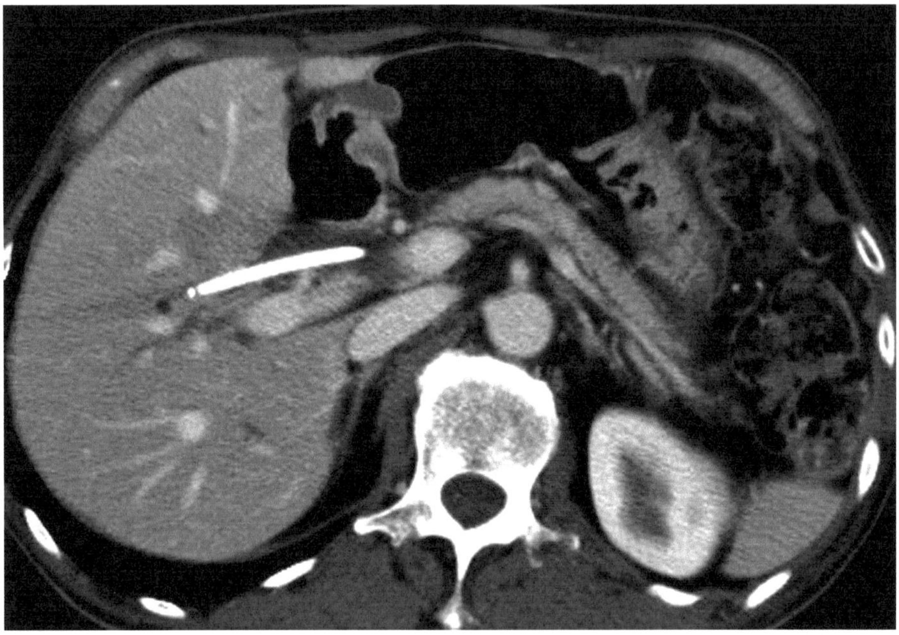

E

E, Axial CT scan shows that enlargement of the pancreas diminished after steroid therapy.

Fig. 1. (E) Images obtained in 58-year-old man with diffuse form of AIP who had jaundice and abdominal pain at presentation.

A diffusely enlarged pancreas can be also seen in diffuse infiltrative pancreatic carcinoma, malignant lymphoma, plasmacytoma, or metastases. However, in most of these conditions, imaging features are usually different from those observed in AIP.

Compared with normal pancreatic parenchyma, diffuse or localized enlargement of the pancreas is seen as low intensity on T1-weighted MR images and high intensity on T2-weighted images (Figure1b). Diffusion-weighted MR images (DWI) are considered useful for detecting AIP and for evaluating the effect of steroid therapy. AIP is seen as high signal intensity on DWI (Figure4c), which improved after steroid treatment. Apparent diffusion coefficients (ADCs) also reflected disease activity (Fiure4d). Thus, DWI is considered a valuable tool for detecting AIP, determining the affected area, and evaluating the effect of treatment (25, 26). In many cases, ADC values are lower in AIP than in pancreatic cancer, so an ADC cut off value is potentially useful for distinguishing AIP from pancreatic cancer (26).

Magnetic resonance cholangiopancreatography (MRCP) is a non-invasive method to evaluate the pancreatic duct and biliary tract, and recently, the imaging quality has increased to almost the equivalent of endoscopic retrograde cholangiopancreatography (ERCP). ERCP is thought to be the most accurate diagnostic modality for AIP, especially when evaluating the pancreatic duct (27). Both MRCP and ERCP show characteristic diffuse narrowing with irregularities or serration along various segments of the main pancreatic duct (Figure1c, 3d). Sometimes, there may be a focal stricture. The intrapancreatic segment of the common bile duct may be focally or segmentally narrowed resulting in dilatation of the proximal bile duct (Figure1d, 3d).

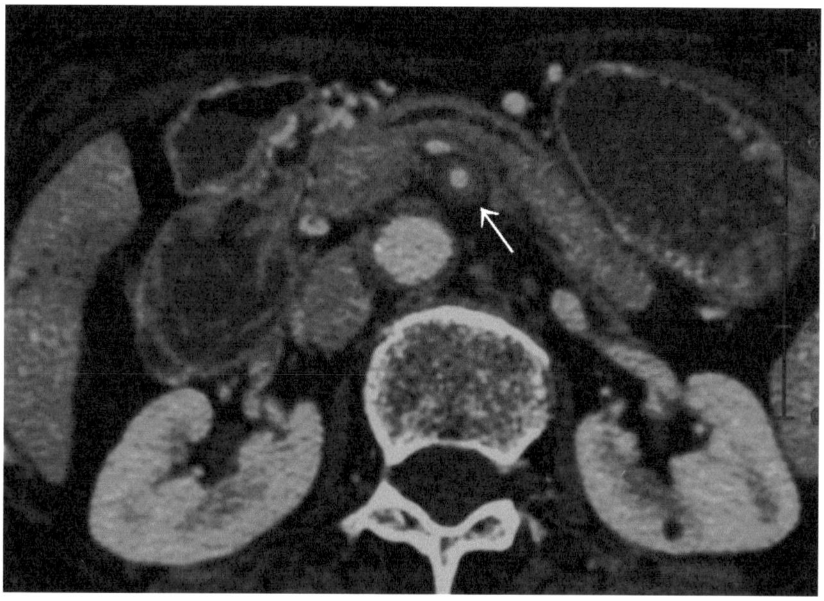

Axial CT scan obtained at the level of the proximal portion of superior mesenteric artery shows circumferential thickening of periarterial soft tissue (arrow) consistent with sclerosing messenteritis.

Fig. 2. 52-year-old man with diffuse form of AIP.

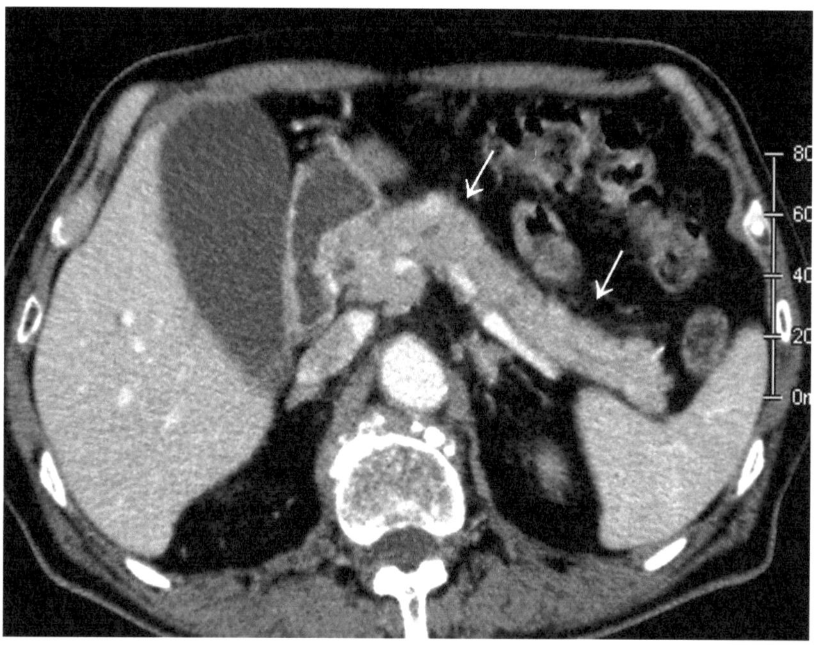

A

A, Contrast enhanced axial CT scan shows diffuse enlargement of the pancreas with sharp borders and minimal peripancreatic stranding (arrow).

Fig. 3. (A) 54-year-old man with diffuse form of AIP.

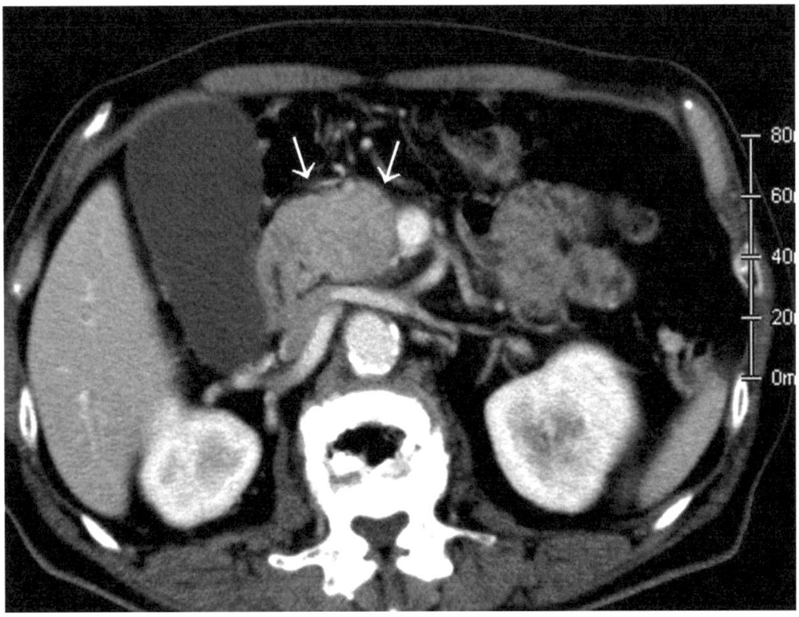

B

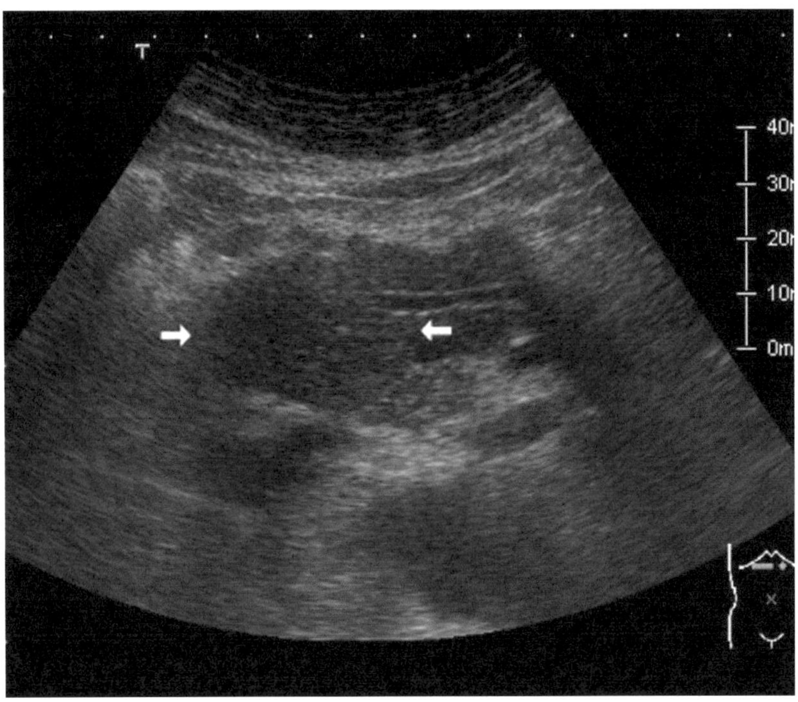

C

B, Swelling of the pancreatic head is also seen (arrow)., C, Transabdominal transverse US image shows enlargement of the pancreatic head with minimal decreased echotexture of pancreas (arrows).

Fig. 3. (B,C) 54-year-old man with diffuse form of AIP.

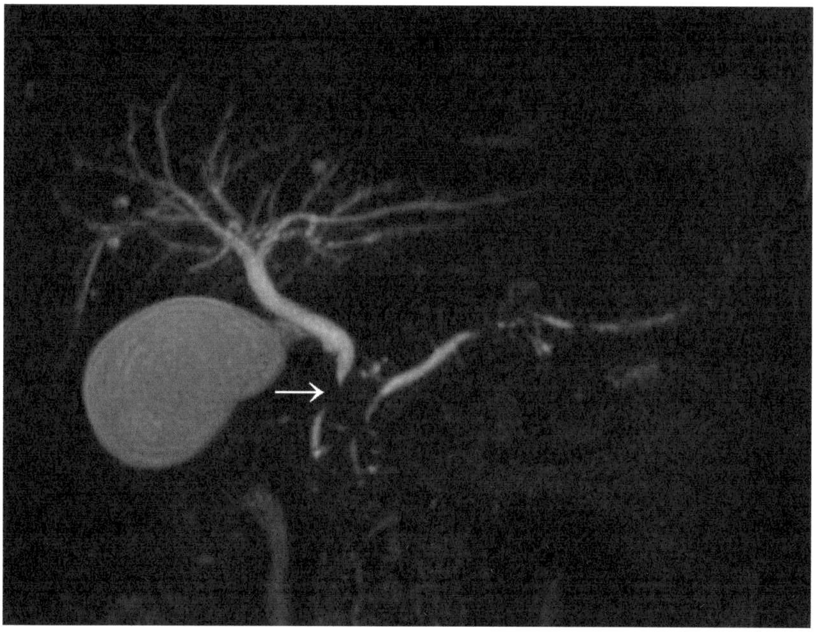

D

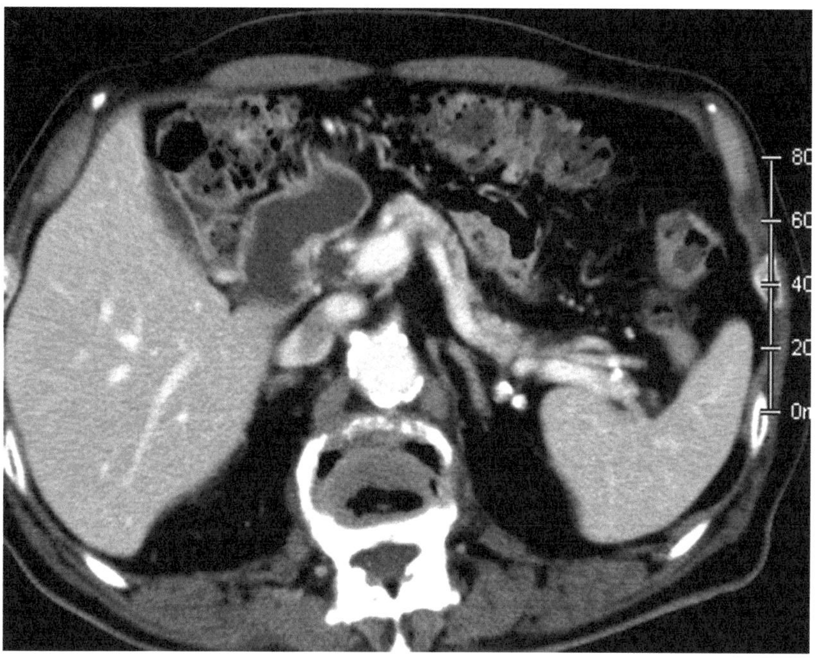

E

D, MRCP image also shows the narrowing of the main pancreatic duct with irregular walls and focal stricture in the distal common bile duct (arrrow),.E, Axial CT scan obtained after steroid therapy shows a normal-appearing pancreas, and enlargement of the pancreas is diminished.

Fig. 3. (D,E) 54-year-old man with diffuse form of AIP.

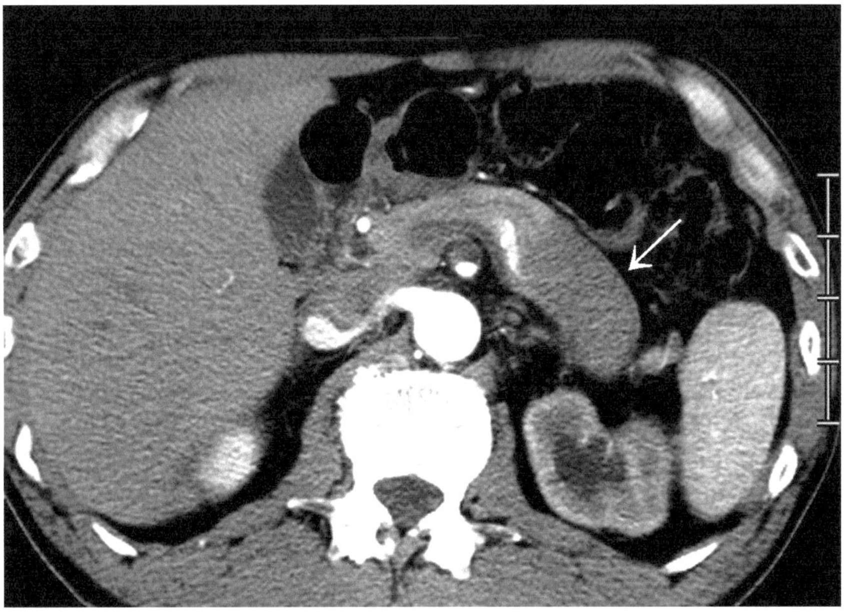

A

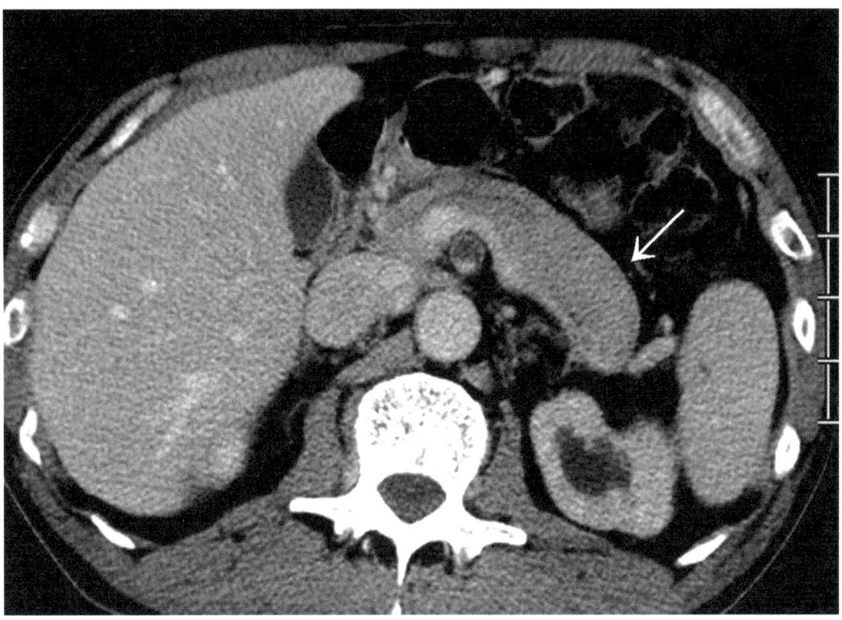

B

Contrast enhanced CT scan shows focal enlargement in the pancreatic body and tail with sharp borders and a thin capsular-like rim. The lesion appears as a relatively low attenuation area compared to normal pancreatic parenchyma on early phase (A), and as an almost iso-attenuation area compared to normal pancreatic parenchyma on delayed phase (B) (arrows). Hydronephrosis on the left is also seen due to concurrent retroperitoneal fibrosis.

Fig. 4. (A,B) 62-year-old man with focal form of AIP.

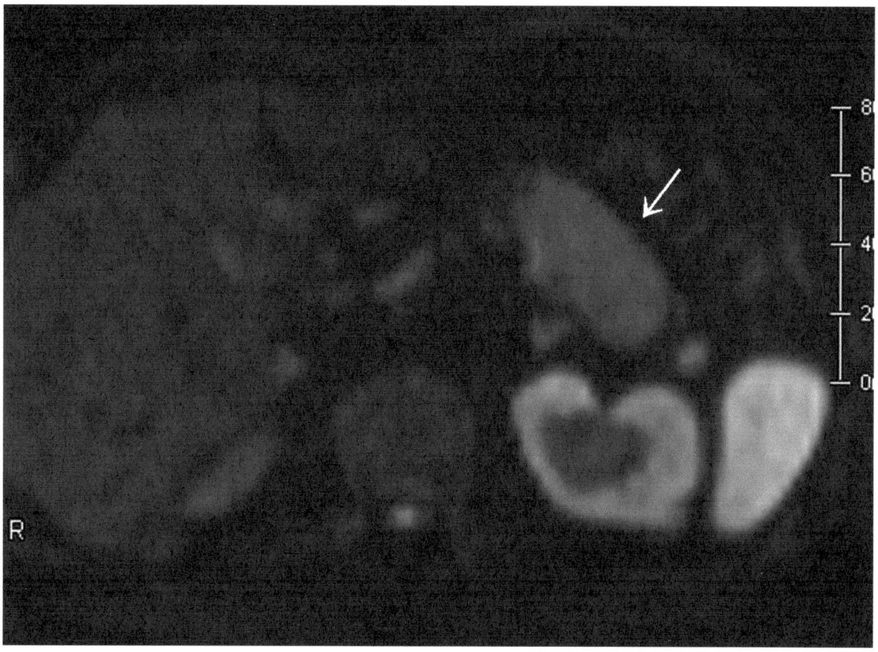

C

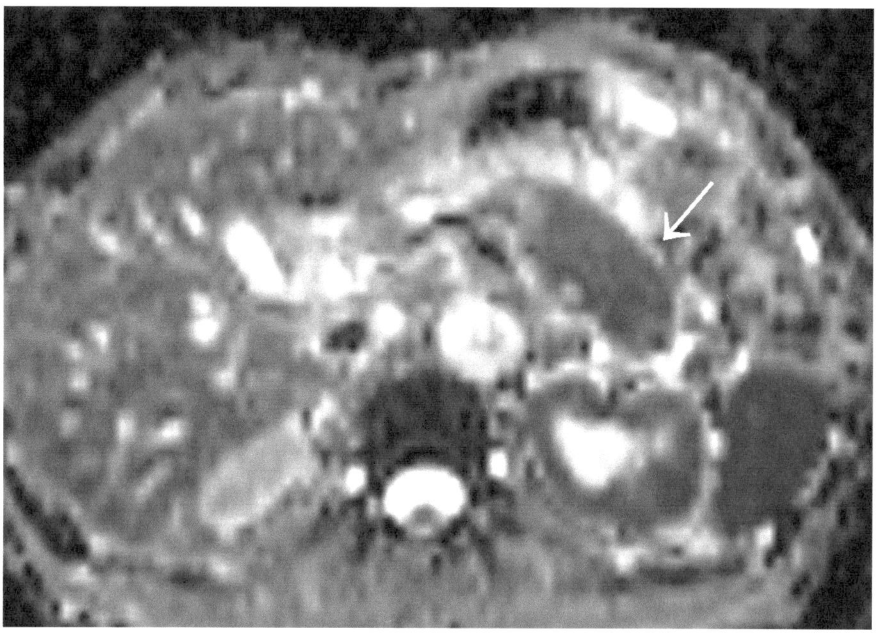

D

C, Diffusion-weighted MR image shows a focal high-intensity area on the pancreatic body and tail (arrow) (b=800mm^2/s). D, ADC map shows low ADC value (1.014x10^{-3}mm^2/sec) on the pancreatic body and tail (arrow) .

Fig. 4. (C,D) 62-year-old man with focal form of AIP.

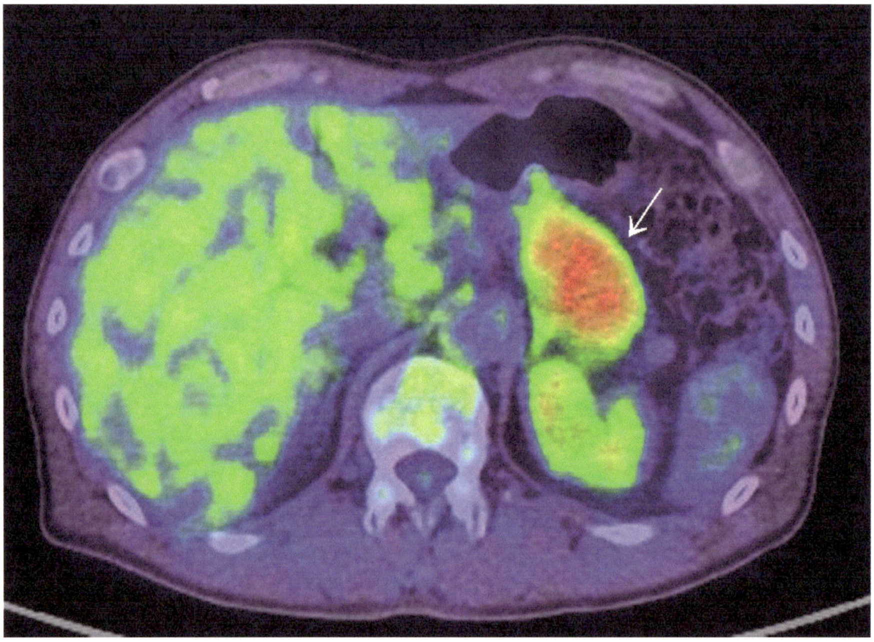

E

E, Combined PET/CT scan shows strong FDG uptake at the pancreatic body and tail (arrow).

Fig. 4. (E) 62-year-old man with focal form of AIP.

FDG-PET/CT is useful for detecting AIP and associated extrapancreatic autoimmune lesions and for monitoring their disease activity. AIP can cause intense FDG uptake in the pancreas (Figure4e). AIP should always be considered when making a diagnosis with FDG-PET in patients with pancreatic disorders. In many cases, differentiation of AIP from pancreatic malignancies is thought to be difficult by PET/CT (28-30). Lee et al reported that in difficult cases, on PET/CT imaging, the presence of diffuse uptake of FDG by the pancreas or concomitant extrapancreatic uptake by the salivary glands may aid in differentiation of autoimmune pancreatitis and pancreatic cancer (29).

3. References

[1] Finkelberg DL, Sahani D, Deshpande V, Brugge WR. Autoimmune pancreatitis. N Engl J Med 2006; 355:2670.

[2] Okazaki K. Autoimmune pancreatitis is increasing in Japan. Gastroenterology 2003; 125:1557.

[3] Kim KP, Kim MH, Lee SS, et al. Autoimmune pancreatitis: it may be a worldwide entity. Gastroenterology 2004; 126:1214.

[4] Kamisawa T, Egawa N, Nakajima H. Autoimmune pancreatitis is a systemic autoimmune disease. Am J Gastroenterol 2003; 98:2811.

[5] Hirano K, Shiratori Y, Komatsu Y, et al. Involvement of the biliary system in autoimmune pancreatitis: a follow-up study. Clin Gastroenterol Hepatol 2003; 1:453.

[6] Shinji A, Sano K, Hamano H, et al. Autoimmune pancreatitis is closely associated with gastric ulcer presenting with abundant IgG4-bearing plasma cell infiltration. Gastrointest Endosc 2004; 59:506.
[7] Takeda S, Haratake J, Kasai T, et al. IgG4-associated idiopathic tubulointerstitial nephritis complicating autoimmune pancreatitis. Nephrol Dial Transplant 2004; 19:474.
[8] Saeki T, Saito A, Hiura T, et al. Lymphoplasmacytic infiltration of multiple organs with immunoreactivity for IgG4: IgG4-related systemic disease. Intern Med 2006; 45:163.
[9] Umemura T, Zen Y, Hamano H, et al. Immunoglobin G4-hepatopathy: association of immunoglobin G4-bearing plasma cells in liver with autoimmune pancreatitis. Hepatology 2007; 46:463.
[10] Ghazale A, Chari ST, Zhang L, et al. Immunoglobulin G4-associated cholangitis: clinical profile and response to therapy. Gastroenterology 2008; 134:706.
[11] Raina A, Yadav D, Krasinskas AM, et al. Evaluation and management of autoimmune pancreatitis: experience at a large US center. Am J Gastroenterol 2009; 104:2295.
[12] Tabata M, Kitayama J, Kanemoto H, et al. Autoimmune pancreatitis presenting as a mass in the head of the pancreas: a diagnosis to differentiate from cancer. Am Surg 2003; 69:363.
[13] Erkelens GW, Vleggaar FP, Lesterhuis W, et al. Sclerosing pancreato-cholangitis responsive to steroid therapy. Lancet 1999; 354:43.
[14] Kojima E, Kimura K, Noda Y, et al. Autoimmune pancreatitis and multiple bile duct strictures treated effectively with steroid. J Gastroenterol 2003; 38:603.
[15] Church NI, Pereira SP, Deheragoda MG, et al. Autoimmune pancreatitis: clinical and radiological features and objective response to steroid therapy in a UK series. Am J Gastroenterol 2007; 102:2417.
[16] Sahani DV, Kalva SP, Farrell J, et al. Autoimmune pancreatitis: imaging features. Radiology 2004; 233:345.
[17] Chari ST, Takahashi N, Levy MJ, et al. A diagnostic strategy to distinguish autoimmune pancreatitis from pancreatic cancer. Clin Gastroenterol Hepatol 2009; 7:1097.
[18] Kamisawa T, Egawa N, Nakajima H, et al. Clinical difficulties in the differentiation of autoimmune pancreatitis and pancreatic carcinoma. Am J Gastroenterol 2003; 98:2694.
[19] Eerens I, Vanbeckevoort D, Vansteenbergen W, Van Hoe L. Autoimmune pancreatitis associated with primary sclerosing cholangitis: MR imaging findings. Eur Radiol 2001; 11:1401.
[20] Irie H, Honda H, Baba S, et al. Autoimmune pancreatitis: CT and MR characteristics. AJR Am J Roentgenol 1998; 170:1323.
[21] Yang DH, Kim KW, Kim TK, et al. Autoimmune pancreatitis: radiologic findings in 20 patients. Abdom Imaging 2006; 31:94.
[22] Nakazawa T, Ohara H, Sano H, et al. Difficulty in diagnosing autoimmune pancreatitis by imaging findings. Gastrointest Endosc 2007; 65:99.
[23] Frulloni L, Scattolini C, Falconi M, et al. Autoimmune pancreatitis: differences between the focal and diffuse forms in 87 patients. Am J Gastroenterol 2009; 104:2288.
[24] Koga Y, Yamaguchi K, Sugitani A, et al. Autoimmune pancreatitis starting as a localized form. J Gastroenterol 2002; 37:133

[25] Differentiation of autoimmune pancreatitis from pancreatic cancer by diffusion-weighted MRI. Kamisawa T, Takuma K, Anjiki H, et al. Am J Gastroenterol. 2010 Aug; 105(8):1870
[26] Diffusion-weighted magnetic resonance imaging in autoimmune pancreatitis. Taniguchi T, Kobayashi H, Nishikawa K, et al. Jpn J Radiol. 2009 Apr; 27(3):138
[27] Horiuchi A, Kawa S, Hamano H, et al. ERCP features in 27 patients with autoimmune pancreatitis. Gastrointest Endosc 2002; 55:494.
[28] The efficacy of whole-body FDG-PET or PET/CT for autoimmune pancreatitis and associated extrapancreatic autoimmune lesions Nakajo M, Jinnouchi S, Fukukura Y et al. European Journal of Nuclear Medicine and Molecular Imaging. 2007. 34(12), 2088.
[29] Utility of 18F-FDG PET/CT for differentiation of autoimmune pancreatitis with atypical pancreatic Imaging findings from pancreatic cancer. Lee TY, Kim MH, Park DH et al. AJR 2009:193(2); 343.

9

Prediction of Post-ERCP Pancreatitis

Takayoshi Nishino[1] and Fumitake Toki[2]
[1]*Institute of Gastroenterology, Department of Medicine, Tokyo Women's Medical University, School of Medicine,*
[2]*Toki Clinic,*
Japan

1. Introduction

Diagnostic accuracy in regard to biliary and pancreatic diseases has improved markedly since the introduction of computed tomography (CT) and magnetic resonance cholangiopancreatography (MRCP)(1,2), but detection of small bile duct cancers and small pancreatic cancers is difficult even by those modalities. Endoscopic retrograde cholangiopancreatography (ERCP) remains the most accurate and reliable procedure for cytodiagnosis and precise staging of biliary and pancreatic neoplasms, and it is indispensable to the endoscopic treatment of biliary and pancreatic diseases.

Pancreatitis remains the most common complication of ERCP and results in substantial morbidity and, occasionally, in death (3-5). The mechanisms responsible for the development of post-ERCP pancreatitis are not fully understood, but they are thought to be multifactorial. A number of specific risk factors have been proposed as predictors of post-ERCP pancreatitis (6-15), and they include patient-, endoscopist-, and procedure-related factors. We therefore think that clear identification of risk factors is facilitated by analyzing the data for diagnostic ERCP and therapeutic ERCP separately.

Early identification of patients who are likely to develop post-procedure pancreatitis is highly desirable in terms of planning long-term follow-up in the hospital and an early therapeutic approach. Hyperamylasemia is common after ERCP, and amylase values have been found to peak between 90 min and 4 h post-ERCP (16,17). Testoni et al. (18) concluded that the serum amylase level measured 4 h after endoscopic sphincterotomy was the most reliable predictor of post-ERCP pancreatitis, and Thomas et al.(19) showed that the 4-h post-procedure amylase level is clinically significant as a predictor of post-ERCP pancreatitis. We therefore hypothesized that the 4-h amylase level is the most accurate amylase value for predicting subsequent pancreatitis.

Several studies (20-24) have demonstrated that the serum lipase level is more sensitive indicator than the serum amylase level for diagnosing other forms of acute pancreatitis, but only a few studies (25-27) have compared measurements of various pancreatic enzymes as a means of predicting post-ERCP pancreatitis. Moreover, it is still unclear whether there are differences in the diagnostic accuracy of pancreatic enzyme levels for predicting post-ERCP pancreatitis according to the procedures, in other words, whether the ERCP is diagnostic or therapeutic. In the present study we evaluated the 4-h post-ERCP serum amylase level and serum lipase level as predictors of pancreatitis, with special focus on comparison of the two as a means of predicting post-ERCP pancreatitis, in a retrospective single-center design in Japan.

2. Patients and methods

We conducted a retrospective study in a single center by reviewing the 1631 consecutive cases in which ERCP was performed between January 1999 and December 2004 and (male:female ratio= 974:657 (1.48/1) ; age range 8-97 years old, median 67 years old). Diagnostic ERCP had been performed in 910 cases (male:female ratio=518:392 (1.32/1); age range 8-90 years old, median 63 years old), and therapeutic ERCP in 721 cases (male: female ratio=456:265 (160/1); age range 19-97 years old, median 67 years old). All patients were enrolled in this study, and there were no exclusion criteria. Diagnostic ERCP included brushing cytology (biliary tract, pancreatic duct) and intraductal ultrasonography (IDUS). Therapeutic ERCP included endoscopic papillary balloon dilatation (EPBD), endoscopic sphicterotomy (EST), stone removal, and bile duct drainage.

All ERCP patients were intravenously infused over 4 hours with one of the following protease inhibitor solutions beginning 30 minutes before the ERCP examination: Gabexate mesilate 200 mg in 0.9% saline, 500 ml, Nafamostat mesilate 20 mg in 0.9 % saline, 500 ml; or Ulinastatin 50,000 U in 0.9 % saline, 500 ml. The choice of inhibitor was at the discretion of the chief physician responsible for the patient's care.

All patients remained in the hospital for at least 24 hours after the procedure to monitor them for clinical manifestations of pancreatitis. Serum amylase and lipase levels were measured before and 4 and 16-18 hours (the next morning) after ERCP. We evaluated 23 variables, including patient-related factors, an endoscopist-related factor, and procedure-related factors that could be analyzed in detail based on information in the patients' charts. We also evaluated and compared the 4-h post-ERCP serum amylase level and serum lipase level as predictors of pancreatitis based on receiver-operator characteristic (ROC) curves. To compare the ROC curves, we analyzed only the data from cases in which both amylase and lipase could be measured, in other words, we made a matched pair comparison. We analyzed the data of a total of 1267 patients, consisting of 65 pancreatitis patients and 1202 non-pancreatitis patients. A total of 688 patients, consisting of 39 pancreatitis patients and 649 non-pancreatitis patients had undergone diagnostic ERCP, and a total of 579 patients, consisting of 26 pancreatitis patients and 553 non-pancreatitis patients, had gone therapeutic ERCP.

Data related to the procedures were gathered in a prospective manner, but the global analysis was performed in a retrospective manner.

2.1 Endoscopists

The 1631 ERCP procedures were performed by 11 different endoscopists (median: 57 procedures per endoscopist, range: 8-423). Four of the endoscopists performed about 84% of the procedures, and each of the 4 had performed more than 200 ERCPs before the study. The other 7 endoscopists had performed fewer than 200 ERCPs each before the study.

2.2 Definition

High levels of emzymes was defined as an amylase level (normal range: 40-125 IU/l) and /or lipase level (normal range 13-49 IU/l) above the upper limit of the normal range. The criteria for the diagnosis of post-ERCP pancreatitis were: (1) abdominal pain that persisted for at least 24 hours; (2) a serum amylase level and/or lipase level measured 16-18 hours after the procedure (next morning) that was more than three times the upper limit of the normal range; (3) pancreatic swelling with or without fluid collection on an abdominal US and/or CT examination the next morning. Fulfillment of criterion 1 plus criterion 2 and/or 3 was required to make the diagnosis. Pancreatitis was graded as follows according to the scoring system proposed by the Ministry of Health, Labour and Welfare of Japan (JPN score) (28,29): mild (0 points); moderate (1 point); severe (2 points or more).

The injection pressure of contrast medium into the pancreatic duct was scored as follows based on the degree of pancreatic duct visualization, according to a modification of the criteria proposed by Tsujino et al. (30): 0, no pancreatic duct visualization; 1, visualization of the main pancreatic duct alone; 2, 1 and visualization of primary branches; 3, 2 and visualization of secondary branches; and 4, 3 and/or visualization of acini (acinarization).

2.3 Statistical analysis

In the first step, a univariate analysis was performed by the chi-square method for each of the potential risk factors. In the second step, factors with a p value <0.2 according to the chi-square analysis were included in a multivariate (logistic regression) analysis performed using Statview 5.0 software. A p value <0.05 was considered statistically significant. The odds ratios are reported with their 95% confidence limits.

ROC curve analyses for the serum amylase and lipase values were performed using Medcalc software. We assessed whether the difference in area under two ROC curves was significant based on the methods proposed by Hanley JA et al (31). In short, the difference in area under two ROC curves derived from the same set of patients is calculated as a critical ratio z by using the formula:

$$z= (A_1-A_2)/\sqrt{(SE_1{}^2+SE_2{}^2-2rSE_1SE_2)},$$

where A1 is the observed area and SE1 is estimated error of the ROC area associated with modality 1, A2 and SE2 are the corresponding values for modality 2, and r is a constant calculated from (A1+A2)/2 and (rn+ra)/2, where rn is the coefficient for the correlation between modality 1 and modality 2 in the control group (non-pancreatitis group in this study), and ra is the coefficient for the correlation between modality 1 and modality 2 in the diseased group (pancreatitis group in this study). This quantity z is then referred to tables of the normal distribution and values of z above a certain cutoff are taken as evidence of a difference between the 'true' ROC areas.

We selected optimal cutoff values for the serum amylase and lipase values as predictors of post-ERCP pancreatitis based on their sensitivity and specificity and especially their positive predictive value (PPV) and negative predictive value (NPV), by using a prior probability value for post-ERCP pancreatitis of 4.2% (incidence rate among the cases in this study as a whole).

3. Results

3.1 Incidence of post-ERCP pancreatitis

Pancreatitis developed after 67 (4.2%) of the 1631 ERCP procedures. According to the JPN scores the pancreatitis was mild after 60 (3.7 %) of the procedures, moderate after 5 (0.3%), and severe after 4 (0.2%). There were no deaths in our series. Pancreatitis developed after 40 (4.4%) of the 910 diagnostic ERCPs, and after 29 (4.0%) of the 721 therapeutic ERCPs. The difference between the incidence of post-ERCP pancreatitis after diagnostic ERCP and after therapeutic ERCP was not statistically significant.

The incidence of post-ERCP pancreatitis after diagnostic ERCP in the Gabexate mesilate group, Nafamostat mesilate group, and Ulinastatin group was 4.7% (31/666), 3.8% (7/184), and 3.3% (2/66), respectively, and there were no statistically significant differences in the incidence of post-ERCP pancreatitis between the three groups. The incidence of post-ERCP pancreatitis after therapeutic ERCP in the Gabexate mesilate group, Nafamostat mesilate group, and Ulinastatin group was 4.4% (19/428), 3.4% (7/209), and 3.6% (3/84), respectively, and there were no statistically significant differences in the incidence of post-ERCP pancreatitis between the three groups.

3.2 Risk factors for post-ERCP pancreatitis

3.2.1 Diagnostic ERCP

3.2.1.1 Univariate analysis

The univariate analysis revealed statistically significant associationss between an increased risk of post-ERCP pancreatitis and 4 of the13 patient-related factors and 4 of the 9 procedure-related factors (Tables 1 and 2). The patient-related factors that significantly increased the risk of pancreatitis were: age 65 years or over, presence of hyperamylasemia and/or hyperlipasemia before ERCP, past or present pancreatitis and IPMN. The significant procedure-related risk factors according to the univariate analysis were: injection of contrast medium into the pancreatic duct score >= 3, brushing cytology in the pancreatic duct, IDUS, and endoscopic nasobiliary drainage (ENBD).

3.2.1.2 Multivariate analysis

Five risk factors were significant according to the multivariate analysis. Two were patient-related factors, age (OR=1.043/1 yr increase in age) and presence of hyperamylasemia and/or hyperlipasemia before ERCP (OR=2.291), and the other three were procedure-related factors, high contrast medium injection pressure into the pancreatic duct (OR=2.406/ 1 point increase), brushing cytology in the pancreatic duct (OR=4.135), and IDUS (OR=4.373). The R-square value was 0.204.

3.2.2 Therapeutic ERCP

3.2.2.1 Univariate analysis

The univariate analysis revealed a statistically significant association between an increased risk of post-ERCP pancreatitis and only one endoscopist-related factor: inexperienced endoscopist (Tables 3 and 4).

Patient-related factors	Pancreatitis (n=40)	Non-pancreatitis (n=870)	p value
Significant			
Age (>=65years/<65years)	26/14	378/492	<0.001
Hyperamylasemia and/or hyperlipasemia (yes/no)	18/22	184/686	<0.001
Past or present pancreatitis (yes/no)	9/31	76/773	0.004
IPMN	12/28	131/739	0.011
Not significant			
Gender (male/female)	17/23	501/369	0.062
Past-post ERCP pancreatitis(yes/no)	1/39	6/864	0.200
Past or presenting cholangitis (yes/no)	1/39	79/791	0.151
Periamupullary diverticulum (yes/no)	3/37	66/804	0.984
Chronic pancreatitis (yes/no)	5/35	97/773	0.791
Pancreatic cancer (yes/no)	2/38	108/762	0.160
Pancreas divisum (yes/no)	1/39	30/840	0.746
Anomalous pancreatic-biliary junction (yes/no)	2/38	25/845	0.438
Bile duct stone (yes/no)	1/39	40/830	0.532

IPMN, intraductal papillary mucinous neoplasia
ERCP: Patient-related Factors (ref 34))

Table 1. Univariate Analysis of Risk Factors for Post-ERCP Pancreatitis after Diagnostic

Endoscopist-related factor and Procedure-related factors	Pancreatitis (n=40)	Non-pancreatitis (n=870)	p value
Significant			
Injection pressure of contrast medium into the pancreatic duct (score 3,4/0-2)	29/11	348/522	<0.001
Brushing cytology in the pancreatic duct (yes/no)	11/29	69/801	<0.001
IDUS (yes/no)	8/32	55/815	<0.001
ENBD (yes/no)	1/39	3/867	0.040
Not significant			
Endoscopist experience (<=200 ERCPs/>200 ERCPs)	9/31	125/745	0.156
EST (yes/no)	0/40	1/869	0.830
EPBD (yes/no)	0/40	0/870	N.E.
Bile duct stone exploration (yes/no)	0/40	0/840	N.E.
Brushing cytology in the bile duct (yes/no)	1/39	44/826	0.466
Biliary stenting (yes/no)	0/40	0/870	N.E.

ERCP: An Endocopist-related Factor and Procedure-related Factors (ref 34))
IDUS, intraductal ultrasonography; EST, endoscopic sphincterotomy; EPBD, endoscopic papillary balloon dilation; ENBD, endoscopic nasobiliary drainage

Table 2. Univariate Analysis of Risk Factors for Post-ERCP Pancreatitis after Diagnostic

Patient-related factors	Pancreatitis (n=29)	Non-pancreatitis (n=692)	p value
Not Significant			
Age (>=65years/<65years)	19/10	391/301	0.337
Gender (male/female)	21/8	435/257	0.300
Hyperamylasemia and/or hyperlipasemia (yes/no)	8/21	207/485	0.788
Past or present pancreatitis(yes/no)	1/28	49/643	0.450
Past-post ERCP pancreatitis(yes/no)	1/39	6/864	0.200
Past or presenting cholangitis (yes/no)	13/16	313/379	0.966
Periamupullary diverticulum (yes/no)	8/21	115/577	0.123
Chronic pancreatitis (yes/no)	1/28	18/674	0.780
Pancreatic cancer (yes/no)	3/26	112/580	0.400
Pancreas divisum (yes/no)	0/29	1/691	0.838
IPMN(yes/no)	0/29	2/690	0.772
Anomalous pancreatic-biliary junction (yes/no)	1/28	6/686	0.165
Bile duct stone (yes/no)	14/15	350/342	0.808

IPMN, intraductal papillary mucinous neoplasia

Table 3. Univariate Analysis of Risk Factors for Post-ERCP Pancreatitis after Therapeutic ERCP: Patient-related Factors (ref34))

Endoscopist-related factor and Procedure-related factors	Pancreatitis (n=29)	Non-pancreatitis (n=692)	p value
Significant			
Endoscopist experience (<=200 ERCPs/>200 ERCPs)	8/21	62/630	<0.001
Not significant			
Injection pressure of contrast medium into the pancreatic duct (score 3,4/0-2)	5/24	59/633	0.106
Brushing cytology in the pancreatic duct (yes/no)	0/29	10/682	0.514
IDUS (yes/no)	0/29	6/686	615
EST (yes/no)	5/24	98/594	0.642
EPBD (yes/no)	8/21	114/578	0.118
Bile duct stone exploration (yes/no)	7/22	156/536	0.841
Brushing cytology in the bile duct (yes/no)	1/28	20/672	0.861
Biliary stenting (yes/no)	4/25	120/572	0.620
ENBD (yes/no)	5/24	231/461	0.070

ERCP: An Endocopist-related Factor and Procedure-related Factors (ref34))
IDUS, intraductal ultrasonography; EST, endoscopic sphincterotomy; EPBD, endoscopic papillary balloon dilation; ENBD, endoscopic nasobiliary drainage

Table 4. Univariate Analysis of Risk Factors for Post-ERCP Pancreatitis after Therapeutic

3.2.2.2 Multivariate analysis

Two risk factors were significant according to the multivariate analysis. One was an endoscopist-related factor, inexperienced endoscopist (OR=4.407), and the other was a procedure-related factor, high contrast medium injection pressure into the pancreatic duct (OR=1.693/ 1 point increase). The R-square value was 0.073.

3.2.2.3 Multivariate analysis of the cases as a whole

Six risk factors were significant according to the multivariate analysis for whole cases. Two were patient-related factors, age (OR=1.038/1 yr increase in age) and presence of hyperamylasemia and/or hyperlipasemia before ERCP (OR=1.807). One was an endoscopist-related factor, inexperienced endoscopist (OR=2.645), and the other three were procedure-related factors, high contrast medium injection into the pancreatic duct (OR=1.608/1 point increase), brushing cytology in the pancreatic duct (OR=2.605), and IDUS (OR=2.602). R-square value was 0.114.

3.2.3 Prediction of pancreatitis following ERCP by the 4-h post-procedure serum amylase level and lipase level

3.2.3.1 Diagnostic ERCP

The receiver-operating characteristics (ROCs) of both the 4-h amylase level and lipase level after diagnostic ERCP showed good test performance, with an area under the curve of 0.88 (95% CI: 0.85-0.91) and 0.94 (95% CI: 0.92-0.96), respectively (Figure 1). The 4-h

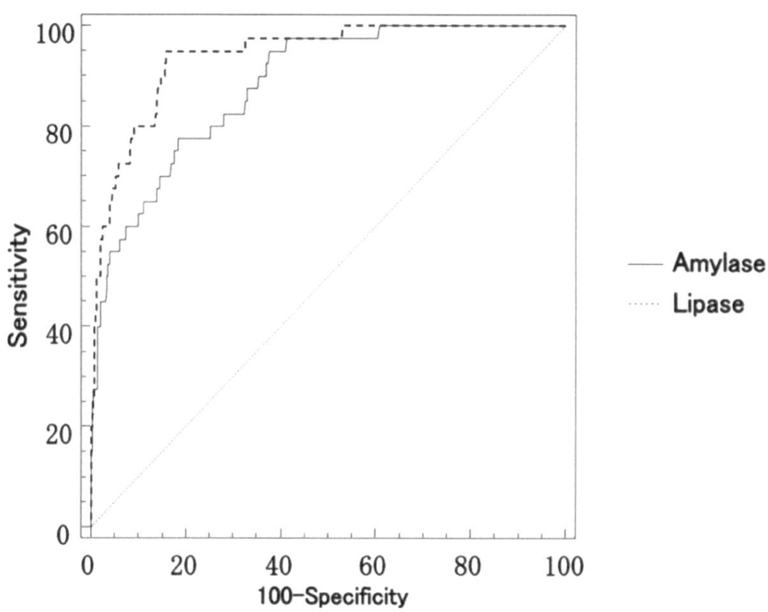

The area under the curve of the amylase levels was 0.88 (95% CI: 0.85-0.91).
The area under the curve of the lipase levels was 0.94 (95% CI: 0.92-0.96).

Fig. 1. ROC curve of the 4-h post-procedure serum amylase levels and lipase levels after diagnostic ERCP.

post-procedure serum lipase level was a more effective predictor of post-ERCP pancreatitis than the amylase level based on the areas under the ROC curves (p=0.025).

3.2.3.2 Therapeutic ERCP

The receiver-operating characteristics (ROCs) of both the 4-h amylase level and lipase level after therapeutic ERCP showed good test performance, with an area under the curve of 0.92 (95% CI: 0.90-0.93) and 0.96 (95% CI: 0.94-0.97), respectively (Figure 2). The 4-h post-procedure serum lipase level was a more effective predictor of post-ERCP pancreatitis than the amylase level, based on the area under the ROC curves (p=0.035).

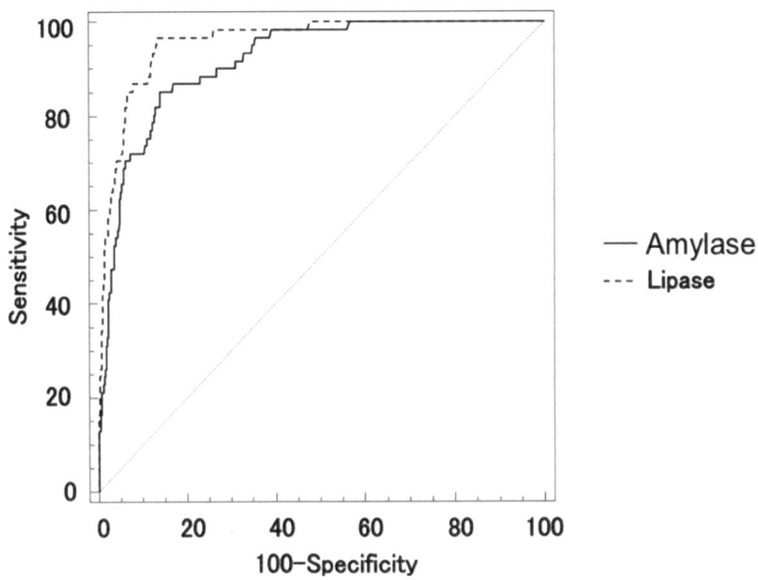

The area under the curve of the amylase levels was 0.92 (95% CI: 0.90-0.93).
The area under the curve of the lipase levels was 0.96 (95% CI: 0.94-0.97).

Fig. 2. ROC curve of the 4-h post-procedure serum amylase levels and lipase levels after therapeutic ERCP.

3.2.3.3 ERCP cases as a whole

The receiver-operating characteristics (ROCs) of both the 4-h amylase level and lipase level after ERCP for the cases as a whole showed good test performance, with an area under the curve of 0.91 (95% CI: 0.89-0.92) and 0.96 (95% CI: 0.94-0.97), respectively (Figures 3). The 4-h post-procedure serum lipase level was a more effective predictor of post-ERCP pancreatitis than the amylase level based on the areas under the ROC curves (p=0.007).

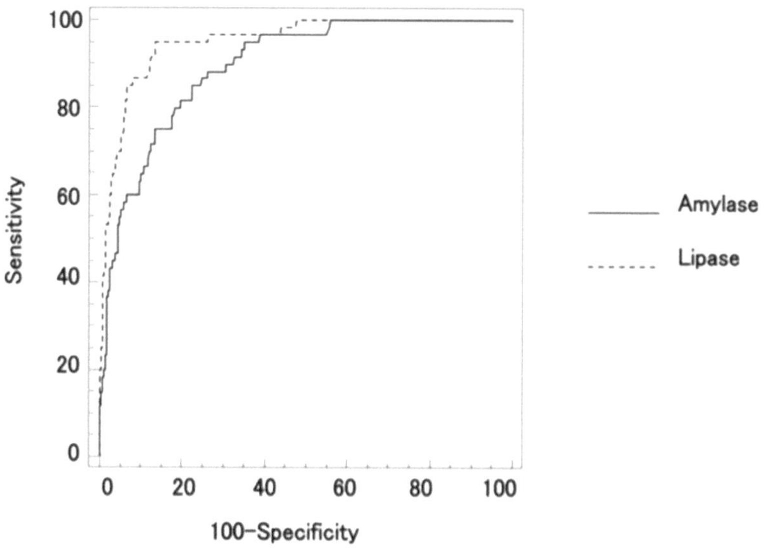

The area under the curve of the amylase levels was 0.91 (95% CI: 0.89-0.92).
The area under the curve of the lipase levels was 0.96 (95% CI: 0.94-0.97).

Fig. 3. ROC curve of the 4-h post-procedure serum amylase levels and lipase levels after ERCP in the cases as a whole.

3.2.3.4 Optimal cutoff values for amylase and lipase

The optimal cutoff values for amylase were five times (625 IU/l) the upper limit of the normal range in the diagnostic ERCP cases, therapeutic ERCP cases, and ERCP cases as a whole based on their sensitivity and specificity and especially on their PPV and NPV (Table 5).

	Amylase level	Sensitivity (%)	Specificity(%)	PPV (%)	NPV (%)	Likelihood ratio
Diagnostic						
	> 3 times	82.5	70.3	10.8	98.9	2.78
	> 4 times	77.5	79.9	14.5	98.8	3.86
	> 5 times	70.0	85.1	17.1	98.5	4.37
Therapeutic						
	> 3 times	90.2	72.4	14.5	99.4	3.26
	> 4 times	86.9	79.7	17.8	99.3	4.29
	> 5 times	85.2	86.1	21.2	99.3	6.13
All cases						
	> 3 times	89.8	72.9	12.7	99.4	3.32
	> 4 times	84.7	80.4	16.0	99.2	4.36
	> 5 times	78.0	85.8	19.5	98.9	5.51

Post-ERCP pancreatitis (ref34)). PPV, positive predictive value; NPV, negative predictive value.

Table 5. Diagnostic Accuracy of Various Amylase Cutoff Levels for Predicting

The optimal cutoff values for lipase were ten times (490 IU/l) the upper limit of the normal range in diagnostic ERCP cases, therapeutic ERCP cases, and ERCP cases as a whole based on their sensitivity and specificity and especially on their PPV and NPV (Table 6).

	Lipase level	Sensitivity (%)	Specificity(%)	PPV (%)	NPV (%)	Likelihood ratio
Diagnostic						
	> 6 times	95.0	73.6	13.6	99.7	3.60
	> 8 times	95.0	82.0	18.8	99.7	5.21
	> 9 times	95.0	83.7	20.1	99.7	5.84
	> 10 times	92.5	84.5	21.2	99.6	5.97
Therapeutic						
	> 6 times	96.7	81.4	18.5	99.8	5.16
	> 8 times	96.7	85.1	22.9	99.8	6.48
	> 9 times	96.7	86.1	24.2	99.8	6.94
	> 10 times	95.1	86.8	26.8	99.8	7.23
All cases						
	> 6 times	96.6	80.8	18.1	99.8	5.05
	> 8 times	96.6	84.8	21.8	99.8	6.34
	> 9 times	96.6	85.9	23.1	98.8	6.85
	> 10 times	94.9	86.4	23.8	99.7	7.04

Table 6. Diagnostic Accuracy of Various Lipase Cut-off Levels for Predicting Post-ERCP pancreatitis (ref34)). PPV, positive predictive value; NPV, negative predictive value..

4. Discussion

Pancreatitis remains the most common complication of ERCP, occurring after 1% to 30% of procedures (4-15), and its reported incidence has varied with the thoroughness of follow-up, the definition used, factors related to patient susceptibility, case mix, types of maneuvers performed, and the endoscopist. Rates of pancreatitis of 2% to 9% have been typical in unselected large prospective series (6-14). The subjects of the present study were consecutive patients who underwent diagnostic or therapeutic ERCP, and the incidence rate of pancreatitis was 4.2% in the subjects as a whole, 4.4 % in the diagnostic ERCP group, 4.0 %. In therapeutic ERCP group. These figures are comparable to those reported in recent prospective studies in which the definition and study population were similar to those in our study.

A number of specific risk factors, acting independently or in concert, have been proposed as predictors of post-ERCP pancreatitis (6-14). The present study assessed 23 risk factors that included patient-related, procedure-related, and endoscopist-related variables. The results of the multivariate analysis showed that older age, hyperamylasemia and/or hyperlipasemia before ERCP, endoscopist experience with fewer than 200 ERCPs, high contrast medium injection pressure into the pancreatic duct, brushing cytology in the pancreatic duct, and IDUS each increased risk independently. The results of this study also demonstrated that the risk of post-ERCP pancreatitis is as much related to patient characteristics as to endoscopic technique and/or maneuvers, as previously reported (6-10,14). However, the limitation of the present study is that it was a retrospective study. In spite of the fact that data were obtained from consecutive ERCP cases, minimal bias must be taken into account.

Previous studies have suggested that early hyperamylasemia is useful as a predictor of post-ERCP pancreatitis (18,19,32,33). Thomas et al. (19) found that a 4-h amylase level threefold higher than normal was a useful predictor of pancreatitis and had a sensitivity and specificity of 70% and 95.3%, respectively. Testoni et al. (18) reported that a serum amylase level fivefold higher than normal 4 h after the procedure is a reliable predictor of post-procedure pancreatitis, with a sensitivity of 68.4%. In the present study the ROC of both the 4-h amylase level and the 4-h lipase level after diagnostic ERCP showed good test performance, with an area under the curve of 0.88 and 0.94, respectively, and the ROC of both the 4-h amylase level and the 4-h lipase level after therapeutic ERCP also showed good test performance, with an area under the curve of 0.92 and 0.96, respectively. In addition, the ROC of both the 4-h amylase and the 4-h lipase level after ERCP in the cases as a whole showed good test performance, with an area under the curve of 0.91 and 0.96, respectively. The optimal cutoff values for the amylase level after diagnostic ERCP, therapeutic ERCP, and ERCP as a whole were 5 times (625 IU/l) the upper limit of the normal range, and the sensitivity and specificity of the cutoff value for the as a whole cases was 78.0% and 85.8%, respectively. The optimal cutoff values for the lipase level after diagnostic ERCP, therapeutic ERCP, and ERCP as a whole cases were 10 times (490 IU/l) the upper limit of the normal range, and their sensitivity and specificity in the cases as a whole were 94.9% and 86.4%. The results of this study confirmed that the 4-h post-procedure serum amylase and lipase level are good predictors of pancreatitis both after diagnostic ERCP and after therapeutic ERCP.

Comparisons of measurements of various pancreatic enzymes as a means of detecting of acute pancreatitis other than post-ERCP pancreatitis have shown that the blood lipase level is almost as sensitive as the total blood amylase level and has better specificity (20). Other studies (21-23) have demonstrated that the blood lipase level is more sensitive than the blood amylase level, and still another study concluded that the blood lipase level is an important diagnostic indicator for acute pancreatitis and that measuring it should be given top priority (24). By contrast, few studies have compared measurements of various pancreatic enzymes as a means of diagnosing post-procedure pancreatitis (25-27). Panteghini et al. (25) found that the serum lipase level increased faster than the levels of the other enzymes measured and that the average peak in lipase level was the highest in post-procedure pancreatitis. Doppl et al. (26) concluded that serum lipase measurement is the most sensitive diagnostic test for post-ERCP pancreatitis. The results of the present large retrospective study demonstrated that serum lipase was a more effective marker than amylase for predicting post-ERCP pancreatitis both after diagnostic ERCP and after therapeutic ERCP, based on the area under the ROC curves. A further prospective study should be performed to confirm the superiority of serum lipase over amylase as a predictor of post-ERCP pancreatitis.

In conclusion, the 4-h post-ERCP serum amylase level and the 4-h post-ERCP lipase level, in particular, were found to be a useful means of predicting pancreatitis both after diagnostic ERCP and after therapeutic ERCP in a large retrospective study in a single center. A prospective study should be undertaken to confirm the usefulness of the 4-h post-ERCP amylase and lipase levels as predictors of post-ERCP pancreatitis.

5. References

[1] Wallner BK, Schumacher KA, Weidenmaie W, Friedrich JM. Dilated biliary tract: evaluation with MR cholangiography with a T2-weighted contrast-enhanced fast sequence. Radiology 1991;181:805-8

[2] Morimoto K, Shimoi M, Shirakawa T, Shirakawa T, Aoki Y, Choi S, et al. Biliary obstruction: evaluation with three-dimensional MR cholangiography. Radiology 1992;183;578-80
[3] Testoni PA, Mariani A, Giussani A, Vailati C, Masci E, Macarri G, et al. Risk factors for post-ERCP pancreatitis in high- and low-volume centers and amon expert and non-expert operators: a prospective multicenter study. Am J Gastroenterol 2010;105:1753-61.
[4] Cotton PB, Garrow DA, Gallagher J, Romagnuolo J. Risk factors fo complications after ERCP; a multivariate analysis of 11,497 procedures over 12 years. Gastrointest Endosc 2009;70:80-8.
[5] Gottlieb K, Sherman S. ERCP and endoscopic biliary sphincterotomy-induced pancreatitis. Gastrointest Endosc Clin N Am 1998;8:87-114
[6] Freeman ML, DaSario JA, Nelson DB, Fennerty MB, Lee JG, Bjorkman DJ, et al. Risk factors for post-ERCP pancreatitis: a prospective, multicenter study. Gastrointest Endosc 2001;54:425-434
[7] Christoforidis E, Goulimaris I, Kanellos I, Tsalis K, Demetriades C, Betsis D. Post-ERCP pancreatitis and hyperamylasemia: patient-related and operative risk factors. Endoscopy 2002;34:286-92
[8] Friedland S, Soetikno RM, Vandervoot J, Montes H, Tham T, Carr-Locke DL. Bedside scoring system to predict the risk of developing pancreatitis following ERCP. Endoscopy 2002;34:483-8
[9] Leperfido S, Angelini G, Benedetti G, Chilovi F, Costan F, De Berardinis F, et al. Major early complications from diagnostic and therapeutic ERCP: a prospective multicenter study. Gastrointest Endosc. 1998;48:1-10
[10] Masci E, Toti G, Mariani A, Curioni S, Lomazzi A, Dinelli M. Complications of diagnostic and therapeutic ERCP: a prospective multicenter study. Am J Gastroenterol 2001;96:417-23
[11] Mehta SN, Pavone E, Barkun JS, Bouchard S, Barkun AN. Predictors of post-ERCP complications in patients with suspected choledocholithiasis. Endoscopy 1998;30:457-63
[12] Rabenstein T, Schneider HT, Bulling D, Nicklas M, Katalinic A, Hahn EG. Analysis of risk factors associated with endoscopic sphincterotomy techniques: preliminary results of a prospective study, with emphasis on reduced risk of acute pancreatitis with low-dose anticoagulation treatment. Endoscopy 2000;32:10-19
[13] Vandervoort J, Soetikno RM, Tham TC, Wong RC, Ferrari AP Jr, Montes H, et al. Risk factors for complications after performance of ERCP. Gastrointest Endosc 2002;56:652-6
[14] Cheng CL, Sherman S, Watkins JL, Barnett J, Freeman M, Geenen J,. Risk factors for post-ERCP pancreatitis: a prospective multicenter study. Am J Gastroenterol 2006;101:139-47
[15] Sherman S, Hawes RH, Rathgaber SW, Uzer MF, Smith MT, Khusro QE, et al. Post-ERCP pancreatitis: randomized, prospective study comparing a low- and high-osmolality contrast agent. Gastrointest Endosc 1994;40:422-7
[16] Thomas P, Sengupta S. Prediction of pancreatitis following retrograde cholangiopancreatography by the 4-h post procedure amylase level. J Gastroenterology and Hepatology 2001;16:923-926.

[17] Ito K, Fujita N, Noda Y, Kobayashi G, Horaguchi J, Takasawa O, et al. Relationship between post-ERCP pancreatitis and the change of serum amylase level after the procedure, World J Gastroenterology 2007;13:3855-60.

[18] Testoni PA, Bagnolo F, Caporuscio S, Lella F. Serum amylase four hours after endoscopic sphincterotomy is a reliable predictor of postprocedure pancreatitis. Am J Gastroenterology 1999; 94:1235-1241.

[19] Thomas P, Sengupta S. Prediction of pancreatitis following retrograde cholangiopancreatography by the 4-h post procedure amylase level. J Gastroenterology and Hepatology 2001;16:923-926.

[20] Apple F, Benson O, Preese L, Eastep S,Bilodeau L, Heiler G. Lipase and pancreatic amylase activities in tissue and in patients with hyperamylasemia. Am J Clin Pathol 1991;96:610-4.

[21] Nordestgaad AG, Wilson SE, Williams RA. Correlation of serum amylase levels with pancreatic pathology and pancreatitis etiology. Pancreas 1988;3:159-61.

[22] Levitt MD, Johnson SG. Is the Cam/CCr rario of value for the diagnosis of pancreatitis? Gastroenterology 1978;75:118-9.

[23] Orebaugh SL. Normal amylase levels in the presentation of acute pancreatitis. Am J Emerg Med 1994;12:21-4.

[24] Koizumi M, Takada T, Kawarada Y, Hirata K, Mayumi T, Yoshida M, et al. JPN guideline for the management of acute pancreatitis: diagnostic criteria for acute pancreatitis. J Hepatobiliary Pancreat Surg 2006;13:25-32.

[25] Panteghini M, Pagani F, Alebardi O, Lancini G, Cestari R. Time course of changes in pancreatic enzymes, isoenzymes, and isoforms in serum after endoscopic retrograde cholangiopancreatography. Clin Chrm 1991;37:1602-5.

[26] Doppl WE, Weber H, Temme H, Klör HU, Federlin K. Evaluation of ERCP- and endoscopic sphincterotomy-induced pancreatic damage: A prospective study on the time course and significance of serum levels of pancreatic secretory enzymes. Eur J Med Res 1996;1:303-11.

[27] Kapetanos D, Kokozidis G, Kinigopoulou P, Xiarchos P, Antonopoulous Z, Proqia E, et al. The value of serum amylase and elastase measurements in the prediction of post-ERCP acute pancreatitis. Hepato-gastroenterology 2007;54:556-560

[28] Ogawa M, Hirota M, Hayakawa T, Matsuno S, Watanabe S, Atomi Y,et al. Development and use of a new staging system for severe acute pancreatitis based on a nationwide survey in Japan. Pancreas 2002;25:325-30

[29] Hirota M, Takada T, Kawarada Y, Hirata K, Mayumi T, Yoshida M, et al. JPN guideline for management of acute pancreatitis: severity assessment of acute pancreatitis. J Hepatobiliary Pancreat Surg 2006;13:33-41.

[30] Tsujino T, Komatsu Y, Isayama H, Hirano K, Sasahira N, Yamamoto N, et al. Ulinastatin for pancreatitis after endoscopic retrograde cholangiopancreatography: A randomized, controlled trial. Clin. Gastroenterology and Hepatology 2005;3:376-83.

[31] Hanley JA, McNeil BJ. A method of comparing the areas under receiver operating characteristic curves derived from the same cases. Radiology 1983;148:839-843.

[32] Gottlieb K, Sherman S, Pezzi J,Esber E, Lehman GA. Early recognition of post-ERCP pancreatitis by clinical assessment and serum pancreatic enzymes. Am J Gastroenterology 1996;91:1553-7.

[33] Testoni PA, Bagnolo F. Pain at 24 hours associated with amylase levels greater than 5 times the upper normal limit as the most reliable indicator of post-ERCP pancreatitis. Gastrointestinal Endoscopy 2001;53:33-9.

[34] Nishino T, Toki F, Oyama H, Shiratori K. More accurate prediction of post-ERCP pancreatitis by 4-H serum lipase levels than amylase levels. Digstive Endoscopy 2008;20:169-177.

Part 4

Treatment

10

Mini Invasive Treatments in Acute Biliary Pancreatitis

Juan Carlos Barbella, Diego L. Dip,
Anzorena Francisco Suarez, Jorge Dodera and Emiliano Monti
Buenos Aires University,
Argentina

1. Introduction

Gallstone disease is one of the most common causes of acute pancreatitis. There are two accepted mechanisms regarding its pathogenesis: reflux of bile into the pancreatic duct and transient ampullary obstruction in the ampulla [1].

Although most episodes are mild and resolve spontaneously, severe pancreatitis with local and systemic complications may lead to death [2]. It is uncertain whether gallstones initiate or also maintain biliary pancreatitis [3].

Since the advent of endoscopic retrograde cholangiopancreatography (ERCP) in 1974, it has replaced conventional surgery with the T-tube as the treatment of choice for common bile duct stones, reducing complications and shortening recovery time.

It is also used to treat a variety of pancreaticobiliary diseases such as biliary strictures, stone removal, and biliary leaks.

This chapter will review the role of endoscopy in acute gallstone pancreatitis and some of its complications.

2. The role of endoscopy in acute gallstone pancreatitis

2.1 Technique

ERCP is performed with a side-viewing duodenoscope, reaching the ampulla of Vater. The bile duct is cannulated selectively under fluoroscopic guidance. There are different cannulation techniques, such as the use of a standard catheter or sphincterotome (Cotton-Cannulatatome II PC Double Lumen Sphincterotome Cook-Medical), guidewire assistance, or a needle knife.

2.2 ERCP in acute gallstone pancreatitis

The management of acute gallstone pancreatitis has been controversial and the major debate has been whether the endoscopic treatment of acute gallstone pancreatitis ameliorates or exacerbates the disease.[4]

One of the most discussed issues in the investigation of acute pancreatitis has been whether enrolled patients would benefit from ERCP, with or without sphincterotomy, and whether it is possible to determine in which cases it would be beneficial.

Increases in serum bilirubin, alkaline phosphatase and/or gamma-glutamyl transferase, and persistent dilatation of the common bile duct [5], suggest that gallstones are the cause of the pancreatic inflammation.

In the majority of patients with mild biliary pancreatitis, bile duct stones have already passed to the duodenum by the time cholangiography is considered, so routine ERCP would be unnecessary [6]; the prevalence of residual choledocholithiasis is less than 30% [7].

Thus, patients with resolving mild acute pancreatitis can undergo laparoscopic cholecystectomy with intraoperative cholangiography, and any remaining bile duct stones can be dealt with by postoperative or intraoperative ERCP [8] . During the last years, several studies have reported that the indication for ERCP has changed from being a diagnostic tool to a therapeutic procedure [9 10], avoiding the risk of complications.

Abdominal ultrasound, magnetic resonance (MR) and endosonography are the imaging techniques of choice.

Although the value of ultrasound is limited due to its low sensitivity, its specificity is high. Dilation of the common bile duct alone is neither sensitive nor specific for the detection of common bile duct stones [8].

MR is known to miss small gallstones 6 mm [1]. The latter are the most frequent cause of acute pancreatitis. Limitations of magnetic resonance imaging include the difficulty in performing this procedure in critically ill or uncooperative patients, and its contraindications such as the presence of pacemakers [8]. In these cases it is advisable to perform a biliary endosonography, with a positive predictive value of 91% to 100% in detecting bile duct stones [7].

EUS is generally considered to be the most accurate method.

Persistent biliary obstruction worsens the outcome and increases the severity of acute pancreatitis. When tests clearly show an alteration in liver function, with images compatible with common bile duct stones, it is undoubtedly advisable to perform endoscopic sphincterotomy and stone removal. Biliary drainage is necessary when bile drainage is incomplete because cholestasis predisposes the patient to cholangitis [9 11].

Routine ERCP should be avoided in patients with low to intermediate suspicion of retained bile duct stones and who are planned to have cholecystectomy [8].

2.3 Acute gallstone pancreatitis at the time of admission

Wirsung duct hypertension and the migration gallstone theory

One of the most prominent theories on the pathophysiology of acute pancreatitis is the common pathway and gallstone migration [12]. In 1974 Acosta et al demonstrated the association between gallstone disease and acute pancreatitis. Gallstones were found in the feces of 34 out of 36 patients with pancreatitis [13]. Transient obstruction of the ampulla of Vater increases pancreatic duct pressure and activates digestive enzymes [11].

Currently, most authors agree that transient obstruction by a migrating gallstone initiates pancreatitis. There is no consensus on the effects that follow stone impaction and the development of pancreatic inflammation. Some studies have questioned the relationship between duration of obstruction and severity of pancreatitis. A randomized trial in 61 patients reported by Acosta et al in 2006 demonstrated that duration of ductal obstruction is a critical factor in determining severity. [14].

2.4 Early descompression of the wirsung duct - ERCP

As a result of the theories proposed for the onset of acute pancreatitis, different studies have questioned the benefit of early decompression of the ampulla of Vater.

There are several randomized studies that compare patients receiving either early endoscopic intervention (EEI) within 72 hours after admission or early conservative management (ECM) [15 14], and which show contradictory conclusions [16 17 3].

A study conducted in Hong Kong by Fan et al included 195 patients with acute pancreatitis: 97 patients underwent ERCP within 24 hours after admission, and 98 received initial conservative treatment. Complications occurred in 18% of patients receiving early ERCP and in 29% of those receiving conservative treatment. The authors concluded that early ERCP is safe and effective in reducing the incidence of biliary sepsis, but removal of stones from the ampulla or from the common bile duct does not completely reverse the damage already done to the pancreas during the first hours or days of the illness [17]. Fan et al and Neoptolemos et al demonstrated a significantly lower rate of complications in patients who had predicted severe pancreatitis and underwent early ERCP [16 17].

In a study performed in Germany in 1997, Folsch et al randomized 126 patients to early ERCP and 112 to conservative treatment. This was a 22-institution multicenter prospective trial, which excluded patients with jaundice or cholangitis. Complications were similar in the two compared groups, but patients in the ERCP group had more respiratory failure. Because the authors found no explanation for this difference, they concluded that early ERCP and papillotomy were not beneficial [3].

A meta-analysis carried out in the USA in 1999 by Sharman and Colin reported statistically significantly fewer overall complications and reduced mortality in patients with acute pancreatitis treated with ERCP + sphincterotomy compared with those treated conservatively. The role of ERCP + ES in patients with mild gallstone pancreatitis should be further evaluated in a large prospective RCT. ERCP + ES should be recommended for all patients with acute biliary pancreatitis and may be particularly beneficial in those with severe disease.

ERCP may not be necessary or beneficial in patients with low likelihood of biliary obstruction [18].

In 2006, Oria et al randomized 103 patients to receive either EEI (n =51) or ECM (n = 52). Their study failed to provide evidence that EEI benefits patients with acute gallstone pancreatitis.

In 2008, Petrov et al conducted a meta-analysis in 450 patients. The results showed that early ERCP in patients with predicted mild and predicted severe ABP without acute cholangitis did not lead to a significant reduction in the risk of overall complications and mortality [1].

One of the most important points is proper patient selection. Larger prospective studies are needed to determine the correct value of ERCP in acute gallstone pancreatitis. Finally, there is no consensus as to which patients should be treated within 72 hours or later. In conclusion, ERCP in acute gallstone pancreatitis is still controversial, except when there is associated cholangitis.

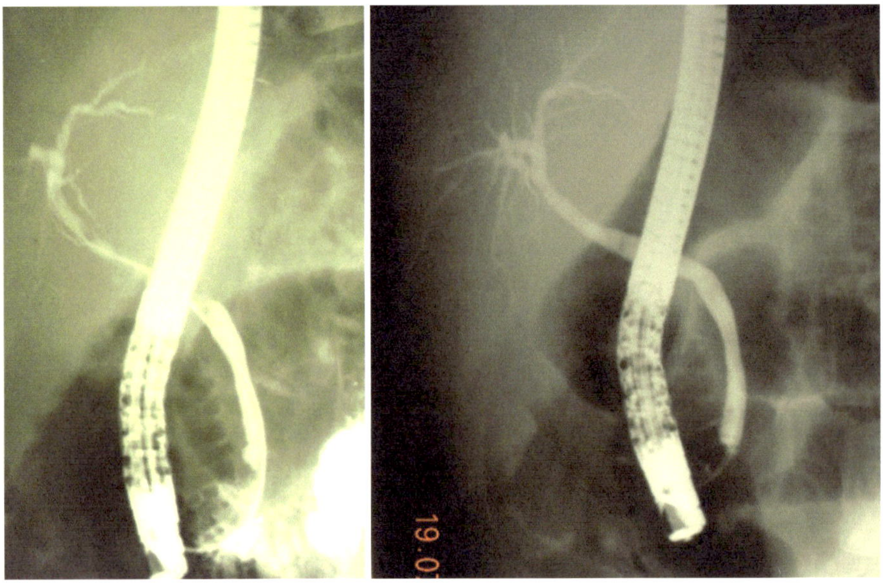

Stone removal with a Dormia Basket.

Figs. 1 - 2. ERCP in acute gallstone pancreatitis

2.5 Cholangitis and acute gallstone pancreatitis

Biliary drainage is indicated within 24h of admission for patients with cholangitis (fever, abdominal pain and jaundice, the classic Charcot's triad) [8].

Clinical presentation ranges from a mild, self-limited process to a serious, life-threatening condition [19] . The most frequent symptoms are fever in 90%, jaundice in 60% and abdominal pain in 70% of cases. It can be associated with hypotension and altered mental status, the so-called Reynold's Pentad Syndrome [20].

Historically, surgery was the treatment of choice.

Currently, endoscopic retrograde cholangiopancreatography is the gold standard treatment.

There are several methods to perform ERCP endoscopy, sphyncterotomy with or without stent placement, or nasobiliary drainage placement. The latter has advantages in that it can be washed and bile culture can be done, but has the disadvantage of patient discomfort [21].

Biliary obstruction promotes bacterial colonization and infection. The most common organisms are *E. coli, Enterococcus* and *Klebsiella*. Biliary obstruction is necessary but not sufficient to cause cholangitis. Partial obstruction is associated with a higher rate of infection than complete obstruction.

It is essential to perform early diagnosis and deliver prompt treatment [19], which should initially include medical therapy, antibiotics and supportive medical care, followed by biliary decompression. The delay or failure in early recognition of cholangitis may be fatal.

An endoscopic biliary stent should be placed if bile duct stones cannot be removed, so as to ensure proper drainage of the bile duct.

Twenty to 40 ml of bile should be aspirated to provide a sample of bile for microbiologic analysis, and adopt the most suitable antibiotic therapy. Endoscopic treatment can only involve stone removal with or without biliary stents, or with a nasobiliary catheter. Stents can be placed in different sizes, from 8.5 to 10 French, and their length shall depend on the length of the bile duct. Several studies have demonstrated no difference in treatment outcomes between biliary stenting and nasobiliary catheter drainage [22 23].

Biliary stents are temporary and are removed after 30 days.

2.5.1 Post ERCP pancreatitis

ERCP complications are pancreatitis, hemorrhage, perforation, cholangitis and cholecystitis. The overall rate of complications is 9.8% [24]. The most frequent is pancreatitis. Young age, a history of pancreatitis, and sphincter of Oddi dysfunction, are risk factors. Thus, the technique and the experience of the endoscopist are important. The mechanisms underlying pancreatitis include intraductal pressure due to overinjection and papillary edema. [25].

Criteria to define ERCP pancreatitis are: acute pain and tenderness in the upper abdomen, elevated pancreatic enzyme levels in blood, and radiologic abnormalities characteristic of acute pancreatitis.

Pancreatitis post ERCP should be classified according to Cotton's staging [6] .

Although there has been controversy regarding the use of pre-cut sphincterotomy, a recent meta-analysis by Cenname et al showed that pre-cut implementation reduces post-ERCP pancreatitis risk [26].

3. Endoscopic treatment of pancreatic pseudocyst

3.1 Introduction

Pancreatic pseudocysts are organized collections of enzyme-rich fluid after an acute pancreatitis, an exacerbation of chronic pancreatitis, or pancreatic trauma [27]. They can be associated with necrotizing pancreatitis in between 2% and 50% of cases [28].

Spontaneous resolution rate is 30% to 50% after a period of 6 weeks.

Pseudocysts larger than 6 cm and persistent more than 6 weeks should be drained.

Two thirds are located in the head of the pancreas [28].

Infection of the pseudocyst results in a pancreatic abscess that can progress to sepsis, so early recognition and prompt intervention are necessary. [27].

Surgical management is performed by internal drainage by cystenteric anastomosis, either in the form of a cystgastrostomy, cystduodenostomy, or cystjejunostomy [29].

The major advantage of endoscopic drainage over surgical drainage is minimal invasiveness, which reduces the duration of hospital stay and improves patient tolerance [30].

Endoscopic transmural drainage is a minimally invasive alternative to surgery [31]. The approach is to create a fistula between the pancreatic collection and the digestive tract. It is a proven treatment and can be performed via a transpapillary and/or transmural approach. The transgastric route is the most preferred.

The risk of perforation is high when luminal compression is not visible at endoscopy [31].

The introduction of endoscopic ultrasonography has allowed a proper selection of the puncture sites, avoiding major gastric vessels and adjacent structures [32].

Morbidity mainly consists of bleeding, infection, and perforation.

Bleeding is the most frequent complication [28]

3.2 Technique

It is very important that the pseudocyst be in close approximation to the enteric wall (less than 1 cm).

The first step is to search for a luminal compression in the stomach or in the duodenum by using the duodenoscope.

When the cyst is not found to bulge, which occurs in almost 50% of cases, endoscopic ultrasound may be used for localization and evaluation of the distance between the two structures and identification of interposed vessels [29].

When a luminal compression is identified, a needle-knife catheter is used to puncture and access the pseudocyst. After access, a 0.035-inch guidewire (Tracer Metro Direct Wilson-Cook Medical) is coiled within the pseudocyst and dilation of the fistula is performed using a 15 mm balloon dilator (CRE balloon; Microvasive) under fluoroscopic guidance.

There are several devices that are used to puncture the gastric or duodenal wall to enter into the cyst cavity[30]. Once inside the pseudocyst, the pancreatic necrosis is removed with a Dormia Basket (Cook Medical WEB-2X4-2X6).

In a randomized trial, Varadarajulu et al demonstrated that success rate of transmural drainage of pancreatic pseudocysts was higher when performed under endosonography guidance. The authors concluded it should be considered as the first-line treatment.

4. Percutaneous approach in necrotizing biliary pancreatitis

4.1 Introduction

About 20% of patients with acute pancreatitis develop pancreatic necrosis associated or not with peri pancreatic necrosis [33]. This is one of the most feared complications of acute pancreatitis due to its high morbidity and mortality. Infection of pancreatic necrosis naturally develops during the second phase of the disease (most commonly in the 2nd and 3rd week after the onset of symptoms) and has been reported in as many as 40–70% of patients with necrotizing pancreatitis. The risk of infection increases with the extent of intra- and extra-pancreatic necrosis [34]. It is crucial to know whether the necrosis is infected or not, since this will determine which treatment is to be performed.

When fever, leukocytosis, and unexpected deterioration appear, infection is suspected[11].

Infected pancreatic necrosis necessitates surgical debridement, while sterile necrosis is managed best non-operativelly (Fig 3.) Infected necrosis constitutes an absolute indication for prompt intervention.

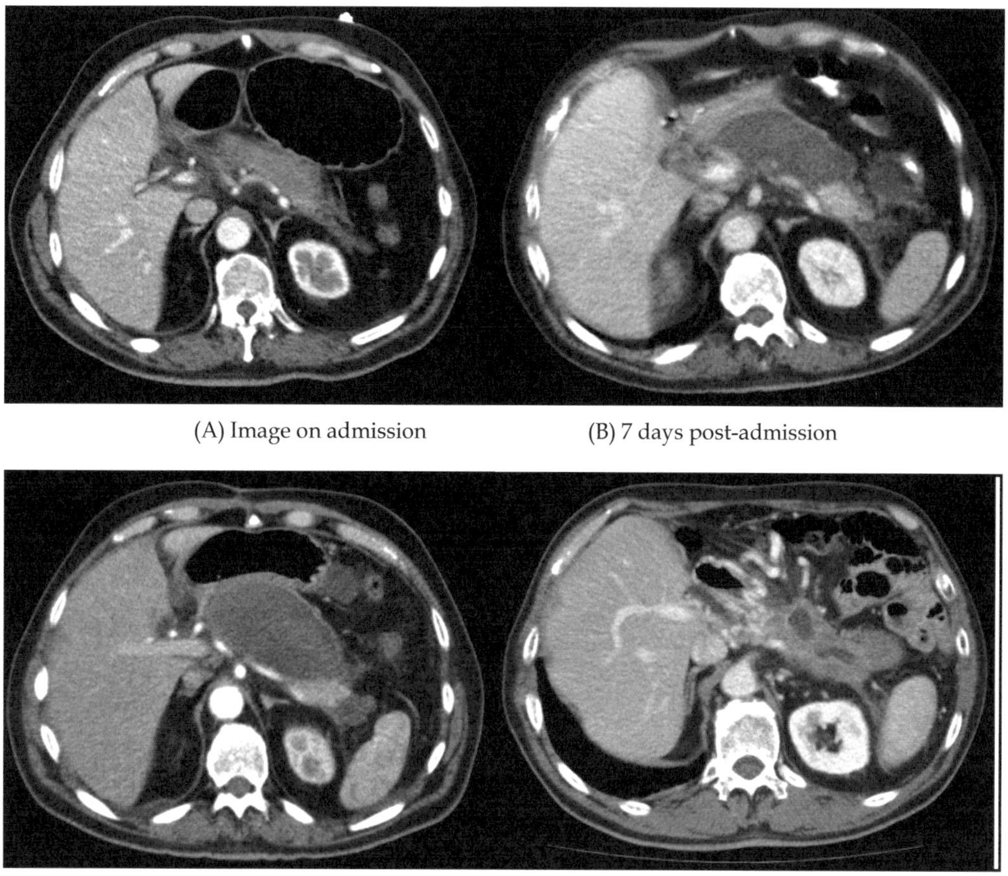

(A) Image on admission

(B) 7 days post-admission

(C) One month post-admission.

(D) At 4 months, without treatment.

Fig. 3. Conservative treatment.

Until recently, the first-choice intervention in infected necrotizing pancreatitis was surgical necrosectomy by laparotomy. This approach is associated with considerable morbidity (34–95%) and mortality (11–39%) [33].

In 1998, Freeny et al published a series of patients who were treated primarily with imaging-guided percutaneous catheter drainage.

Since Van Sonnenberg and D'agostino et al's first reports, intervention strategies in acute pancreatitis have been used for over fifteen years in patients not amenable to surgical treatment.

There are various techniques of necrosectomy: surgical, endoscopic and endoscopic necrosectomy. Treatments are multidisciplinary and tend to be conservative.

Retroperitoneoscopy, endoscopy and laparoscopy are minimally invasive techniques and have prompted the use of mini-invasive or step-up treatment strategies.

Both surgical and percutaneous drainage are associated with a significant risk of pancreatico-cutaneous fistula formation[35].

This chapter will address only percutaneous necrosectomy

Percutaneous treatments for resolution of the complications of acute pancreatitis

- Ultrasound-guided diagnostic puncture.
- CT-guided diagnostic puncture.
- Single or multiple percutaneous drainage under ultrasound guidance.
- Single or multiple percutaneous drainage with CT guidance.
- Replacement of catheters up to 30 Fr with fluoroscopic guidance.
- Retroperitoneal lavage under fluoroscopic guidance.
- Retroperitoneoscopy under fluoroscopic guidance.
- Catheter replacement under fluoroscopic guidance.

Infected pancreatic necrosis is uniformly fatal if untreated and even after aggressive surgical intervention [36]

The time point for surgical or interventional procedures has changed in the last years. Mortality rate of patients undergoing early surgical necrosectomy reached 65%. Ideally, necrosectomy should be performed on day 30 after onset of symptoms. Delayed necrosectomy allows demarcation of the necrotic tissue [37]. One of the most difficult tasks is choosing the right time for intervention.

The evolution and advances in radiologic imaging and new developments of interventional radiology have demonstrated the advantages of mini-invasive treatment.

Percutaneous treatment in severe acute pancreatitis is directed at addressing local complications, such as abscesses, peripancreatic collections and infected necrosis, to postpone surgical intervention or even to obviate the need for surgical necrosectomy[33].

Percutaneous endoscopic necrosectomy requires insertion of a catheter under CT guidance into the necrotic retroperitoneal collection. The drain tract is dilated to 28 to 30 F to allow piecemeal necrosectomy at multiple endoscopic sessions with acceptable success and mortality rates [38].

The procedure is best suited for the stable patient but can be attempted in the critically ill patient as well [39].

In addition to catheter debridement, these patients also require care from a multidisciplinary team involving collaboration by internists and surgeons, as well as interventional radiologists, to manage their complex clinical picture [36].

4.2 Fine needle aspiration

Elevations in white blood count and temperature occur in both sterile and infected necrosis. Hence, it is not possible to distinguish these conditions clinically unless CT scan shows evidence of air in the retroperitoneum, but this is a rare findings [40 41 42] .

The use of FNA is controversial. It has been the practice of some authors to advocate early FNA to identify infection and determine which patients will benefit from necrosectomy.

Treatment strategies based on the presence of infection have led to the widespread advocacy for early fine needle aspiration (FNA) of the necrotic pancreas [37,41,43].

FNA can be guided by either computed tomography or ultrasonography and should be performed in patients who develop significant pancreatic necrosis and clinical signs of sepsis.

Bacterial tests including gram staining and culture of the aspiration material have a diagnostic sensitivity and specificity of 88 and 90%, respectively.

It is important that only those patients who develop clinical signs of sepsis should undergo FNA, since the procedure bears a potential risk of secondary infection [34,37,44]

Haney, Pappas et al. consider that clinical presentation is sufficient to make an operative determination. They argue that to examine the appropriate role of FNA, one must consider the timing of surgical intervention. Although early necrosectomy was once advocated, numerous more recent studies have confirmed that delayed surgical intervention is associated with better outcomes. The current consensus is for delayed surgical intervention, even in the setting of infected necrosis [37,41].

The critical argument against routine FNA, then, is that during this delay, the clinical course of the patient will readily predict who will need debridement and who will not [41].

4.3 Ultrasound - Guided puncture

This procedure is performed in patients in poor general condition in intensive care units with progressive deterioration of their general condition and suspected infected collection.

The puncture approach depends on the ultrasound, and should be performed using the best acoustic window possible. The needles used in the procedure are thin because they are only for diagnostic purposes.

When the puncture yields purulent fluid percutaneous drainage can be placed following the Seldinger technique.

4.4 CT guided puncture

It is performed in patients with progressive deterioration of general condition and suspected infected pancreatic fluid collection. An advantage of CT guided puncture is that it can be performed by different approaches: anterior, posterior, right or left lateral, or transgastric, according to the location of collections.

It is the method of choice in the presence of abdominal distention and deep fluid collection.

The aim of the procedure is to extract as much necrotic tissue as possible.

Catheters are removed when cavity size is small at fluoroscopy, no collection is noted on scan tomography, and catheter output has decreased to 15-30 mL per day.

4.5 Placement of drains

The placement of drains with ultrasound or CT guidance depends on the usage and customs of each operator. Undoubtedly, in the presence of abdominal distention and deep fluid collection the method of choice is computer-tomography guided puncture.

Indication for the procedure is the presence of infection in the collection that has been confirmed either by the presence of pus or a positive culture from the puncture.

Drainage site selection depends on the location of the infected collections; this decision can be made at the time of drainage or during the course of treatment. The size and number of catheters depends on the consistency of content and its location. Eight Fr or 8.5 Fr catheters can be used initially and be replaced with catheters up to 30 Fr; this replacement can be performed with fluoroscopic guidance.

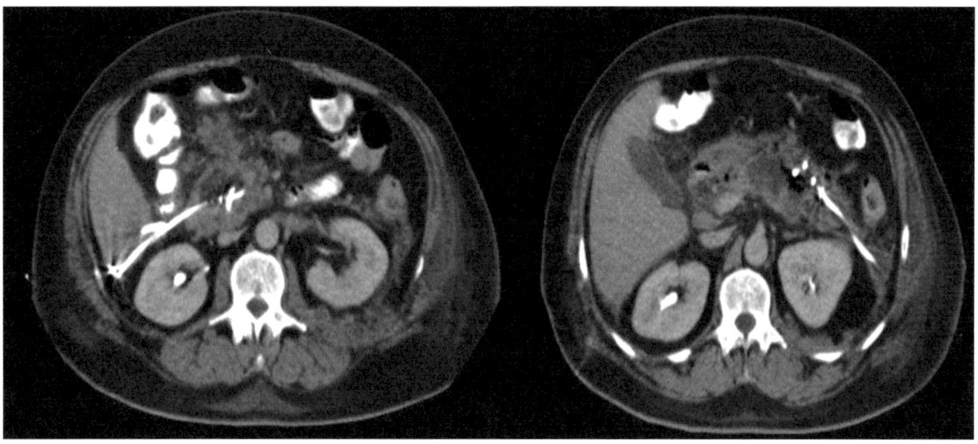

(A) Right lateral drainage (B) Left lateral drainage

Fig. 4.

4.6 Replacement of catheters up to 30 Fr with fluoroscopic guidance

It is important to assess the effectiveness of drainage catheters. When there are poor drainage areas, larger caliber drainage catheters up to 30 Fr can be placed under fluoroscopic guidance. They should be examined constantly according to the patient's clinical course and washed with saline when necessary. Performing a sonogram is useful. Dye is injected through the catheter; drainage catheters are considered sufficiently effective if the dye is evacuated completely leaving no residue.

When debris or poor drainage persists, the procedure should be attempted using catheters of increasing caliber, to reach 30 Fr diameter. A rigid Amplatz-type guidewire is placed through the existing catheter using the set of Amplatz dilators up to 30 Fr. The catheters are then fixed following the regular technique and can be flushed with saline solution when necessary.

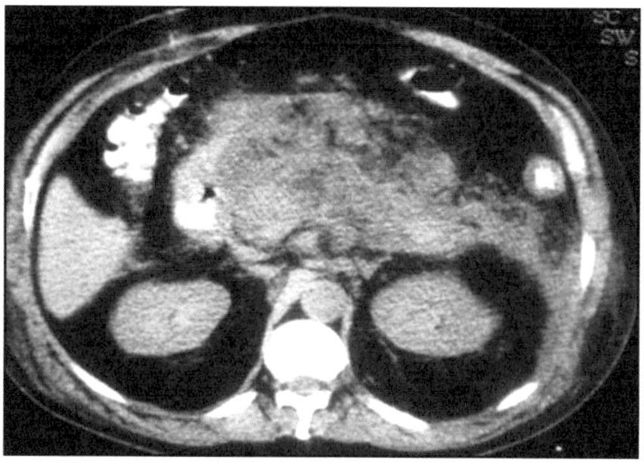

(A) CT on admission.

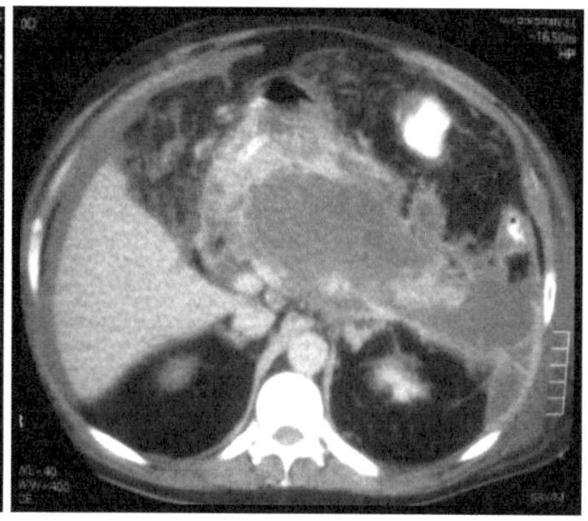

(B) 17 days post-admission

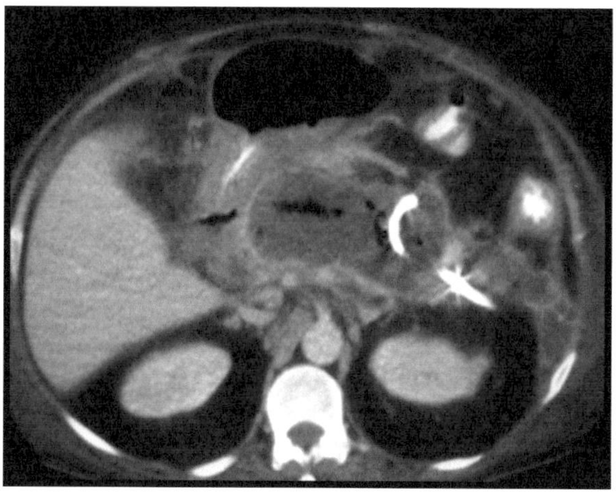

(C) Drainage at 34 days

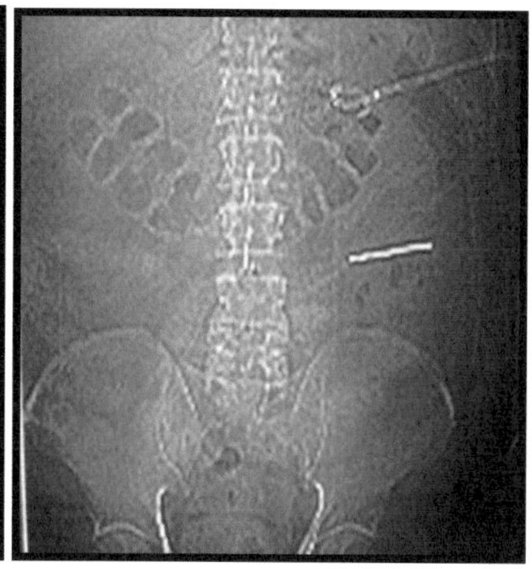

(D) 8.5 Fr Catheter

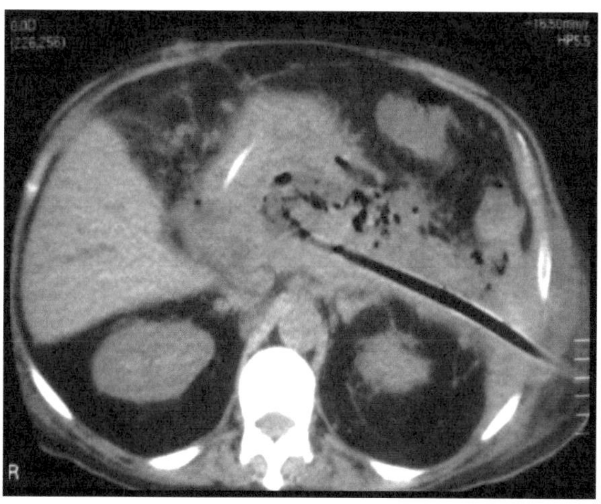

(E) At 58 days

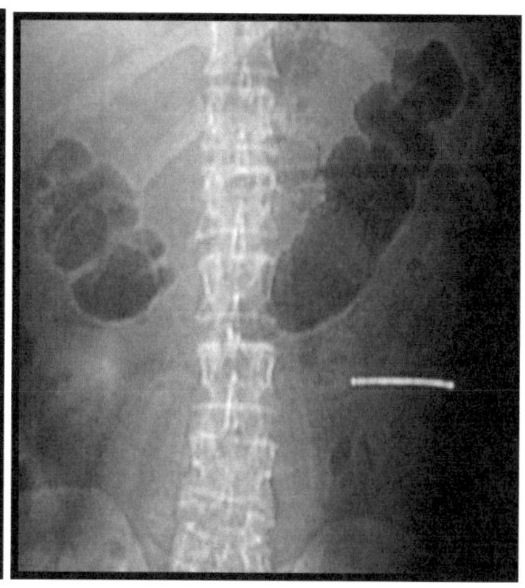

(F) 30 Fr Catheter

Fig. 5.

4.7 Multiple percutaneous Catheter Technique

Multiple catheters are often used simultaneously (Fig 5). One to five 10 to 16 Fr catheters are inserted under CT guidance into the pancreatic necrotic tissue. Aggressive irrigation is performed with saline when necessary, while the debris is removed by syringe suction. Lavage fluid is injected to fill the cavity and aspirated until all fluid is removed. When the catheter becomes occluded, it is removed under syringe suction [36] .

Stone baskets are used to remove large pieces of debris. This is repeated until the fluid becomes clear. Finally, a self-retaining catheter is left in the drainage cavity. The session is repeated 2 to 3 times per week [39]. The aim of the procedure is to extract as much necrotic tissue as possible.

All patients receive intravenous antibiotics appropriate to the organism grown in culture of the pancreatic fluid.

Catheters are removed when cavity size is small at fluoroscopy, no collection is noted on scan tomography, and catheter output has decreased to 15-30 mL per day.

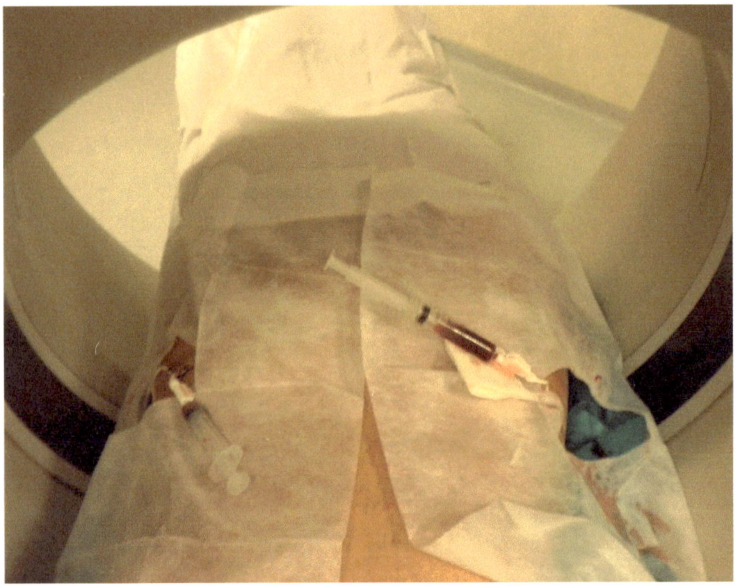

Fig. 6. Multiple drainage performed under CT scan guidance

4.8 Retroperitoneoscopy under fluoroscopic guidance

When collection persists after drainage, catheters can be replaced under fluoroscopic guidance. The procedure is performed under sedation following the Seldinger technique. A nephroscope equipped with two channels for viewing the inside the pancreatic collection is used. It is placed with a video camera connected to a monitor, and tweezers are inserted through the working-channel to remove necrotic and devitalized tissue. The major risk is hemorrhage. It is useful to perform the procedure under direct vision and fluoroscopic guidance, to view how far the ureterescope has reached. On completion of the session, the necrotic cavity is flushed and a 30Fr catheter is inserted.

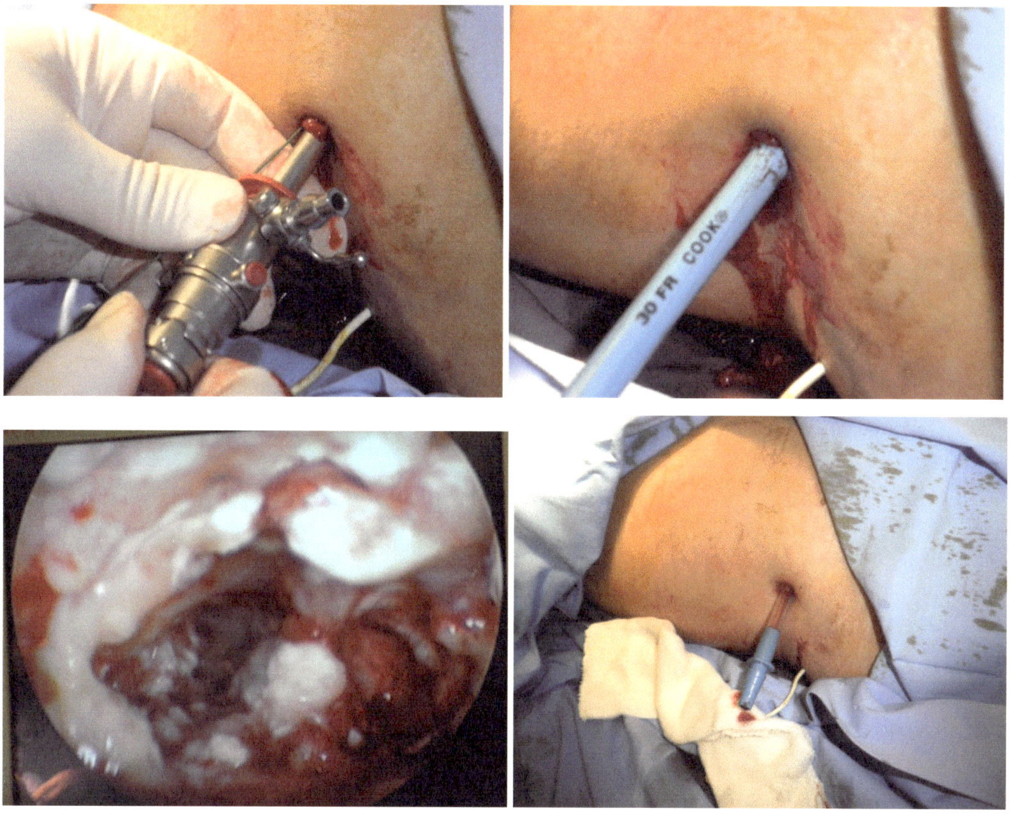

Fig. 7.

5. References

[1] Petrov MS, van Santvoort HC, Besselink MG, van der Heijden GJ, van Erpecum KJ, Gooszen HG. Early endoscopic retrograde cholangiopancreatography versus conservative management in acute biliary pancreatitis without cholangitis: a meta-analysis of randomized trials. Annals of surgery 2008;247:250-7.

[2] Cohen SA, Siegel JH. Endoscopic retrograde cholangiopancreatography and the pancreas: when and why? Surg Clin North Am 2001;81:321-8, x.

[3] Folsch UR, Nitsche R, Ludtke R, Hilgers RA, Creutzfeldt W. Early ERCP and papillotomy compared with conservative treatment for acute biliary pancreatitis. The German Study Group on Acute Biliary Pancreatitis. N Engl J Med 1997;336:237-42.

[4] Kozarek R. Role of ERCP in acute pancreatitis. Gastrointest Endosc 2002;56:S231-S6.

[5] Roston AD, Jacobson IM. Evaluation of the pattern of liver tests and yield of cholangiography in symptomatic choledocholithiasis: a prospective study. Gastrointest Endosc 1997;45:394-9.

[6] Cotton PB, Lehman G, Vennes J, et al. Endoscopic sphincterotomy complications and their management: an attempt at consensus. YMGE 1991;37:383-93.

[7] Romagnuolo J, Currie G. Noninvasive vs. selective invasive biliary imaging for acute biliary pancreatitis: an economic evaluation by using decision tree analysis. Gastrointest Endosc 2005;61:86-97.
[8] Banks PA, Freeman ML, Gastroenterology tPPCotACo. Practice Guidelines in Acute Pancreatitis. Am J Gastroenterol 2006;101:2379-400.
[9] Canlas KR, Branch MS. Role of endoscopic retrograde cholangiopancreatography in acute pancreatitis. World J Gastroenterol 2007;13:6314-20.
[10] Attasaranya S, Abdelaziz A, Lehman G. Endoscopic Management of Acute and Chronic Pancreatitis. Surgical Clinics of North America 2007;87:1379-402.
[11] Whitcomb DC. Clinical practice. Acute pancreatitis. N Engl J Med 2006;354:2142-50.
[12] Wang GJ, Gao CF, Wei D, Wang C, Ding SQ. Acute pancreatitis: etiology and common pathogenesis. World J Gastroenterol 2009;15:1427-30.
[13] Acosta JM, Ledesma CL. Gallstone migration as a cause of acute pancreatitis. N Engl J Med 1974;290:484-7.
[14] Acosta JM, Katkhouda N, Debian KA, Groshen SG, Tsao-Wei DD, Berne TV. Early Ductal Decompression Versus Conservative Management for Gallstone Pancreatitis With Ampullary Obstruction. Annals of Surgery 2006;243:33-40.
[15] Oria A, Cimmino D, Ocampo C, et al. Early endoscopic intervention versus early conservative management in patients with acute gallstone pancreatitis and biliopancreatic obstruction: a randomized clinical trial. Annals of surgery 2007;245:10-7.
[16] Neoptolemos JP, Carr-Locke DL, London NJ, Bailey IA, James D, Fossard DP. Controlled trial of urgent endoscopic retrograde cholangiopancreatography and endoscopic sphincterotomy versus conservative treatment for acute pancreatitis due to gallstones. Lancet 1988;2:979-83.
[17] Fan ST, Lai EC, Mok FP, Lo CM, Zheng SS, Wong J. Early treatment of acute biliary pancreatitis by endoscopic papillotomy. N Engl J Med 1993;328:228-32.
[18] Mark DH, Lefevre F, Flamm CR, Aronson N. Evidence-based assessment of ERCP in the treatment of pancreatitis. Gastrointest Endosc 2002;56:S249-S54.
[19] Attasaranya S, Fogel EL, Lehman GA. Choledocholithiasis, Ascending Cholangitis, and Gallstone Pancreatitis. Medical Clinics of North America 2008;92:925-60.
[20] Yusoff IF, Barkun JS, Barkun AN. Diagnosis and management of cholecystitis and cholangitis. Gastroenterol Clin North Am 2003;32:1145-68.
[21] Park SY, Park CH, Cho SB, et al. The safety and effectiveness of endoscopic biliary decompression by plastic stent placement in acute suppurative cholangitis compared with nasobiliary drainage. Gastrointest Endosc 2008;68:1076-80.
[22] Lee DW, Chan AC, Lam YH, et al. Biliary decompression by nasobiliary catheter or biliary stent in acute suppurative cholangitis: a prospective randomized trial. Gastrointest Endosc 2002;56:361-5.
[23] Sharma BC, Kumar R, Agarwal N, Sarin SK. Endoscopic biliary drainage by nasobiliary drain or by stent placement in patients with acute cholangitis. Endoscopy 2005;37:439-43.
[24] Freeman ML, Nelson DB, Sherman S, et al. Complications of endoscopic biliary sphincterotomy. N Engl J Med 1996;335:909-18.

[25] Akashi R, Kiyozumi T, Tanaka T, Sakurai K, Oda Y, Sagara K. Mechanism of pancreatitis caused by ERCP. Gastrointest Endosc 2002;55:50-4.
[26] Cennamo V, Fuccio L, Zagari RM, et al. Can early precut implementation reduce endoscopic retrograde cholangiopancreatography-related complication risk? Meta-analysis of randomized controlled trials. Endoscopy 2010;42:381-8.
[27] Cannon JW, Callery MP, Vollmer CM, Jr. Diagnosis and management of pancreatic pseudocysts: what is the evidence? J Am Coll Surg 2009;209:385-93.
[28] Barthet M, Lamblin G, Gasmi M, Vitton V, Desjeux A, Grimaud JC. Clinical usefulness of a treatment algorithm for pancreatic pseudocysts. Gastrointest Endosc 2008;67:245-52.
[29] Bergman S, Melvin WS. Operative and nonoperative management of pancreatic pseudocysts. Surg Clin North Am 2007;87:1447-60, ix.
[30] Reddy DN, Gupta R, Lakhtakia S, Jalal PK, Rao GV. Use of a novel transluminal balloon accessotome in transmural drainage of pancreatic pseudocyst (with video). Gastrointest Endosc 2008;68:362-5.
[31] Varadarajulu S, Christein JD, Tamhane A, Drelichman ER, Wilcox CM. Prospective randomized trial comparing EUS and EGD for transmural drainage of pancreatic pseudocysts (with videos). Gastrointest Endosc 2008;68:1102-11.
[32] Antillon MR, Shah RJ, Stiegmann G, Chen YK. Single-step EUS-guided transmural drainage of simple and complicated pancreatic pseudocysts. Gastrointest Endosc 2006;63:797-803.
[33] Van Baal MC, van Santvoort HC, Bollen TL, Bakker OJ, Besselink MG, Gooszen HG. Systematic review of percutaneous catheter drainage as primary treatment for necrotizing pancreatitis. The British journal of surgery 2011;98:18-27.
[34] Uhl W, Warshaw A, Imrie C, et al. IAP Guidelines for the Surgical Management of Acute Pancreatitis. Pancreatology 2002; 2:565-73.
[35] Ross A, Gluck M, Irani S, et al. Combined endoscopic and percutaneous drainage of organized pancreatic necrosis. Gastrointest Endosc 2010;71:79-84.
[36] Echenique AM, Sleeman D, Yrizarry J, et al. Percutaneous catheter-directed debridement of infected pancreatic necrosis: results in 20 patients. J Vasc Interv Radiol 1998;9:565-71.
[37] Schneider L, Buchler MW, Werner J. Acute pancreatitis with an emphasis on infection. Infect Dis Clin North Am 2010;24:921-41, viii.
[38] Fotoohi M, Traverso LW. Pancreatic necrosis: paradigm of a multidisciplinary team. Adv Surg 2006;40:107-18.
[39] Sleeman D, Levi DM, Cheung MC, et al. Percutaneous lavage as primary treatment for infected pancreatic necrosis. J Am Coll Surg 2011;212:748-52; discussion 52-4.
[40] Banks PA, Freeman ML. Practice guidelines in acute pancreatitis. Am J Gastroenterol 2006;101:2379-400.
[41] Haney JC, Pappas TN. Necrotizing pancreatitis: diagnosis and management. Surg Clin North Am 2007;87:1431-46, ix.
[42] Jury RP, Tariq N. Minimally invasive and standard surgical therapy for complications of pancreatitis and for benign tumors of the pancreas and duodenal papilla. Med Clin North Am 2008;92:961-82, x.

[43] Wada K, Takada T, Hirata K, et al. Treatment strategy for acute pancreatitis. J Hepatobiliary Pancreat Sci 2010;17:79-86.

[44] Cappell MS. Acute Pancreatitis: Etiology, Clinical Presentation, Diagnosis, and Therapy. Medical Clinics of North America 2008;92:889-923.

11

Intra-Abdominal Hypertension and Abdominal Compartment Syndrome in Critically Ill Surgical Patients (Special Findings in Severe Acute Pancreatitis)

Zsolt Bodnár
Department of General Surgery, Hospital de Torrevieja, Spain

„...a clinical entity that had been ignored for far too long"
(Ivatury RR-Sugerman HJ)

1. Introduction

Intra-abdominal hypertension (IAH) and abdominal compartment syndrome (ACS) are very frequent findings in patients with severe acute pancreatitis. The causing factors are the retroperitoneal inflammation, paralytic ileus, ascites and the serious visceral edema due to massive fluid resuscitation, which leads to increased intra-abdominal pressure (IAP), early organ disfunction with IAH and finally ACS. Several publications conclude that this clinical entity can appear in high-risk surgical patients (severe acute pancreatitis) within the first 12 hours of the admission to intensive care unit. In these cases the mortality rate is extremely high. That is why we have to pay attention to make the correct and early diagnosis, treatment and follow-up of the severe acute pancreatitis (1-2).

The ACS is a rediscovered life threatening clinical entity. The aim of this chapter is to show the definitions, ethiology, pathophysiology, diagnosis and treatment of this serious, not only surgical problem.

The mortality due to the abdominal compartment syndrome is extremely high (38-71%). It can be defined as adverse physiologic consequences that occur as a result of an acute increase in the IAP. The most common causes are retroperitoneal haemorrhage, visceral oedema, pancreatitis, bowel obstruction, tense ascites, peritonitis, tumor. The affected systems are cardiovascular, pulmonary, renal, central nervous systems and splanchnic organs. The gold standard diagnostic method is the continuous intra-abdominal pressure monitoring. The fundamental ways of the treatment are the adequate fluid resuscitation and surgical decompression (1-2).

Finally we would like to show the special findings of the IAH and ACS according to the problem of severe acute pancreatitis.

2. Historical highlights

There are three big eras in the history of ACS.

The first is the evolution in the understanding of the pathophysiology of the compartment syndrome in general. (The first case of the muscular compartment syndrome was described by Hamilton in 1850.)

The second was the era of the experimental studies for measure the IAP. (different devices and techniques by different locations, for example through the bladder (uterus or rectum).

The third is the era of the understanding and management of the basic problem which was started with the work of Sir Heneage Ogilvie who performed the first laparostomies and described the beneficial effect of this process in the management of giant abdominal war wounds (3).

The real story of ACS started in the second part of the XIX. century (4-5). First, in 1863 Marey published his experiences about the increased abdominal pressure's effects. In 1865 the first intra-abdominal pressure measurement via rectum was performed in Germany. Between 1870 and 1900 numerous attempts were carried out to measure IAP and to study its influence to vital functions (Bert, Schroeder, Schatz, Wendt, Quinke, Heinricius).

In 1911 Emerson published his article titled "The intra-abdominal pressure" (6). In 1940 the first laparostomy was performed to reduce the increased IAP (Ogilvie). The first description of the importance of staged abdominal closure was published in 1948. (Gross). In 1951 Baggot claimed that abdominal closure in case of distension can cause death.

In the 70's several teams carried out investigations on laparoscopy and effects of pneumoperitoneum on IAP. In 1982 Harman and his team proved the harmful effects of IAP on renal function and significance of decompression in these cases. In 1984 Kron was the first who described the compartment syndrome but didn't use the definition itself (4). Also he used the method of pressure measurement via urinary catheter that became commonly used in 1989 though the base of this method was described by Oderbrecht 100 years earlier. Later this technique was developed by several scientists (Iberti, Sugrue, Malbrain, Balogh and their colleagues) (7-11). In 1989 terminus technicus "abdominal compartment syndrome" was created by Fietsam and his team (5). The two articles that had opened the decade of ACS were published in 1995 and 1996 (12-13). In the previous ten years several teams started to investigate the monitoring techniques of intra-abdominal pressure. The first worldwide conference was organized 6-8 December 2004, in Noosa (Queensland) in Australia and WSACS (World Society of Abdominal Compartment Syndrome) was established at the same time. This society now counts numerous members from all over the world.

3. Definitions

3.1 Consensus definitions

To understand perfectly the question of the ACS it is very important to make clear of the basic concepts. The below mentioned consensus definitions were made by the 2004 International ACS Consensus Definitions Conference of the WSACS firstly in December of 2004 in Noosa (Australia) and they were rediscussed in 2007 in the Antwerp (Belgium) during the Third World Congress of the Abdominal Compartment Syndrome (WCACS):

Intra-abdominal pressure (IAP): is the steady-state pressure concealed within the abdominal cavity. (14-15)

Intra-abdominal hypertension (IAH): is defined by a sustained or repeated pathological elevation in IAP ≥ 12 mmHg. (14-15)

Abdominal Compartment Syndrome (ACS): is defined as a sustained IAP > 20 mmHg (with or without an APP < 60 mmHg, where APP = MAP - IAP and APP = abdominal perfusion pressure; MAP = mean arterial pressure) that is associated with new organ dysfunction / failure. (14-15)

(The normal range of the IAP is between the 0 and 5 mmHg, and it significantly depends on Body Mass Index (BMI) (9,16).)

3.2 Classification

IAH is graded as follows:

- grade I. 12-15 mm Hg
- grade II. 16-20 mm Hg
- grade III. 21-25 mm Hg
- grade IV. IAP > 25 mm Hg

(IAP may be defined with several units. To avoid misunderstanding IAP is measured in mmHg according to the international consensus (1 mmHg = 1.36 $H_2$0cm = 0.13 kPa)). (1-2)

3.3 Etiopathogenesis

Primary ACS: is a condition associated with injury or disease in the abdominopelvic region that frequently requiers early surgical or radiological intervention. (for example: peritonitis, pancreatitis, bowel obstruction, haemorrhage, trauma, etc.) (1-2)

Secundary ACS: conditions that do not originate from the abdominal cavity, generaly caused by surgical activity (for example: abdominal closure under distension, extremely large abdominal hernias, operation of bowel obstruction). (1-2)

The incidency of IAH is 2-30% and of the ACS is 1-16% in general surgical syndromes and in the ethiopathogenesis are acute and chronic causes:

Acute (1-2):

- **spontaneous:** peritonitis, abdominal abscess, bowel obstruction, ruptured aortic aneurysm, tension pneumoperitoneum, acute pancreatitis, mesenteric thrombosis
- **postoperative:** peritonitis, abscessus, bowel obstruction, intra-abdominal haemorrhage
- **trauma:** intraperitoneal and retroperitoneal haemorrhage, visceral oedema after cardiopulmonary resuscitation
- **iatrogenic:** laparoscopy, abdominal closure under distension

Chronic (1-2):

ascites, enlarged intra-abdominal cyst, long term peritoneal dialysis, pregnancy, extreme obesity

Chronic and slow increasing of IAP can be compensated by the human organism and the abdomen adaptates for increased load, so ACS won't develop in this case.

Incidency

Incidency of IAH is 2 - 30 % (10,18) in general surgical syndromes and the incidency of ACS is 1 - 16 % (17-19). If intensive care unit (ICU) treatment is necessary, the development of ACS is expectable in the first 12 hours (11,18).

Risk factors for IAH / ACS (14-15)

Diminished abdominal wall compliance:

- acute respiratory failure, especially with elevated intrathoracic pressure
- abdominal surgery with primary fascial or tight closure
- major trauma / burns
- prone positioning, head of bed > 30 degrees
- high body mass index (BMI), central obesity

Increased intra-luminal contents:

- gastroparesis
- ileus
- colonic pseudo-obstruction

Increased abdominal contents:

- hemoperitoneum / pneumoperitoneum
- ascites / liver dysfunction

Capillary leak / fluid resuscitation:

- acidosis (pH < 7.2)
- hypotension
- hypothermia (core temperature < 33 C°)
- polytransfusion (> 10 units of blood / 24 h)
- coagulopathy (platelets < 55000 / mm^3 or prothrombin time (PT) > 15 seconds or partial thromboplastin time (PTT) > 2 times normal or international standardised ratio (INR) > 1.5)
- massive fluid resuscitation (> 5 l / 24 h)
- pancreatitis
- oliguria
- sepsis
- major trauma /burns
- damage control laparotomy

4. Pathophysiological changes during the increased IAP

IAH can cause serious complications in any organ (**Table 1**). Without effective therapy / intervention it can occurr multi organ failure (MOF) by affected cardiovascular, respiratory, central nervous system and renal function. De Waele and his colleagues published that there was a 94% incidence of respiratory, 94% cardiovascular and 89% of renal failure among patients with IAH (where IAP > 12 mmHg). (1,2,12,13,16,18):

Cardiovascular system

The increased IAP reduces the cardiac functions. The increased pressure lowers the end-diastolic volume as well as the venous return from the inferior caval vein, portal vein and superior caval vein. The systemic vascular resistency increases because of the compressed capillary system and the afterload will be consequently elevated. All of these effects result cardiac insufficiency and compensatoric tachycardia (19,20).

IAP = 0-9 mmHg	IAP = 10-15 mmHg	IAP = 16-25 mmHg	IAP = 26-40 mmHg
cytokines release	circulation of the abdominal wall decreases with 42%	significant reduction of splanchnic circulation and venous return	„hemodinamic collapse"
increased capillary permeability	significant reduction in the circulation of other abdominal organs	increase in systemic vascular resistance (SVR), central venous pressure (CVP), peak airway pressure (PAWP)	fatal acidosis
fluid content of the „third space" expands	local acidosis	total respiratory capacity (TRC), vital capacity (VC) lowered due to pulmonary compression	hypoxia hypercapnia
decreased venous return as well as preload	free radical release	hypoxia hypercapnia	anuria
early effects on the central nervous system	bacterial translocation throught intestinal mucosa	circulation of intestinal mucosa decreases with 61%	circulation of coeliac artery is reduced to 58%
		increasing acidosis	circulation of superior mesenteric artery is reduced to 39%
		renal failure: oliguria, anuria	circulation of renal artery is reduced to 30%
		disturbance of central nervous system	circulation of abdominal muscles lowered with 80% (infection, wound-healing disturbances)

Table 1. Physiological changes during increased IAP (Wolfe, 2005)

Respiratory system

Due to the increased IAP the diaphragm will be shifted to cranial direction on both sides causing the reduction of pulmonary volume and cardiac function. Without intervention acidosis and hypoxia will occur (12,19,20).

Renal function

The renal perfusion decreases related to the reduced cardiac function and direct compression of renal arteries and kidneys, with consequent oligo- and anuria. IAP 15 - 20 mmHg results in oliguria, and above 30 mmHg it causes anuria (13,19,20,21).

Splanchnic circu1ation

The splanchnic, mesenteric and hepatic perfusion decreases above 15 mmHg of IAP. It is a well-known and proved fact that splanchnic and hepatic circulation has an autoregulation. The basis of this autoregulation is the renin-angiotensin system, the HABR (hepatic arterial buffer response) and vasopressin. Though numerous clinical studies proved that this complex system could compensate the consequencies of insuffient arterial circulation, venous return, decreased preload due to the increased IAP only for few hours. When it worns out it causes irreversible destruction of the intestinal mucosa and the liver. This is why decompression is essential in the ACS's therapy! The reduced circulation results in a mucosal ischaemia and bacterial translocations. Intestinal bacteria and their toxic products result sepsis and multiple organ failure (MOF) (22-24) (**Figure 1**). Endotoxins or exotoxins cause a chain reaction of mediators that can damage either the pathogen and the human organism and if it becomes irreversible can cause death. This progressive clinical syndrome is a manifestation of multiple organic dysfunction or failure (ARDS - Adult Respiratory Distress Syndrome, renal failure, DIC -Disseminant Intravascular Coagulation). If it progresses the symptoms of multiple organ failure and septic shock with hypotonia will appear. Since this phenomenon occurs as a consequence of not only infections but pancreatitis, burning and ACS, the definition of SIRS (Systemic Inflammatory Response Syndrome) was introduced in the 90's (22).

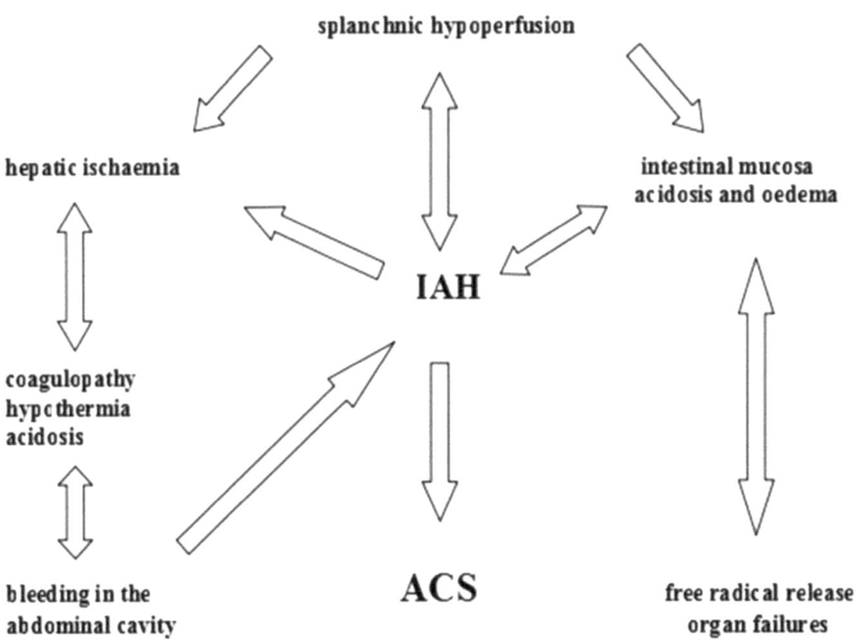

Fig. 1. Effects of increased intra-abdominal pressure on the splanchnic circulation (IAH = intra-abdominal hypertension, ACS = abdominal compartment syndrome)

Abdominal wall circulation

The reduced abdominal wall circulation results in insufficient wound-healing, higher possibility of inflammation and dehiscency (25).

Central Nervous System

The increased IAP lowers the intracranial pressure secondarily due to the compression of jugular venous system and of the thoracic region (26).

5. Laboratory changes of inflammatory markers during the increased IAP in patients with acute pancreatitis

The technique of IAP measurement is accurate, precise, reproducible and cost-effective. However laboratory measures for monitoring of IAH have not been defined. The immunological changes were examined in a study group of 65 patients with acute pancreatitis (IAP > 12 mmHg) in one of our studies. Serum adenosine, IL-1β, IL-2, IL-4, IL-10, TNFα and IFNγ were measured. Significant correlations were found among IAP-adenosine values and IAP-IL-10 values providing new tools for the laboratory monitoring of IAH as well as further understanding of the pathomechanism contributing to ACS.

We present here the historical diagram **(Figure 2)** from one of our preliminary studies which shows the very important correlation between IAP and adenosine:

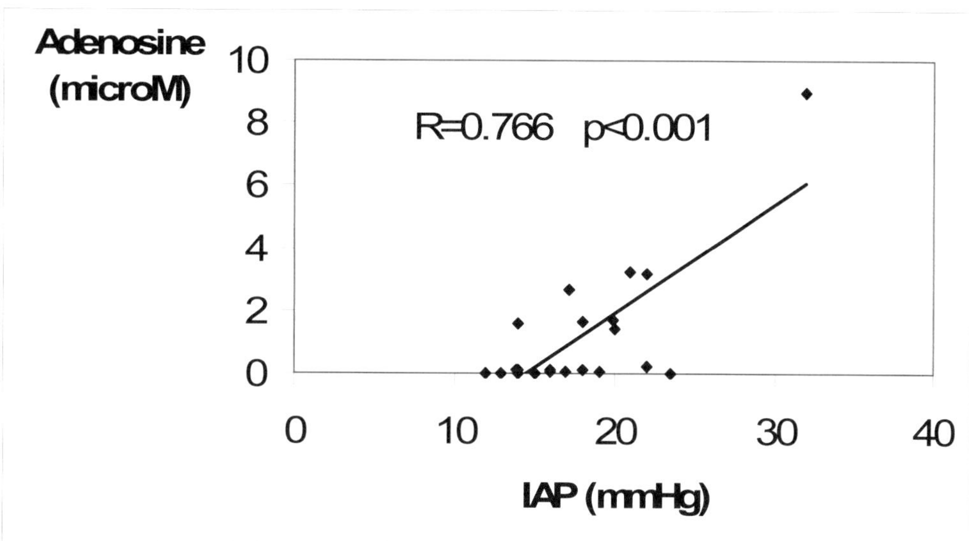

Fig. 2. Significant correlations between IAP and adenosine level

The pathophysiology of IAP is still poorly understood, including the contributions of adenosine and cytokines (27). Adenosine contributes to the maintenance of hepatosplachnic blood flow (28) and hypoxia results in increased serum adenosine concentrations (22,29). Such alterations may result in enlargement of the abdominal organ blood volume and potentially contribute to the pathology associated with increased IAP and ACS. In addition to its contribution to maintenance of hepatosplanchnic blood flow, adenosine is an endogenous regulator of cellular functions including neurotransmission (30), local circulation (31) and the modulation of inflammation (32-35).

Previous studies in porcine and rabbit models demonstrated that increased IAP was associated with reduced gastric intramucosal pH (36) and increased levels of IL-1β, IL-6, TNFα, and CRP (37).

In our own studies, we investigated the associations of serum levels of adenosine, C-reactive protein (CRP) and various cytokines (interleukin 1β [IL-1β], IL-2, IL-4, IL-10, tumour necrosis factor α [TNFα] and interferon γ [IFNγ]) with IAP in surgical patients with or without elevated IAP.

Our observations derive from surgical patients being treated in an intensive care unit and therefore, likely represents the greater degree of individual variation expected in human populations as compared to homogeneous experimental models. Thus, while cytokines such as IL-1β, IL-6, TNFα and CRP may have been significantly associated with IAP in animal models (37), they were not significantly related in our study. On the other hand, our results showed a highly significant relationship of both IL-10 and adenosine with IAP in a heterogeneous human population, suggesting that they may be better indicators of IAP in this case.

We found a robust linear correlation between IAP $\geq$15 mmHg and serum levels of adenosine and IL-10. While we believe that this relationship may be helpful in monitoring the effects of IAP lowering therapies, we also believe that the increase in serum adenosine level may directly contribute to the development and maintenance of IAH-ACS.

We propose that a strong relationship may exist between the advancement of hypoxia and splanchnic ischemia, inducing the release of adenosine from the hypoxaemic tissues of the gut (22,28,29), resulting in splanchnic vasodilatation and subsequent increase in IAP. This relationship is cyclic in nature and if left undisturbed, results in a 'vitious circle' leading ultimately to ACS. Thus, while adenosine itself is a very potent anti-inflammatory molecule (33-35), in the development of IAH-ACS, elevated adenosine concentrations cause renal arterial dysfunction (38), ultimately causing collapse of kidney function manifested by decreased renin production and blood pressure and increased blood urea and creatinine concentrations (39-40). In this context, the renal failure resulting from increased adenosine concentrations is a main cause of multi-organ failure (41-42) and damage of vegetative splanchnic ganglia (43-44). The elevated serum IL-10 levels appear partly to be the direct consequence of adenosine stimulating monocyte secretion of IL-10 (34), but IL-10 can be produced also by other inflammatory cells. In the **Figure 3** we propose a model describing the potential role of adenosine in the pathomechanism of IAH-ACS.

Our observations show that the laboratory determination of serum adenosine and/or IL-10 may be helpful for initial screening or grading of IAH as well as for monitoring progress in therapeutic reduction of IAP. As the determination of IL-10 by ELISA is an easily automated method, it may be preferred to the measurement of adenosine by HPLC, particularly, during follow-up of surgical, trauma or medical patients with high risk of IAH or ACS.

In conclusion, we report that plasma/serum concentrations of adenosine and IL-10 are strongly and linearly correlated to the values of IAP >15 mmHg (Grade II IAH) in surgical patients. Thus, monitoring of serum adenosine and IL-10 concentrations may offer significant insights into the progression and treatment of IAP, particularly, in patient populations at risk of IAH and ACS. The role of adenosine in the pathomechanism of IAH-ACS offers a new insight into this severe clinical syndrome (45-46).

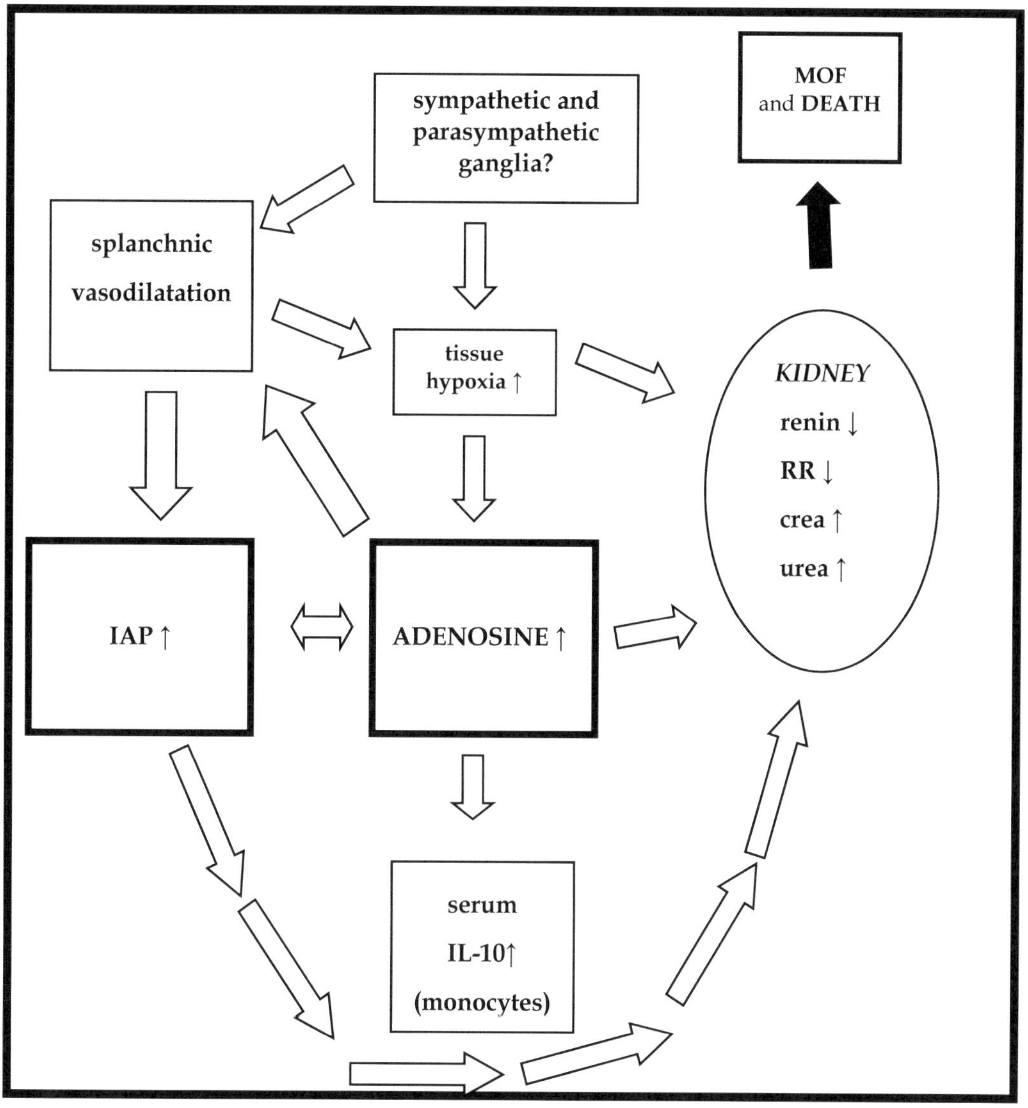

(RR = Riva Rocci (blood tension), Crea = creatinine, MOF = multi organ failure)

Fig. 3. The role of adenosine in the proposed model of the pathomechanism of ACS

6. Diagnostic methods

Numerous investigations proved that only the physical examination of the abdomen to recognise ACS is inappropriate (11). Detection of ACS and elevated intra-abdominal pressure is based on standardized measurements of IAP. Practically IAP is detectable in every region of the abdomen (12,16,47,48).

Direct technique:

- during laparoscopy (laparo-insufflator)
- with an intraperitoneal cateter and transducer
- with a metal cannula lead into the intraperitoneal space and connected to a manometer

Indirect technique:

- pressure measurement of inferior caval vein
- measurement throught nasogastric tube
- measurement of vaginal pressure
- measurement of rectal pressure
- measurement of urinary bladder's pressure

It seems that the most reliable and the less invasive method is the transvesical technique (7,8,13). It is based on the fact that IAP is equal with intravesical pressure. Filling the urinary bladder with 50 ml saline serum ensures that the pressure will be translocated to the catheter wich is clamped during the procedure. The pressure inside the catheter measurable by connecting a T-tube or inserting a sterile needle (Sugrue technique) (12). The T-tube is connected to a monitor via a transducer or to the system used to measure the central venous pressure (pressure of the liquid column). The intravesical technique's results correlated with the direct (laparoscopic insufflator) method. The intravesical way of measuring was more accurate than the gastric or rectal way which are very position depending. Animal-testing proved that the pressure of inferior caval vein is correlating with the vesical pressure but it is much more invasive and can be the source of serious complications - like other direct methods. Additionally urinary catheter is required in all critically ill patients. The intravesical method for measuring IAP was originally described by Kron (4), and then validated by Iberti and his team (8). It was simplificated by Sugrue and his team: a T-tube was inserted to the catheter. Since in this method it is unnecessary to prick the aperture, the number of infectious complications decreased. This method is simple but may be time consuming - because in case of critical patients approximately 7 minutes are needed for the procedure at least four times a day. Having intermittent character the standard IAP measuring is unable to give information about the length of IAH. To eliminate insufficiencies (like labour-intensive, fluctuating character) Balogh and his colleagues developed and validated the continuous abdominal pressure measurement (CIAPM) technique (11). Continuous intra-abdominal pressure measurement requires only a three-way catheter and a transducer, and it is unnecessary to clamp the catheter and fill the urinary bladder („Balogh-Sugrue technique"). This method is used successfully to follow up critically ill patients in our department.

7. Treatment

To solve the problem of this serious clinical entity there are two opportunities: non-surgical (evacuate intraluminal contents and intra-abdominal space occupying lesions, improve abdominal wall compliance, optimize fluid administration and systemic/regional perfusion) and surgical (early decompression) management.

Non-surgical management (14-15)

The treatment of ACS always means surgical decompression, but sometimes or if we have to treat only IAH we have the possibility for non-surgical way. The success is strongly depends on the etiology of the current IAH / ACS.

The main fields of the conservative management are:

- **evacuate intraluminal contents:** insert nasogastric and / or rectal tube
  initiate gastro- / coloprokinetic agents
  minimize enteral nutrition
  administration of enemas
  consider colonoscopic decompression
  discontinue enteral nutrition
- **evacuate intra-abdominal space occupying lesions:** abdominal ultrasound to identify
  abdominal CT to identify
  percutaneous catheter drainage
  consider surgical evacuation
- **improve abdominal wall compliance:** ensure adequate sedation / analgesia
  remove constrictive dressings
  avoid prone position, head of bed > 20 degree
  consider reverse Trendelenberg position
  consider neuromuscular blockade
- **optimize fluid administration:** avoid excessive fluid resuscitation
  aim for zero to negative fluid balance by day 3
  resuscitate using hypertonic fluids, colloids
  fluid removal through judicious diuresis
  consider hemodialysis / ultrafiltration
- **optimize systemic / regional perfusion**: goal-directed fluid resuscitation
  maintain APP (APP > 60 mmHg)
  hemodynamic monitoring to guide resuscitation
  vasoactive medications to keep APP > 60 mmHg

If IAP > 25 mmHg (and/or APP < 50 mmHg) and new organ dysfunction is present, patient's IAH / ACS is refractory to medical management. Strongly consider surgical abdominal decompression.

During the non-surgical management the CIAPM is strongly recommended!

Surgical management (14-15)

The surgical management of the IAH / ACS always means decompressing laparotomy with temporary abdominal closure.

If the patient has etiology for IAH / ACS it is very important to check the IAP continuously. When we have the criteria of ACS (see in the consensus definitions) we have to make the urgent decompression.

From now on it is important to continue with medical treatments and fluid resuscitation to reduce IAP and stabilize our patient. Having APP more than 60 mmHg and IAP < 12 mmHg consistently means that IAH has resolved.

If we have APP > 60 mmHg and IAP > 12 mmHg we have to go on with the non-surgical way. But in case of APP < 60 mmHg we have to perform / revise decompression again.

During the non-surgical management the CIAPM is strongly recommended!

Reconstruction after open abdomen management

After decompression it is necessary to consider the way and the time of closure.

The main possibilities (13,16,49,50,51):

- **primer closure**
- **primer skin or fascial closure** (Towel Clip Closure, direct suture)
- **temporary abdominal closure (TAC) technique**: let the abdomen open replacing it with tissue friendly mesh or other material temporarily (Bogota bag, VAC-Pac / vacuum-assisted closure, Gore-Tex patch, Whitman patch, biological patches, skin graft)
- **covering the abdominal organs with omentum** which may be epithelized in the future
- **staged abdominal closure** (elective hernias)

The closure is possible when the general condition is stable (24-48 hours) or after the definitive recovering (sometimes 6-12 months later).

The aim is to prevent abdominal distension, though an enormous elective hernia will be generated.

8. Special field: Pancreatitis and the ACS

In the last few decades the intra-abdominal hypertension and the abdominal compartment syndrome has arrived to get a special attendence in non-traumatologic patients. One of these cases is the ACS caused by severe acut pancreatitis. By the recent publications the number of acute and chronic pancreatitis is increasing. On one hand it is due to evaluation of the radiological diagnostic techniques, on the other hand we have more possibility to treat the severe cases. In spite of the fact, the successfull management of severe acut pancreatitis still needs an interdiscipline cooperation.

Clinical course

The aim of this chapter is not describing the clinics, diagnosis and treatment of acute pancreatitis, it is done by the authors of other chapters. But to understand the relation between IAH / ACS and pancreatitis I would like to shortly summarise the leading findings in the clinical picture:

The main symptom is the abdominal pain that usually starts in the gastric region but rapidly spreads to the complete abdomen. Often accompained with nausea, vomiting and paralytic ileus. Treating with minor analgesics often fails. In serious cases signs of shock like hypotension, tachycardia and cold sweat can be present. The paralytic ileus starts from the duodenum and jejunum and expand to the colon due to intensive fat necrosis and venous bowel congestion. Liberation of active pancreatic enzymes causes alterations in liver, kidneys and lungs and as the consequence of shock we face with acute renal failure.

A serious complication of pancreatitis is acute lung failure. The frequency depends on the severity of the basic disease.

Patients with imminent and manifest severe cases must be under continuous observation in the intensive care unit. The circulatory parameters, blood pressure and pulse rate, palpation and auscultation of the abdomen, supervision of fluid intake and output, central venous pressure and laboratory values of haemoglobin and haematocrit, the number of leucocytes, amylase levels in the serum and urine and/or lipase in the serum, serum calcium, blood glucose daily profile, serum potassium, urea, creatinine in the serum, arterial pO_2 pressure, acid-base-balance and sonography of the upper abdomen, the latter in 1-3 day intervals, are especially suitable for patient monitoring.

Although the acute necrotizing inflammation (except biliary causes) can be controlled by conservative treatments in most cases, surgical intervention often becomes necessary under emergency conditions.

The indication for early surgery applies upon failure of conservative treatment: the leading clinical symptoms during therapy inferred are: peritonitis, ileus, septic shock, MOF, incontrolable pain.

Due to an increase in the intra-abdominal volume the diaphragm is pushed upward. Compression of the thoracic space results in a restrictive ventilatory disorder. (And we are facing with Abdominal Compartment Syndrome!!!)

As the transverse colon is particulary affected and toxins from the large bowel can have adverse affects on the course of the disease.

In these cases of the ACS urgent laparostomy is recommended. The laparotomy remains wide open and is only covered by a foil (Bogota Bag or VAC-Pac). This allows repeated peritoneal lavage and necrosectomy too. The prolonged inflammatory process in the abdomen and the risk of recurrent ACS favors the use of gradual closure or delayed reconstruction of the abdominal wall. The early recognition of the syndrome and the wide decompression are crucial factors of the treatment of this very serious clinical enthity (52).

Although the above mentioned clinical findings of the severe acute pancreatitis are almost the same as we can see in patients suffering from ACS but do not confuse ACS with acute pancreatitis while it is only one of the possible causes of this serious symptoms. The two entities are very similar, this is the cause why the ACS is often late diagnosed and untreated which leads to early organ failure.

The current estimate of the prevalence of IAH in severe acute pancreatitis is about 40%, with about 10% overall progressing to ACS associated with increased hospital mortality rates. In the majority of cases, the development of IAH is rapid. The agressive fluid resuscitation and the inflammatory process in the retroperitoneum leading to the development of visceral edema and pancreatic ascites within days or even hours from admission.

The agressive fluid resuscitation is a „doble-edged weapon" : without strict control can induce the progress to ACS itself but it is proved that in the early phase the correct fluid therapy combined with prophylactic antibiotic treatment, surgical intervention, monitoring and management of organ dysfunctions, enteral nutrition and early endoscopic spincterotomy in patients with common bile duct gallstone-induced pancreatitis have improved survival.

Loosing patients in the early phase is frequently due to not recognised and not treated ACS.

The presence of IAH can also be used as a predictor of the severity of acute pancreatitis, because by some clinical trials there is correlation with the increased IAP and severity of pancreatitis, mortality, peripancreatic infection rate, and need for surgical intervention (53).

The true prevalence of IAH in patients with severe acute pancreatitis is not known. We can find numerous studies in the bibliography of the prevalence of IAH among the patients treated by severe acute pancreatitis. De Waele and his team described in their study that 44% of the 41 study patients had IAP levels higher than 12 mmHg, and 4 patients (10%) had IAP levels higher than 25 mmHg with severe organ disfunction and undergoing surgical decompression (54). Keskinen treated 37 patients in the ICU for acute pancreatitis and 27% of the patients (n=10) had IAP levels higher than 25 mmHg (55). In a study of 297 patients from China presented that the overall incidence of IAH was 36% (56).

Severe acute pancreatitis is one of the most common diseases associated with IAH in the ICU environment.

Thus, it can be estimated that the overall prevalence of IAH in patients with severe acute pancreatitis is about 40%, and the frequency of ACS requiring surgical decompression is about 10% (53-56).

In a study comparing patients with or without ACS (IAP > 25 mmHg) treated in the ICU for severe acute pancreatitis the hospital mortality rate for patients with ACS was 50% compared with 15% in patients without ACS (55).

The following case reports from patientes treated in our department are to point out the importance of measurement of IAP:

First patient:

33-year-old man was taken to ICU with signs of acute pancreatitis after alcoholic abuse. Conservative treatment was started but on the second day the conditions of the man were getting worse. IAP measurement was started and we found IAP = 12 mmHg which rised to 26 mmHg during the next 3 days and developed MOF. During the intervention we found the tipical clinical picture of acute necrotizing pancreatitis with retroperitoneal necrosis. Although the decompression with Bogota Bag insertion was performed we lost the patient 2 days later. Concluding this case it is very important to pay attention to the early signs of IAP / ACS and the timing of the decompression.

Second patient:

37-year-old woman was taken to our hospital after alimentary abuse and with consequent abdominal pain. Examinations proved acute pancreatitis. Despite the appropriate conservative therapy her condition worsened, IAP reached 20 mmHg, respiratory distress and oliguria developed.

Laparotomy, lavage, drainage was performed. To prevent abdominal distension the abdomen was left open and organs were covered with a sterile urinary drainage bag (Bogota Bag). In the ICU 12 operations were performed during 108 nursing days. The IAP was monitored permanently and when it reached the critical value necrectomy and lavage was performed. On the 116th nursing day she was sent home without complaints.

Her abdomen was covered with epithelized omentum which will be solved by a further operation (1-2).

9. Discussion

IAH and ACS are one of the major causes of organ failure and increased mortality (ACS with extremely high 38-71% mortality) among a wide variety of patient populations.

The pathophysiology of IAH and ACS is based on the chain reaction of physiological processes generated by the increased abdominal pressure which affects almost every organ and it could be fatal without correct diagnosis and treatment. It was originally noticed in traumatological cases (gunshot and stab wounds, intra-abdominal haemorrhage) when the extreme abdominal distension was related with a rapidly worsening condition and ended in ARDS, MOF and toxic shock. The same process is taking place in general surgical patients in spite of the different etiology. The leading etiological factor among general surgical critically ill patients is the acute pancreatitis. The cause of this phenomenon is the extremely increased IAP. The diagnosis was supported by the improved methods of monitoring IAP because the physical examination of the abdomen is far from accurate with a sensitivity of only 40%. The gold standard of the IAP monitoring is the CIAPM ensures diagnosis of ACS and the appropriate indication of the operation. The treatment consists of adequate fluid resuscitation and surgical decompression.

Intra-abdominal hypertension and abdominal compartment syndrome are frequent clinical findings among acute general surgical patients. Patients with comparable demographics and acute severity of illness are more likely to die if intra-abdominal hypertension or abdominal compartment syndrome is present. We conclude that the early recognition and surgical decompression is urgent.

„We must study and learn from the past and, at the same time, proactively „invent" the future. The future of IAH and ACS is in our hands. It is time to pay attention." (Cheatham, Ivatury, Malbrain, Sugrue) (53)

10. References

[1] Bodnar Zs, Sipka S, Hajdu Z (2008) The Abdominal Compartment Syndrome (ACS) in General Surgery. Hepato-Gastroenterology. 55:2033-2038.

[2] Bodnar Zs, Bulyovszky I, Tóth D, Kathy S, Hajdu Z (2006) The abdominal compartment syndrome (ACS) in general surgery. Hung. J. Surg. 59:152-159.

[3] Ogilvie WH (1940) The late complications of abdominal war wounds. Lancet. 2: 253-256.

[4] Kron IL, Harman PK, Nolan SP (1984) The measurement of intraabdominal pressure as a criterion for abdominal reexploration. Ann. Surg. 199:28-30.

[5] Fietsam RJr, Villalba M, Glover IL, Clark K (1989) Intraabdominal compartment syndrome as a complication of ruptured abdominal aortic aneurysm repair. Ann. Surg. 55:396-402.

[6] Emerson H (1911) Intra-abdominal pressures. Arch. Intern. Med. 7:754-784.

[7] Iberti TJ, Lieber CE, Benjamin E (1989) Determination of intraabdominal pressure using a transurethral bladder catheter: clinical validation of the technique. Anesthesiology. 70:47-50.
[8] Iberti TJ, Kelly KM, Gentili DR, Hirsch S, Benjamin E (1987) A simple technique to accurately determine intra-abdominal pressure. Crit. Care Med. 15:1140-1142.
[9] Sugrue M (1995) Intra-abdominal pressure. Clin. Intensive Care 6:76-79.
[10] Malbrain MNLG (1999) Abdominal pressure in the critically ill: measurement and clinical relevance. Int. Care Med. 25:1453-1458.
[11] Balogh Zs, Jones F, D'Amours S, Parr M, Sugrue M (2004) Continuous intra-abdominal pressure measurement technique. Am. J. Surg. 188:679-684.
[12] Schein M, Wittmann DH, Aprahamian CC, Condon RE (1995) The abdominal compartment syndrome: the physiological and clinical consequences of elevated intra-abdominal pressure. J. Am. Coll. Surg. 180:745-753.
[13] Burch IM, Moore EE, Moore FA, Franciose R (1996) The abdominal compartment syndrome. Surg. Clin. North. Am. 76:833-842.
[14] Malbrain MLNG, Cheatham ML, Kirkpatrick A, Sugrue M, Parr M, De Waele J, Balogh Zs, Leppaniemi A, Olvera C, Ivatury R, D'Amours S, Wendon J, Hillman K, Johansson K, Kolkman K, Wilmer A (2006) Results from the International Conference of Experts on Intra-abdominal Hypertension and Abdominal Compartment Syndrome. I. Definitions. Int. Care. Med. 32: 1722-1732.
[15] Cheatham ML, Malbrain MLNG, Kirkpatrick A, Sugrue M, Parr M, De Waele J, Balogh Zs, Leppaniemi A, Olvera C, Ivatury R, D'Amours S, Wendon J, Hillman K, Wilmer A (2007) Results from the International Conference of Experts on Intra-abdominal Hypertension and Abdominal Compartment Syndrome. II. Recommendations. Int. Care. Med. 33: 951-962.
[16] Malbrain MLNG, Chiumello D, Pelosi P, et al (2005) Incidence and prognosis of intraabdominal hypertension in a mixed population of critically ill patients: a multiple-center epidemiological study. Crit Care Med. 33:315-322.
[17] Tóns Ch, Schachtrupp A, Rau M, Mumme Th, Schumpelick V (2000) Abdominelles Kompartment Syndrom: Vermeidung und Behandlung. Chirurg. 71:918-926.
[18] Malbrain MNLG, Chiumello D, Pelosi P, Bihari D, Innes R, Ranieri VM et al (2005) Incidence and prognosis of intraabdominal hypertension in a mixed population of critically ill patients: A multiple-center epidemiological study. Crit. Careo Med. 33:315-322.
[19] Chen H, Li F, Sun JB, Jia JG (2008) Abdominal compartment syndrome in patients with severe acute pancreatitis in early stage. World J Gastroenterol. 14:3541-3548.
[20] Balogh Zs, McKinley BA, Holcomb JB et al (2003) Both primary and secondary abdominal compartment syndrome (ACS) can be predicted early and are harbingers of multiple organ failure. J. Trauma. 54:848-861.
[21] Sugrue M, Balogh Zs, Malbrain M (2004) Intra-abdominal hypertension and renal failure. ANZ J. Surg. 74:78.
[22] Jakob SM (2002) Clinical review: Splanchnic ischaemia. Crit. Care 6:306-312.
[23] Diebel LN, Dulchavsky SA, Brown WJ (1997) Splanchnic ischaemia and bacterial translocation in the abdominal compartment syndrome. J. Trauma. 43:852-855.

[24] Diebel LN, Dulchavsky SA, Willson RF (1992) Effect ofincreased intra-abdominal pressure on mesenteric arterial and intestinal mucosal blood flow. J. Trauma. 33:45-49.,

[25] Diebel L, Saxe J, Dulchavsky SA (1992) Effect of intra-abdominal pressure on abdominal blood flow. Am. Surg. 58:573-575.

[26] Vegar-Brozovic V, Brezak J, Brozovic I (2008) Intra-abdominal hypertension: pulmonary and cerebral complications. Transplant Proc. 40:1190-1192.

[27] Waele JJ, Leppaniemi AK (2009) Intra-abdominal hypertension in acute pancreatitis. World J Surg 33:1128–1133

[28] Motew SJ, Mourelatos MG, Miller RN et al (1997) Evidence that adenosine contributes to the maintenance of hepatosplanchnic blood flow during peritoneal sepsis in rats. Shock 7:439–446

[29] Eltzschig HK, Thompson LF, Karhausen J, Cotta RJ, Ibla JC, Robson SC, Colgan SP (2004) Endogenous adenosine produced during hypoxia attenuates neutrophil accumulation: coordination by extracellular nucleotide metabolism. Blood 104:3986–3992

[30] Housley GD, Bringmann A, Reichenbach A (2009) Purinergic signalling in special senses. Trends Neurosci 32:128–141

[31] Berne RM, Knabb RM, Ely SW, Rubio R (1983) Adenosine in the local regulation of blood flow: a brief review. Fed Proc 42:3136–3142

[32] McCallion K, Harkin DW, Gardiner KR (2004) Role of adenosine in immunomodulation: review of the literature. Crit Care Med 32:273–277

[33] Sipka S, Kovács I, Szántó S et al (2005) Adenosine inhibits the release of interleukine-1β in activated human peripheral mononuclear cells. Cytokine 31:258–263

[34] Le Moine O, Stordeur P, Schanane L et al (1996) Adenosine enhances IL-10 secretion by human monocytes. J Immunol 156:4408–4414

[35] Mosser DM, Zhang X (2008) Interleukin 10: new perspectives on an old cytokine. Immun Rev 226:205–218

[36] Paraskevi M, Sidiropovlov T, Pandazi A, Batistaki C, Matiatov S, Panagiotou GK (2007) Changes of gastric intramucosal pH in obese patients undergoing laparoscopic and open cholecystectomy. Arch Med Sci 3 (3):223-228

[37] Ozmen MM, Zulfikarogly B, Col C, Cinel I, Isman FK, Cinel L, Besler TH (2009) Effect of increased abdominal pressure on cytokines (IL-1 β, IL-6, TNFα) C-reactive protein (CRP), free radicals (NO, NDA), and histology. Surg Laparosc Endosc Percutan Tech 19:142–147

[38] Hansen PB, Hashimoto S, Oppermann M, Huang Y, Briggs JP, Schnermann L (2005) Vasoconstrictor and vasodilator effects of adenosine in the mouse kidney due to preferential activation of A1 or A2 adenosine receptors. J Pharmacol Exp Ther 315:1150–1157

[39] De Laet I, Malbrain MLNG, Jadoul JL, Rogiers P, Sugrue M (2007) Renal implications of decreased intra-abdominal pressure: are the kidneys the canary for abdominal hypertension? Acta Clin Belg Suppl 62:119–130

[40] De Waele JJ, De laet I (2007) Intra-abdominal hypertension and the effect of renal function. Acta Clin Belg 62(Suppl):371–374

[41] Vallon V, Mühlbauer B, Osswald H (2006) Adenosine and kidney function. Physiol Rev 86:901–940

[42] Wauters J, Claus P, Brosens N, McLaughlin MM, Wilmer A (2009) Pathophysiology of renal hemodynamics and renal cortical microcirculation in a porcine model of elevated intra-abdominal pressure. J Trauma 66:713–719

[43] Imai K, Furuya K, Kawada M et al (2006) Human pelvic extramural ganglion cells: a semiquantitative and immunohistochemical study. Surg Radiol Anat 28:596–605

[44] De Laet I, Hoste E, Verholen E, Waele D (2007) The effect of neuromuscular blockers in patients with intra-abdominal hypertension. Intensive Care Med 33:1811–1814

[45] Bodnar Zs, Keresztes T, Kovács I, Hajdu Z, Boissonneault GA, Sipka S (2010) Increased serum adenosine and interleukin 10 levels as new laboratory markers of increased intra-abdominal pressure. Langenbecks Arch Surg. 395: 969-972.

[46] Bodnar Zs, Szentkereszty Z, Hajdu Z, Boissonneault GA, Sipka S (2011) Beneficial effects of theophylline infusions in surgical patients with intra-abdominal hypertension. Langenbecks Arch Surg. (Published Online: 03 June 2011)

[47] Malbrain MLNG (2004) Different techniques to measure intra-abdominal pressure (IAP): time for a critical re-appraisal. Int. Care Med. 30:357-371.

[48] Davis PJ, Koottayi S, Taylor A, Butt WW, (2005) Comparison of indirect methods of measuring intra-abdominal pressure in children. Int. Care Med. 31:471-475.

[49] Balogh Zs, McKinley BA, Cocanour CS et al (2003) Supranormal trauma resuscitation causes more cases of abdominal compartment syndrome. Arch. Surg. 138:637-643.

[50] Howdiesholl TR, Proctor CD, Sternberg E, Cué JI, Mondy JS, Hawkins ML (2004) Temporary abdominal closure followed by definitive abdominal wall reconstruction of the abdomen. Am. J. Surg. 188:301-306.

[51] Vargo D (2004) Component separation in the management of the difficult abdominal wall. Am. J. Surg. 188:633-637.

[52] Young SP, Thompson JP (2008) Severe acute pancreatitis. Contin Educ Anaesth Crit Care Pain. 8 (4): 125-128.

[53] Ivatury RR, Cheatham ML, Malbrain MLN, Sugrue M (2006) Abdominal Compartment Syndrome. Landes Bioscience. Texas (USA)

[54] De Waele J, Hoste E, Blot S et al (2004) Intraabdominal hypertension and severe acute pancreatitis. Inaugural WCACS, Noosa (Australia)

[55] Keskinen P, Leppaniemi A, Pettila V et al (2004) Intra-abdominal pressure in acute necrotizing pancreatitis. Inaugural WCACS, Noosa (Australia)

[56] Tao HQ, Zhang JX, Zou SC (2004) Clinical characteristics and management of patients with early acute severe pancreatitis: Experience from a medical center in China. World J Gastroenterol. 10: 919-921.

12

Traumatic Pancreatitis – Endoscopic and Surgical Management

Hirotaka Okamoto[1,2] and Hideki Fujii[2]
[1]*Department of Surgery, Tsuru Municipal Hospital,*
[2]*Department of Gastrointestinal, Breast & Endocrine Surgery, Faculty of Medicine, University of Yamanashi*
Japan

1. Introduction

Acute pancreatitis is inflammation of the pancreas that occurs suddenly and usually resolves in a few days with treatment. Acute pancreatitis can be a life-threatening illness with severe complications. The most common cause of acute pancreatitis is the presence of small gallstones that cause inflammation of the pancreas as they pass through the common bile duct. Chronic heavy alcohol use is also a common cause. Acute pancreatitis can occur within hours or as long as 2 days after consuming alcohol. Other causes of acute pancreatitis include abdominal trauma, medications, infections, tumors, and genetic abnormalities of the pancreas.

Pancreatic trauma is uncommon, accounting for only 0.2-6% of all injuries resulting from abdominal trauma, and is associated with a high mortality rate of 13.8-31% (Leppäniemi et al., 1988). The high mortality rate is due to the frequent occurrence of associated abdominal injuries. In addition, blunt abdominal trauma is considered to be the cause of one fifth of all cases of traumatic pancreatitis and it may result in contusion, parenchymal fracture, or ductal disruption (Portis et al., 1994). These injuries to the pancreas are typically caused by compression of the organ against the vertebral column, mostly in traffic related-accidents. Blunt trauma to the epigastrium is caused by steering wheels, handlebars, seatbelts, or directly. Other mechanisms of injury include sporting accidents, such as direct hits from a ball or a blunt blow.

Therapeutic decisions for pancreatic trauma are based on the injury site and status of the pancreatic ductal system. When pancreatic ductal disruption exists or when duodenal injury cannot be ruled out, surgical exploration is usually required; however, surgery carries considerable morbidity and mortality risks. In this chapter, we discuss the management of pancreatic trauma and acute pancreatitis, including therapeutic endoscopy and surgical exploration.

2. Amatomy and physiology

The pancreas grows rapidly during a child's first five years of life with a slower growth rate up to the age of 18 years of age (Spiegel et al., 1997). It is a large complex gland that lies outside the walls of the alimentary tract parallel to the stomach at the level of the first and second lumbar vertebrae. It is surrounded anteriorly by the upper abdominal intraperitoneal organs and posteriorly by the thick paraspinal muscles. The lobules of the pancreas drain into the main pancreatic duct of Wirsungs which traverses the length of the gland and joins the common bile duct, emptying into the duodenum through the ampulla of Vater. The minor duct of Santorini usually branches off from the main pancreatic duct and also empties into the duodenum. The gland is not encapsulated; therefore, tears in pancreatic tissues permit pancreatic digestive enzymes to invade the peripancreatic tissue and leak into the peritoneal cavity.

3. Pathogenesis

The mechanism of blunt pancreatic trauma usually involves anterior compressive forces applied to the pancreas, which lies over the vertebral column. The pancreas is relatively fixed so that during blunt impact, the pancreas is not displaced and absorbs the full amount of force applied (**Rawls, 2001**).

4. Classification

Classically, according to Lucas's classification of pancreatic injury, injuries without MPD disruption are designated Class I, while Class II or III injuries involve MPD disruption (Lucas, 1977). The Organ Injury Scaling Committee of the American Association for the Surgery of Trauma has proposed a pancreatic organ injury scale that is widely used and is based on the extent of parenchymal damage as well as the presence or absence of pancreatic duct injury (Moore et al., 1990). Minor contusions or superficial lacerations of the pancreas without duct involvement are classified as grade I injury. Grade II injuries are major contusions or lacerations without duct disruption. Distal transection of the pancreas or major parenchymal injuries with duct injuries is described as grade III. Grade IV injuries are proximal transections or any proximal parenchymal injuries involving the ampulla. Grade V injuries describe massive destructions of the pancreas head (**Table 1**).

Grade	Injury Description
I	Minor contusion or superficial laceration wihtout duct injury
II	Major contusion or laceration without duct injury or tissue loss
III	Distal transection or parenchymal injury with duct injury
IV	Proximal transection or parenchymal injury involving ampulla
V	Massive disruption of pancreas head

Table 1. Pancreatic injury severity scale (Moore et al., 1990)

5. Diagnosis

5.1 Laboratory data

It is generally reported that laboratory findings are relatively insensitive and non-specific in diagnosing pancreatic injury (Arkovitz et al., 1997; Bradley et al., 1998; Jobst et al., 1999). Serum amylase evaluation can suggest pancreatic injury; however, amylase levels have failed to predict or correlate with the degree of injury or disclose potential ductal disruption, especially when obtained in the early post-trauma period (Simon et al., 1994).

Serum lipase is often based clinically in the setting of acute pancreatitis, but after blunt trauma, elevated serum lipase levels may be nonspecific and a poor indication of injury (Buechter et al., 1990). Because of their low sensitivity and specificity for pancreatic trauma, serum amylase and lipase have limited diagnostic value, but elevated levels may provide a clue to a severe injury requiring further investigation.

5.2 Ultrasound

An ultrasound examination will usually be performed to enable the diagnosis of free abdominal fluid or gross damage to the liver or spleen. The pancreas is not easily identified and examined to its full extent; therefore, pancreatic injuries, parenchymal or ductal, will frequently be missed. However, routine abdominal ultrasound examination in the emergency room will establish the diagnosis of an intra-abdominal injury and therefore establish the need for an urgent explorative laparotomy. To disclose main pancreatic duct injury in blunt and penetration pancreatic trauma, intraoperative ultrasonography has proven to be helpful (Hikida et al., 2004).

5.3 Computed tomography

When initially evaluating for injury, CT scanning is a simple, noninvasive means of evaluating the pancreas. New-generation helical CT scanners quickly enable an overview of abdominal injuries in severely traumatic patients. CT was reported to have 90% sensitivity in detecting pancreatic disruption (Teh et al., 2007). Furthermore, CT allows additional assessment of the severity and extent of pancreatic tissue damage and concomitant injuries (Bigattini et al. 1999).

5.4 Magnetic resonance cholangiopancreatography

Magnetic resonance cholangiopancreatography (MRCP) is another non-invasive diagnostic tool that allows the evaluation of pancreatic injuries with high sensitivity and specificity. Particularly in stable patients with suspected pancreatic injury, MRCP enables the non-invasive detection or exclusion of pancreatic duct trauma and pancreatic specific complications. It may therefore provide information that can be used to guide management decisions in the further course of pancreatic trauma patients; however, its purely diagnostic nature and its inability to provide real-time visualization of ductal findings and extravasation are two of its disadvantages (Fulcher et al., 2000). Recently, secretin-stimulated MRCP was also reported to be a safe, non-invasive test that can provide additional useful information about duct integrity and facilitate management (Gillams AR et al., 2006).

5.5 Endoscopic retrograde cholangiopancreatography

Endoscopic retrograde cholangiopancreatography (ERCP) was documented to be a useful diagnostic tool, displaying sensitivity and specificity of 100% for pancreatic duct injury (Gougeon et al., 1976; Doctor et al., 1995). ERCP was also reported to be the definitive test for pancreatic duct injury, particularly, to demonstrate clearly the site of duct disruption and the grade of duct injury, whether the branch or main duct and partial or complete disruption of the main pancreatic duct MPD (Kim et al., 2001).

Recently, ERCP has been shown not only to provide sufficient information for conclusive diagnosis but also to be an effective and safe non-operative treatment tool (Bendahan et al., 1995; Huckfeldt et al., 1996; Kim et al., 2001; Cay et al., 2005; Houben et al., 2007). In certain cases of leakages of the pancreatic duct, transpapillary stent insertion might seal the injury and stabilize it in a way that eventually leads to resolution of the leakage

6. Therapy

Isolated pancreatic trauma is rare and usually results from direct trauma to the epigastrium, for example from the handle bars in bicycle accidents or in sports, typically in children or adolescents. Most patients with pancreatic lesions will present with multiple injuries, some of them hemodynamically unstable, and concomitant abdominal injuries; therefore, unstable patients may require initial damage control and correct assessment of the extent of pancreatic injury. On the other hand, in stable patients, ERCP plays an important role in the diagnosis, but also in the treatment of pancreatic duct injuries. Reports on the transpapillary stenting of duct lesions are very encouraging and justify the extensive use of ERCP (Canty et al., 2001).

6.1 Case of endoscopic treatment

A 17-year-old man was brought to the emergency department of our hospital with severe upper abdominal pain following a blow received in a rugby game. Emergency computed tomography (CT) revealed severe pancreatic neck injury. Forty-eight hours later, follow-up enhanced CT revealed that the pancreas was clearly lacerated and that the amount of peri-

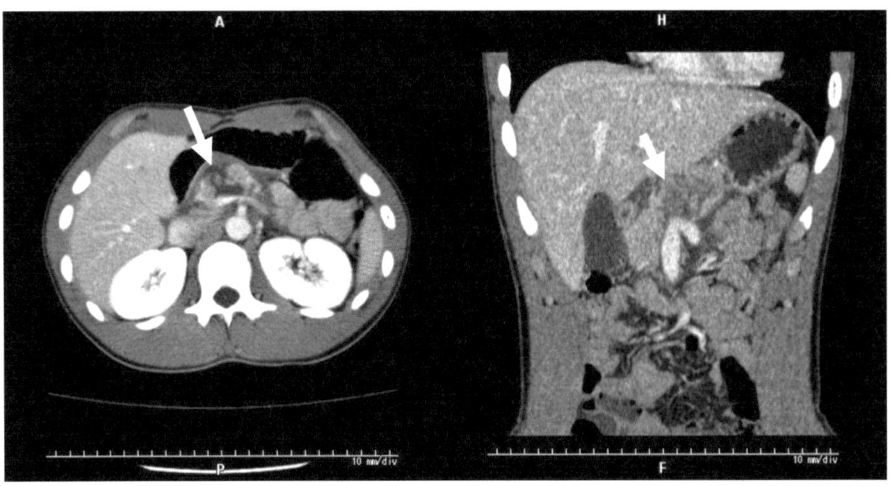

Fig. 1. Enhanced CT revealed an obvious laceration of the pancreas neck. (white arrow)

pancreatic fluid was increasing (**Fig. 1**); furthermore, serum amylase and elastase levels were elevated. ERP (endoscopic retrograde pancreatography) revealed that contrast medium in the main pancreatic duct (MPD) had leaked into the parenchyma, indicating MPD injury (**Fig. 2**). To prevent the traumatic pancreatitis from worsening, a stent was inserted endoscopically at a site distal to the injured portion of the MPD (**Fig. 3**). Thereafter, the patient's complaint was markedly reduced, and his serum amylase levels returned to normal. In addition, the apparent pancreatic edema and peripheral fluid were decreased on CT (Okamoto et al., 2010).

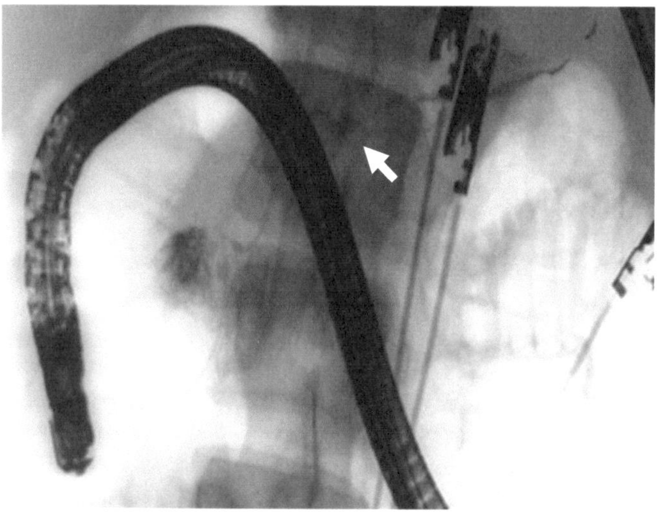

Fig. 2. Endoscopic pancreatography (ERP) revealed leakage of contrast medium.(white arrow)

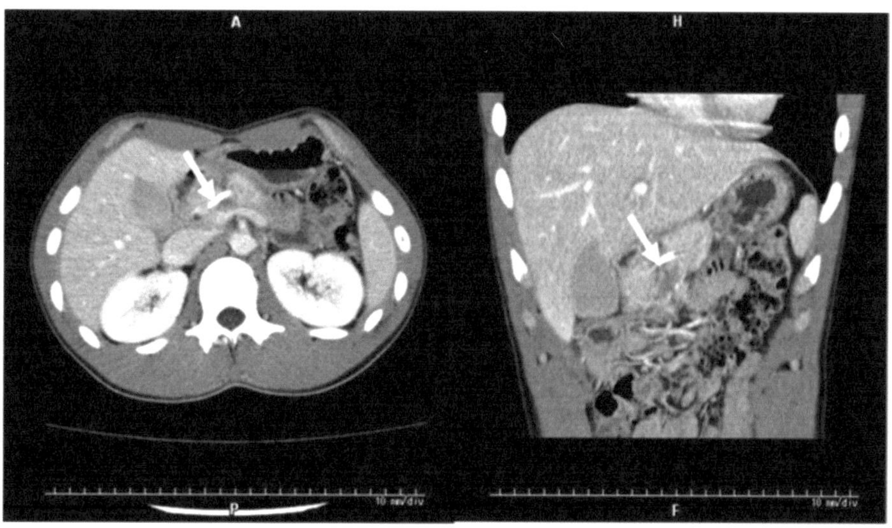

Fig. 3. Enhanced CT revealed the inserted pancreatic stent and disappearance of pancreas peripheral fluid. (white arrow)

6.2 Endoscopic pancreatic duct stent treatment

Endoscopic transpapillary stent insertion by literature review is summarized in **Table 2**.

	Age	Gender	Trauma	Initial S-Amy (IU/L	CT findings	Time to ERCP	ERCP findings	Disrupted portion	Outcome	References
1	22	M	Stabbed injury	n.d.	(Emergent operation)	3d	Duct disruption	Proximal	Recoverd	Bendahan J., et al., 1995
2	27	F	Car accident	127	Irregular order of the pancreas tail	3-4hr	Extravasation of the contrast from MPD	Neck (isthmus)	Recovered	Huckfeldt R, et al. 1996
3	9	F	Bike fall	436	Partial disruption of pancreatic parenchyma	1d	Extravasation of the contrast from MPD	Body	Recovered	Cantly T.G., et al., 2001
4	8	M	Traffic accident	126	Disruption of the distal pancreas	1d	Extravasation of the contrast from MPD	Tail	Recovered, mild MPD stricture	Cantly T.G., et al., 2001
5	46	M	n.d.	234	Head swelling	1d	Extravasation from tail of MPD	Head	Recovered	Kim HS, et al., 20001
6	35	M	n.d.	390	Pancreas fracture	4d	Intracapsular leakage from MPD	n.d.	Recovered, pseudocyst	Kim HS, et al., 20001
7	40	F	n.d.	742	Body swelling	1d	Intracapsular leakage from MPD	Body	Recovered, pseudocyst	Kim HS, et al., 20001
8	60	M	Car accident	536	Pancreas disruption and pseudocyst	5d	Extravasation of the contrast from MPD	Proximal	Recovered	Hashimoto A., et al., 2003
9	37	F	Steering wheel	2467	Hematoma over pancreatic head	22d	Stricture at the head with contrast extravasation	Head	Recovered, stent migration	Lin B.C., et al.,2006
10	35	M	Steering wheel	435	n.d.	19d	Stricture at the head with contrast extravasation	Head	Recovered, MPD stricture	Lin B.C., et al.,2006
11	36	M	Steering wheel	417	Pancreatic neck laceration	8d	Contrast extravasation at the body and tail	Body	Recovered, MPD stricture	Lin B.C., et al.,2006
12	61	F	Steering wheel	2270	Pancreatic body laceration	1d	Contrast extravasation at the body with retroperiton	Body	Sepsis, Death	Lin B.C., et al.,2006
13	18	M	Steering wheel	366	Pancreatic body laceration	8h	Contrast extravasation at the body	Body	Recovered, MPD stricture	Lin B.C., et al.,2006
14	28	M	Steering wheel	231	Pancreatic head laceration	16h	Contrast extravasation at the head	Head	Recovered, mild MPD stricture	Lin B.C., et al.,2006
15	8	M	Handlebar	n.d.	n.d.	28d	Incomplete disruption	Body	Recovered	Houben C.H., et al., 2007
16	11	M	Hit lamppost	n.d.	n.d.	4d	Transection of MPD	Neck	Recovered	Houben C.H., et al., 2007
17	10	F	Handlebar	n.d.	n.d.	2d	Incomplete disruption	Body	Recovered	Houben C.H., et al., 2007
18	11	M	Handlebar	n.d.	n.d.	2d	Transection of MPD	Neck	Recovered	Houben C.H., et al., 2007
19	11	F	Fall from seesaw	n.d.	n.d.	2d	Transection of MPD	Body	Recovered	Houben C.H., et al., 2007
20	7	M	Handlebar	n.d.	n.d.	9d	Transection of MPD	Neck	Recovered	Houben C.H., et al., 2007
21	10	M	Handlebar	n.d.	n.d.	7d	Transection of MPD	Neck	Recovered	Houben C.H., et al., 2007
22	12	M	Trivial fall	n.d.	n.d.	3d	Transection of MPD	Neck	Recovered	Houben C.H., et al., 2007
23	9	M	Trivial fall	n.d.	n.d.	4d	Transection of MPD	Neck	Recevered	Houben C.H., et al., 2007
24	28	M	Gun shot	406	Pancreatic injuruy involving the head, neck	1m	Leakage of the contrast	Head	Recovered	Rastogi M, et al., 2009
25	31	F	Bicycle accident	406	Pancreatic edema	0d	Disrupted unicinate branch	Unicinate process	Recovered	Rogers S.J., et al., 2009
26	49	M	Car accident	L 7121	Pancreatic edema	0d	Disrupted MPD	Body	Recovered	Rogers S.J., et al., 2009
27	41	F	Car accident	L 480	Pancreatc edema	15d	Disrupted unicinate branch	Unicinate process	Recovered	Rogers S.J., et al., 2009
28	41	F	Car accident	235	Distal pancreatic tear	10d	Disrupted unicinate branch	Unicinate process	Recovered	Rogers S.J., et al., 2009
29	18	F	Skiing fall	L 844	Peripancreatic edema, possible laceration	2d	Transection of MPD	Tail	Recovered	Rogers S.J., et al., 2009
30	54	M	Gun shot	L 583	IVC laceration, retroperitoneal fluid	1d	Extravasation MPD	Head	Recovered	Rogers S.J., et al., 2009
31	17	M	Sport	437	Pancreas disruption and pseudocyst	2d	Leakage from MPD	Neck	Recovered	Okamoto H., et al., 2010

n.d.: not determined, h: hour, d: day, m: month, L: lipase

Table 2. Summary of reported pancreatic duct stent treatment cases

This summary indicates that endoscopic transpapillary stent insertion is an effective technique for managing certain pancreatic traumatic injuries. A significant improvement in outcome was found for patients with stent therapy. Pancreatic stents are known to be associated with minor damage to the duct including ductal irregularity, stenosis, and side branch ectasia (Kozarek et al., 1991). These changes can occur even if the stent is patent, and they can persist or resolve after stent removal (Huckfeldt et al., 1996). A long-term study of a small group showed that 4 of 6 cases were complicated by ductal stricture, although stent therapy could avoid surgery in the acute trauma stage (Lin et al., 2006). Endo- and exocrine function were not examined. Further accumulated experiences are needed to clarify the significance of stent therapy.

6.2.1 Case of surgical treatment

A 34-year-old man was transferred to our hospital 18 hours after blunt abdominal trauma caused by impact against an automobile steering wheel. Emergent CT showed laceration of the pancreatic head and surrounding hematoma. Emergent laparotomy was carried out. Intraoperative pancreatography revealed injury of the proximal main pancreatic duct.

Because stenosis of the main pancreatic duct was predicted as a complication, cholecystectomy, external drainage of the common bile duct, and external abdominal drainage were carried out. He was discharged with a pancreatic fistula 4 months postoperatively. Three months later, pancreatic juice output through the drainage tube decreased, and patient developed acute pancreatitis. CT revealed dilatation of the main pancreatic duct and atrophy of the pancreas distal to the site of injury (**Fig. 4**). A second operation was planed to perform to preserve pancreatic function after the patient's general condition improved. ERP demonstrated ductal stricture of the main pancreatic duct in the head of the pancreas and upstream dilatation of the pancreatic duct. A diagnosis of chronic obstructive pancreatitis was made, and in order to preserve the function of the distal pancreas, longitudinal pancreatojejunostomy with Roux-en-Y anastomosis was performed 10 months after the initial operation. After the second operation, the patient's pancreatic function and pancreatic atrophy improved (Matsuda et al., 1999).

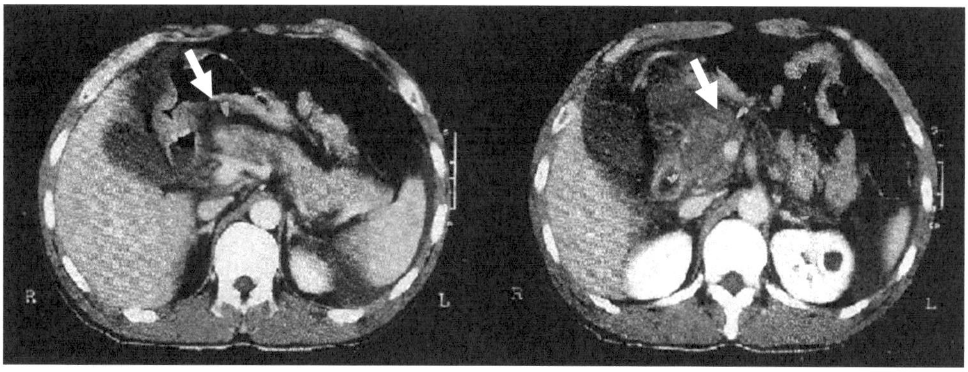

Fig. 4. Enhanced CT revealed a laceration of pancreatic head (left, white arrow) and a hematoma near pancreas head (right, white arrow).

6.2.2 Surgical treatment

Isolated pancreatic injuries are rare and most patients will present with multiple injuries, some of them hemodynamically unstable, and concomitant abdominal injuries; therefore, unstable patients may require initial damage control and correct assessment of the extent of pancreatic injury. This usually allows delayed definitive treatment of complex injuries, especially of the head of the pancreas. With regard to treatment, external drainage alone has been proposed for grade I and II injuries, while surgical intervention, including distal pancreatectomy or pancreaticojejunostomy, is usually performed for grade III, IV, and V injuries.

6.3 Nonoperative management

Conservative management of pancreatic trauma in the absence of a ductal injury (grade I and II) is widely accepted and practiced as the majority are contusions that usually resolve spontaneously after conservative treatment (Rescorla et al., 1995; Keller et al., 1997; Meier et al., 2001; Canty et al., 2001). Nonoperative management of a pancreatic injury consists of bowel arrest, total parental nutrition, and serial imaging with either CT scans or ultrasound to follow injury resolution.

Octreotide, a synthetic somatostatin analogue that inhibits pancreatic secretions has been shown in adults to reduce the incidence of postsurgical pancreatitis after pancreatic surgery. The benefits of octreotide in pancreatic trauma are controversial, and in particular its role in pediatric trauma is still undefined (Amirara et al., 1994; Nwariaku et al., 1995; Mulligan et al., 1995; Cavallini et al., 2001), however, there are few reported cases of octreotide administration being effective for traumatic pancreatic injury (Morali et al.,1991; Shan et al., 2002). Further accumulated evidence is required to prove this effect.

7. Treatment algorithm

We proposed an early treatment algorithm for endoscopic and surgical therapy, based on the presence or absence of a major pancreatic duct lesion.

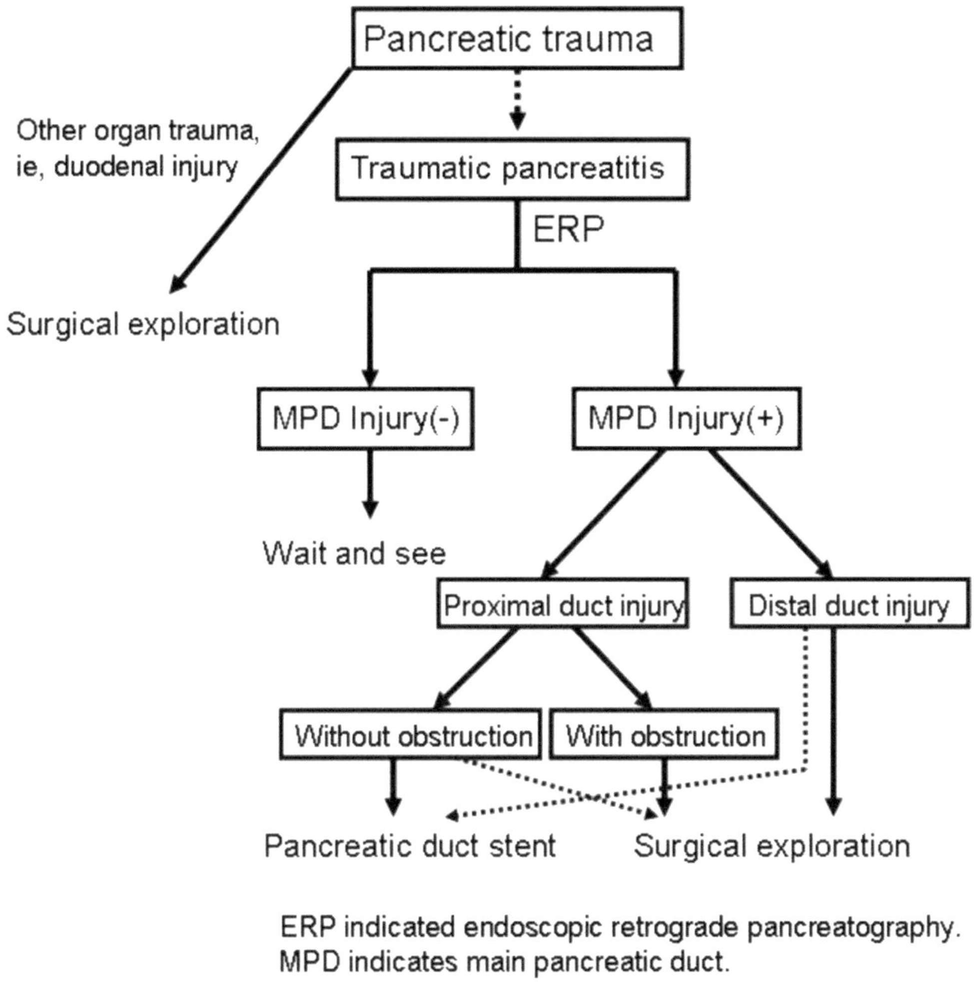

Fig. 4. Proposed early treatment algorithm for endoscopic and/or surgical therapy.

7.1 Proximal duct injury

Incomplete disruption of the MPD or complete disruption of the MPD without duct obstruction is the best candidate for the pancreatic duct stent therapy. Transductal pancreatic stent allows internal drainage of the pancreatic secretion and re-establishment of duct continuity (Bendahan et al., 1995; Huckfeldt et al., 1996; Cantly et al., 2001; Kim et al., 2001; Lin et al., 2006; Houben et al., 2007; Rogers et al., 2009).

Complete disruption of the MPD with duct obstruction increases the difficulty of stent placement beyond the fracture site. Disruption or complex injuries of the pancreatic head involving the ampulla, or devitalizing injuries of the pancreas head and duodenum usually are non-reconstructable injuries. In stable patients, pancreaticoduodenectomy is the best definite treatment for grade IV injuries. In unstable patients, exploration and placing of external drainage may be the best choice for damage control. Definitive treatment of the lesion can be achieved later, after the patient has been stabilized.

7.2 Distal duct injury

Distal pancreatic injury with duct involvement include major or stab wounds in the body or tail of the pancreas with an obvious duct injury or transection of more than half the width of the pancreas. If the clinical condition of the patient allows it, these grade III injuries are best treated by distal pancreatectomy even in emergency situations. In some cases, such as complete transection of the pancreatic body from the head, a distal pancreaticojejunostomy and closure of the proximal end of the pancreas rupture as in the Letton & Wilson procedure, may even become necessary if an organ-preserving approach is attempted (Letton et al., 1959). It has been documented that 19 patients were treated by distal pancreatectomy with splenectomy, 8 by pancreatectomy with preserving the spleen, and 2 by placing a pancreatic duct stent in a series of 32 grade III patients (Lin et al., 2004). Major distal duct injuries have been managed mainly by surgical exploration.

8. Complications and outcome

The complication rate of any pancreatic injury is not only associated with concomitant injuries, but also with the severity of the pancreatic injury. As is widely accepted, the grade of pancreatic injury is an independent predictor of both pancreas-associated morbidity and mortality. Complications following pancreatic trauma include fistula, pancreatic abscess, pseudocyst formation, and sepsis. The American Association for the Surgery Trauma Organ Injury Score has been shown to predict the development of complications and mortality after pancreatic injury (Kao et al., 2003).

Pancreatic abscesses have been treated interventionally by percutaneous drainage, but are frequently infected by multiple resistant bacteria, leading to sepsis. The treatment of pancreatic pseudocysts is interventional drainage and sealing, endoscopic gastrocystostomy, and operative enteric drainage.

9. Conclusion

Endoscopic transpapillary pancreatic duct stent is effective and safe management for pancreatic duct disruption, especially for proximal duct injury in selected patients. It may avoid emergent surgery in the acute trauma stage; however, long-term ductal stricture should be carefully investigated during long-term follow-up.

10. References

Amirata, E., Livingston, D.H., Elcavage, J.: Octreotide acetate decreases pancreatic complications after pancreatic trauma. *Am J Surg* 1994; 168:345-347,1994.

Arkovitz, M.S., Johnson, N., Grasia, V.E.: Pancreatic trauma in children: mechanisms of injury. *J Trauma* 1997; 42(1): 49-53.

Bendahan, J., Van Rewsburg, C.J., Van Vuren, B., Muller, R.: Endoscopic intrapancreatic stent for traumatic duct injury. *Injury* 1995; 26:553-554.

Bigattini, D., Boverie, J.H., Dondelinger, R.F.: Ct of blunt trauma of the pancreas in adults. *Eur Radiol* 1999; 9:244-249.

Buechter, K.J., Arnold, M., Steele, B., Martin, L., Byers, P., Gomez, G., Zeppa, R., Augenstein, J.: The use of serum amylase and lipase in evaluating and managing blunt abdominal trauma. *Am Surg* 1990; 56:104-208.

Bradley, E.L., 3rd, Young, P.R., Jr., Chang, M.C., Allen, J.E., Baker, C.C., Meredith, W., Reed, L., Thomason, M.: Diagnosis and initial management of blunt pancreatic trauma: guide lines from a multiinstitutional review. *Ann Surg* 1998; 227(6):861-869.

Cay, A., Imamoglu, M., Bektas, O., Ozdemir, O., Arslan, M., Sarihan, H.: Nonoperative treatment of traumatic pancreatic duct disruption in child with an endoscopically placed stent. *J Pediatr Surg* 2005; 40:9-12.

Canty, T.G., Weinman, D.: Management of major pancreatic duct injuries in children. *J Trauma* 2001; 50:1001-1007.

Cavallini, G., Frulloni, L.: Somatostatin and octreotide in acute pancreatitis: the never-ending story. *Digest Liver Dis* 2001;33:192-201.

Doctor, N., Dooley, J.S., Davidson, B.R.: Assessment of pancreatic duct damange following trauma: is endoscopy retrograde cholangiopancreatography the gold standard? *Postgrad Med J* 1995; 71:116-117.

Fulcher, A.S., Turner, M.A., Yelon, J.A., McClain, L.C., Broderick T., Ivatury R.R., Sugerman H.J.: Magnetic resonance cholangiopancreatography (MRCP) in the assessment of pancreatic duct trauma and its sequelae: preliminary findings. *J Trauma* 2000; 48:1001-1007.

Gillams,,A.R., Kurzawinski, T., Lees, W.R.: Diagnosis of duct disruption and assessment of pancreatic leak with dynamic secretion-stimulated MR cholangiopancreatography. *AJR* 2006; 186:499-506.

Gougeon, F.W., Legros, G., Archambault, A., Bessette, G., Bastien, E.: Pancreatic trauma: a new diagnostic approach. *Am J Surg* 1976; 132:400-402.

Hikida, S., Sakamoto, T., Higaki, K., Hata, H., Maeshiro, K., Yamauchi, K., Kimura, Y.N., Egawa, N., Mizote, H., Shirouzu, K. () intraoperative ultrasonography is useful for diagnosing pancreatic duct injury and adjacent tissue damage in a patient with penetrating pancreas trauma.: *J Hepatobiliary Pancreat Surg* 2004; 11:272-275.

Huckfeldt, R., Agee, C., Nicholas, W.K., Barthel, J.: Nonoperative treatment of traumatic pancreatic duct disruption using an endoscopically placed stent. *J Trauma* 1996; 41:143-144.

Houben, C.H., Ade-Ajayi, N., Patel, S., Kane, S., Karan,i J., Devlin, J., Harrison, P., Davenport, M.: Traumatic pancreatic duct injury in children: minimal invasive approach to management. *J Pediatr Surg* 2007; 42:629-635.

Jobst, M.A., Canty, T.G., Sr., Lynch, F.P.: Mangement of pancreatic injury in pediatric blunt abdominal trauma. *J Pediatr Surg* 1999; 34(5):818-824.

Kao L.S., Bulger E.M., Parks D.L., Byrd G.F., Jurkovich G.J.: Predictors of morbidity after traumatic pancreatic injury. *J Trauma* 2003; 55:898-905.

Keller, M.S., Stafford, P.W., Vane, D.W.: Conservative management of pancreatic trauma in children. *J Trauma* 1997; 42:1097-1100.

Kim, H.S., Lee, D.K., Kim, I.W., Baik, S.K., Kwon, S.O., Park, J.W., Cho, N.C., Rhoe, B.S.: The role of endoscopic retrograde pancreatography in the treatment of traumatic pancreatic duct injury. *Gastrointest Endosc* 2001; 54:49-55.

Kozarek, R.A., Ball,T.J., Patterson, D.J., Freeny, P.C., Ryan, J.A., Traverso, L.W.: Endoscopic transpapillary therapy for disrupted pancreatic duct and peripancreatic fluid collections. *Gastroenterology* 1991; 100:1362-1370.

Leppäniemi, A., Haapiainen, R., Kiviluoto, T., Lempienen, M.: Pancreatic trauma: acute and late manifestations. *Br J Surg* 1988; 75:165-167.

Letton, A.H., Wilson, J.P.: Traumatic severance of pancreas treated by Roux-Y anastomosis. *Surg Gynecol Obstet* 1959; 109:473-478.

Lin, B.C., Chen, R.D., Fang, J.F., Hsu, J.F., Kao, Y.C., Kao, J.L.: Management of blunt major pancreatic injury. *J Trauma* 2004; 56:774-778.

Lin, B.C., Lin, N.J., Fang, J.F., Kao, Y.C.: Long-term results of endoscopic stent in the management of blunt major pancreatic duct injury. *Surg Endosc* 2006; 20:1551-1555.

Lucas, C.E., () Diagnosis and treatment of pancreatic and duodenal injury.: *Surg Clin North Am* 1977; 57:49-65.

Matsuda, M., Fujii, H., Mogaki, M., Miyasaka, Y., Maeda, Y., & Matsumoto, Y.: Initial treatment of a case of pancreatic trauma with injured main pancreatic duct in the head of pancreas-concept of preserving total pamcreatic function. *Suizou, (in Japanese, English abstract)* 1999; 14:387-393.

Meier, D.E., Coln, C.D., Hicks, B.A., Guzzetta, P.C.: Early operation in child with pancreas transaction. *J Pediatr Surg* 2001; 36:341-344.

Moore, E.E., Cogbill, T.H., Malangoni, M.A., Jurkovich, G.J., Champion, H.R., Gennarelli, T.A., McAninch, J.W., Pachter, H.L., Schackford, S.R., & Trafton P.G.: Organ injury scaling II: pancreas, duodenum, small bowel, colon, and rectum. *J Trauma* 1990; 57:49-65.

Morali, G.A., Braverman, D.L., Shemesh, D., Abramovitz, Z., Jaccobsohn, W.Z.: Successful treatment of pancreatic pseudocyst with a somatostatin analogue and catheter drainage. *Am J Gastroenterol* 1991; 86:515-518.

Mulligan, C., Howell, C., Hartley, R., Martindale, R., Clark, J.: Conservative management of pancreatic psuedocyst using octreotide acetate. *Am Surg* 1995; 61:206-209.

Nwariaku, F.E., Terracina, A., Mileski, W.J., Minei, J.P.,Carrico, C.J.: Is octreotid beneficial following pancreatic injury? *Am J Surg* 1995; 170:582-585.

Okamoto, H., Hosaka, M., Fujii, H., Wakana, H., Kawashima, K., & Fukasawa, T.: Successful management of a blunt pancreatic trauma by endoscopic stent placement. *Clin J Gastroenterol* 2010; 3:204-208.

Portis, M., Meyers, P., McDonald, J.C., & Gholson, C.F.: Traumatic pancreatitis in a patient with pancreas divism: Clinical and radiographic features. *Abdom Imaging* 1994; 19(2):162-164.

Rawls, D.E. & Custer, M.D.: Pancreatic trauma: an unusual soccer injury. *South Med J* 2001;94(7):741-743.

Rescorla, F.J., Plumley, D.A., Sherman, S., Scherer, L.R., 3rd, West, K.W., Grosfeld, J.L.: The efficacy of early ERCP in pediatric pancreatic trauma. *J Pediatr Surg* 1995; 30: 336-340.

Shan, Y.H., Sy E.D., Tsai. H.M., Liou C.S., Lin, P.W.: Nonsurgical management of main pancreatic duct transaction associated with psuedocyst after blunt abdominal injury. *Pancreas* 2002; 25(2):210-215.

Simon, H.K., Muehlberg, A., Linakis J.G.: Serum amylase determinations in pediatric patients presenting to the ED with acute abdominal pain or trauma. *Am J Emerg Med* 1994; 12:292-295.

Spiegel, M.J., & Sivit, C.J.: Pancreatic emergencies. *Radiol Clin North Am* 1997; 35(4):814-830.

The, S.H., Sheppard, B.C, Mullins, R.J., Schreiber, M.A., Mayberry, J.C.: Diagnosis and management of blunt pancreatic ductal injury in the era of high-resolution computed axial tomography. *Am J Surg* 2007; 193:641-643.

Part 5

Complications

13

Pancreatic Ascites and Pleural Effusion

K. Prakash
PVS Memorial Hospital,
Kaloor, Kochi, Kerala,
India

1. Introduction

Pancreatic ascites or internal pancreatic fistulae and pancreatic pleural effusion are rare complications of pancreatitis. This can occur in the clinical setting of an acute pancreatitis and more commonly as a complication of chronic pancreatitis[1]. This is an uncommon clinical condition; often the patients are sick and nutritionally compromised. Pancreatic ascites was first reported in the literature in 1953 when Smith described two cases of ascites associated with chronic pancreatitis[2].

2. Definition

Exact definition to diagnose this condition is not clear in the literature. Pancreatic ascites /pleural effusion is characterised by accumulation of high amylase fluid in the peritoneal cavity/pleural cavity due to leakage of pancreatic juice from a disrupted pancreatic duct and a diagnosis is usually made once the aspirated fluid is high in protein (>3g/dl) and high in amylase (>1000 IU/L)[3].

3. Aetiology and pathogenesis

Pancreatic ascites/pleural effusion can occur due to a) rupture of a pseudocyst into peritoneal cavity or to mediastinum and pleura or b) due to the disruption of a main pancreatic duct during the natural course of chronic pancreatitis[3]. Pancreatic leak occurs in 3.5% of patients with chronic pancreatitis and 6% to 14% of patients with pancreatic pseudocyst [4, 5]. The pathogenesis of the serous cavity effusion is different in acute and chronic pancreatitis setting. In acute pancreatitis, mostly in alcoholic pancreatitis, there is enough inflammatory reaction around the pancreas with neighbouring structures like stomach and transverse colon to form a pseudocyst. This can rupture into peritoneal cavity or mediastinum and to pleural cavity subsequently to produce ascites or pleural effusion respectively. Similar type of duct disruptions may also occur in acute setting in blunt abdominal trauma, biliary pancreatitis, and rupture of duplication cyst and rarely after pancreatic surgery or splenectomy[1, 6].

In the setting of chronic pancreatitis, leakage is seen in up to 80% of cases from a communicating pseudocyst due to ductal stricture and less commonly (20%) due to duct disruption itself[3, 7]. This has also been described in the setting of tropical calcific pancreatitis as well from duct disruptions and leaking pseudocyst[8]. Once the amylase rich fluid enters serous cavity, since the enzymes are not activated it does not produce digestion, instead it produces irritation resulting in outpouring of albumin resulting in high-albumin ascites. This accumulation of amylase rich fluid is usually massive before it produces symptoms due to its pressure effects. The amylase in the fluid can get reabsorbed into the blood stream and produce elevation of serum amylase as well. It has been also reported in one series that pancreatic ascites or effusions may present with indolent symptoms and up to 42% of patients gave no history of pancreatic disease[9].

4. Diagnosis and evaluation

Aim of the investigations in patients with pancreatic ascites are a). Overall assessment of patient's general and nutritional status and b). To delineate the pancreatic ductal anatomy and to locate the possible site of leak. These patients should have a haemogram, serum protein, and albumin and amylase value and coagulation profile. Upper GI endoscopy to rule out peptic ulcer or periampullary malignant disease and ultrasonography should be done. The diagnosis is usually confirmed with ascitic fluid assay. Usually the ascitic/pleural fluid contains high protein >3g/dl and high amylase >1000 IU/ml. Ascitic fluid assay should also be done to rule out other differential diagnosis like cirrhosis of liver or disseminated malignancy.

The localization of site of rupture or leak of main pancreatic duct is essential for planning therapy. Earlier, intraoperative pancreatography was the mainstay of localisation which is superseded largely by Endoscopic Retrograde Pancreatography (ERP) in recent years. However, these procedures are invasive and correct delineation of the duct anatomy and leak may not be feasible in all cases due to strictures or due to technical reasons. Demonstration of pancreatic duct leak by non invasive methods offer advantages like avoiding a sedation or anaesthesia, avoiding risk of introducing infection during injection of dye to the pancreatic duct. Non invasive investigations like CT scan helps in indentifying peripancreatic collections and details of the parenchyma of the pancreas. The details of pancreatic parenchyma, duct size, stones, strictures and psuedocysts are well displayed in a CT scan. The identification of site of leak from the pancreatic duct is possible in nearly half of the patients[10]. Magnetic Resonance Imaging (MRI) has also been reported to give good details of pancreatic parenchyma, details of the duct and details of the fistula[11, 12]. In MRP, high signal intensity of static or slowly flowing liquids is observed in T2 weighted images. Hence the pancreatic duct and the fistulous tract is displayed as high-signal intensity structure which helps in identifying the communication like pancreaticopleural fistula. The details of the pancreatic parenchyma and duct structural changes are also well displayed in MRI. Moreover, in MRI no contrast material is injected and there is no risk of infection in comparison with ERP. In a recent study[13], the ability of helical CT scan and Magnetic Resonance Pancreatography (MRP) when performed alone in identifying the site of duct disruption were 50 and 67% respectively. When these two modalities were combined the exact site of rupture of duct was observed in 94% of cases. Hence, a combination of imaging modalities helps to improve the details of the duct disruption,the site of leak and the details of the pancreatic parenchyma which is essential in planning of therapy.

5. Management

Management of these patients are challenging due to the compromised nutritional state, generalized weakness, diabetes mellitus and disease related factors like multiple strictures, large stones and inflammatory mass. All patients with a diagnosis of pancreatic ascites or pleural effusion should be assessed for their nutritional status. This is important as the morbidity and mortality of the various modes of treatment is related to the patient's general condition. These patients may be managed by conservative approach, endoscopic therapy and by surgical therapy. This may be done in using an algorithm depending upon patient's clinical condition[8]. (Table 1)

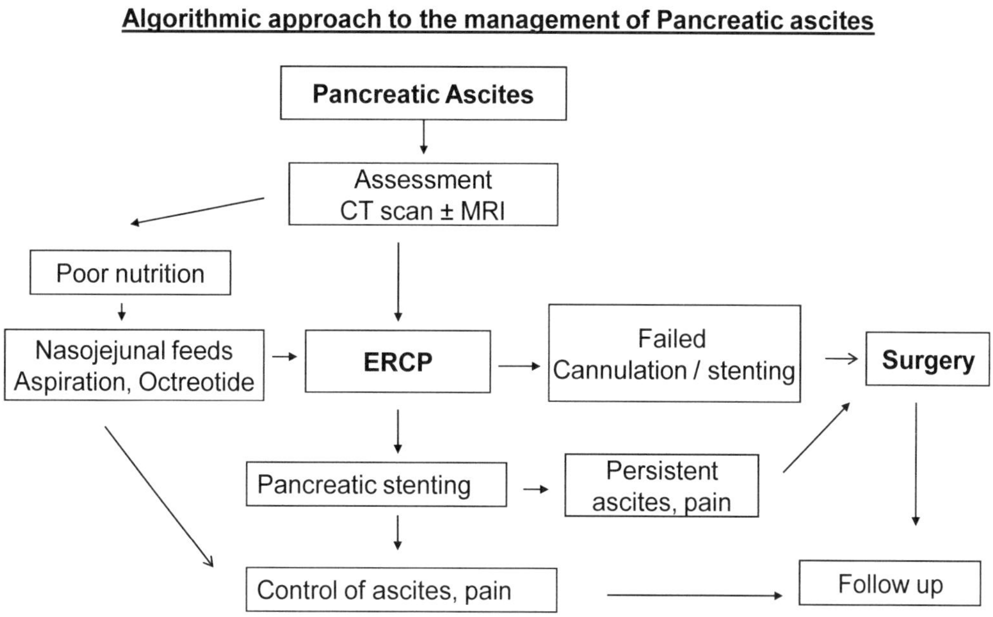

Table 1. Algorithmic approach to the management of pancreatic ascites.

6. Conservative treatment

Initial trial of conservative treatment is indicated in almost all patients. It was generally believed that there is high risk for mortality while the patients are on conservative therapy, which is due to poor nutritional management and assessment in the initial reports. Though an old series[14] had reported high mortality with conservative therapy, the progress of the patient can be safely monitored on conservative therapy in current daily practice. The key steps in the conservative management of the pancreatic ascites or pleural effusion are a). Rest to the pancreas and to limit pancreatic exocrine stimulation by keeping the patients nil orally, b). Nutritional support by means of nasojejunal feeds or by Total Parenteral Nutrition (TPN), c). Use of drugs likes to decrease pancreatic secretion d). Drainage of fluid by aspiration, drainage of ascites or by tube thoracocentesis. So patients are kept nil per oral and nutritional support should be planned on case to case basis. There is no significant difference between enteral or parenteral feeds on pancreatic exocrine secretion clinically[15]. However, these patients are often nutritionally compromised and have nausea, anorexia and poor tolerance to feeds due to exocrine insufficiency. Enteral nutritional support should be attempted whenever possible as it maintains mucosal integrity and prevents bacterial translocation. Nasojejunal feeds have a theoretic benefit as it prevents stimulation of pancreas and minimises fistula output. In patients who do not tolerate enteral feeds well or those with catabolic response TPN should be used either alone or along with enteral feeds.

Serous cavities should be emptied to promote approximation of serosal surfaces by drainage of ascitic/pleural fluid. Repeated aspiration of ascites or drainage of the ascites with the tube near the pseudocyst helps to drain the fluid by a controlled fistula. Similarly, aspiration or tube drainage should be done according to be patient's symptoms. Along with above measures, use of drugs with the aim to decrease the pancreatic exocrine secretion like somatostatin or octreotide also have a role in improving the pancreatic leak[15-17]. These drugs have been noted to decrease the fistula output (often within 24 hours of treatment) and accelerate the fistula closure. Depending upon the clinical situation a conservative therapy with above measures for 3-4 weeks helps in resolution of pancreatic leak in 25 - 60% of cases[17,18]. Patients with low sodium levels, albumin levels and those with a high fluid to serum protein levels had high chance for treatment failure[18]. Other agents attempted in closure of pancreatic leak are fibrin glue and nafamostat mesilate with variable results. Patients those who fails to respond to conservative measures or those patients who are symptomatic should undergo endotherapy or surgery.

7. Endotherapy

Endoscopic Retrograde Pancreatography (ERP) is the key step in planning of endoscopic treatment. ERP helps to delineate the anatomy of the duct, presence of strictures and site pancreatic leak (Figure 1). The principles of endotherapy include pancreatic sphincterotomy and placement of a transduodenal pancreatic stent across the site of ductal leak. This helps to obliterate the high-pressure gradient at the pancreatic sphincter, allowing preferential flow of pancreatic secretions along a low resistance path to the duodenum, thereby allowing the site of leak to heal. This has been reported in many series[6, 8,13,19,20]. It has been observed that a sphincterotomy and placement of stent close to the fistula, even if the stent could not be advance beyond the site of leak helps to heal the fistula or stabilizes patients clinical condition[8]. Other endoscopic approaches which are practised are endoscopic placement of nasopancreatic drainage[21] and endosonography guided pancreatogastrostomy[22]. Nasopancreatic drainage alone has been used instead of placement of pancreatic duct stenting in treatment of pancreatic ascites[22]. The authors have reported nearly 90% of success in placement of nasopancreatic drain and disappearance of pseudocyst and ascites were observed on 4-6 weeks. Nasopancreatic drains allow repeated pancreatography to assess the progress of therapy and healing of the duct. This method provides the option of flushing of the drain to clear the blocks and allows removal of the drain once the duct disruption is healed. The disadvantages of this method are the discomfort to the patients due to the nasal tube and risk of accidental dislodgement.

The success of endotherapy ranges from 50-90% depending upon the duct changes[8, 19-21]. Success of endoscopic treatment was based on three factors in this study a) ability to pass the stent across the site of disruption of the duct, b) absence of strictures and stones and c) ability to traverse the stricture. Those patients who had only partial relief of symptoms and those with failed endotherapy would require surgery.

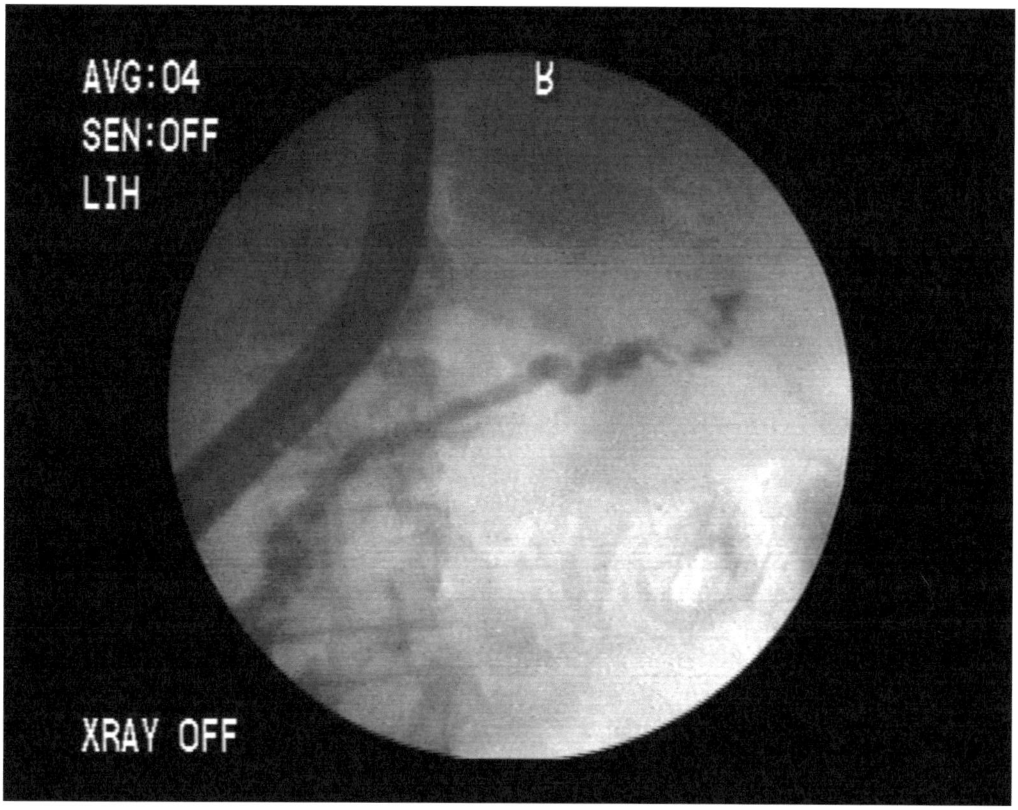

Fig. 1. Endoscopic retrograde pancreatography showing leak of dye from tail duct.

8. Surgery

The surgical intervention is planned according to the ductal anatomy and site of leak (figure 2). Aims of the surgery in patients with chronic pancreatitis with pancreatic ascites are to a) wide drainage of pancreatic duct, often with a Lateral Pancreatojejunostomy (LPJ) b) removal of pancreatic stones and ductal strictures and c) drainage of the cysts and external drainage of abscess.

Patients with chronic pancreatitis with large duct (>7mm) should undergo wide drainage of pancreatic duct often with a lateral panctreatojejunostomy and removal of pancreatic stones and ductal strictures[5, 7, 8]. Specific repair of the site or disruption is often unnecessary; however the area of disruption should be included in the anastomosis. Similarly, a mature pseudocyst also can be incorporated in the anastomosis. In patients with normal sized duct, identification of the site of leak is very important. In those with distal leak, a distal pancreatectomy with or without splenectomy is a good option. Spleen preservation is often difficult in these patients due to dense adhesions and inflammatory process. If the inflammation and fibrosis is significant a medial to lateral approach in distal pancreatectomy may be used to avoid excessive bleeding.

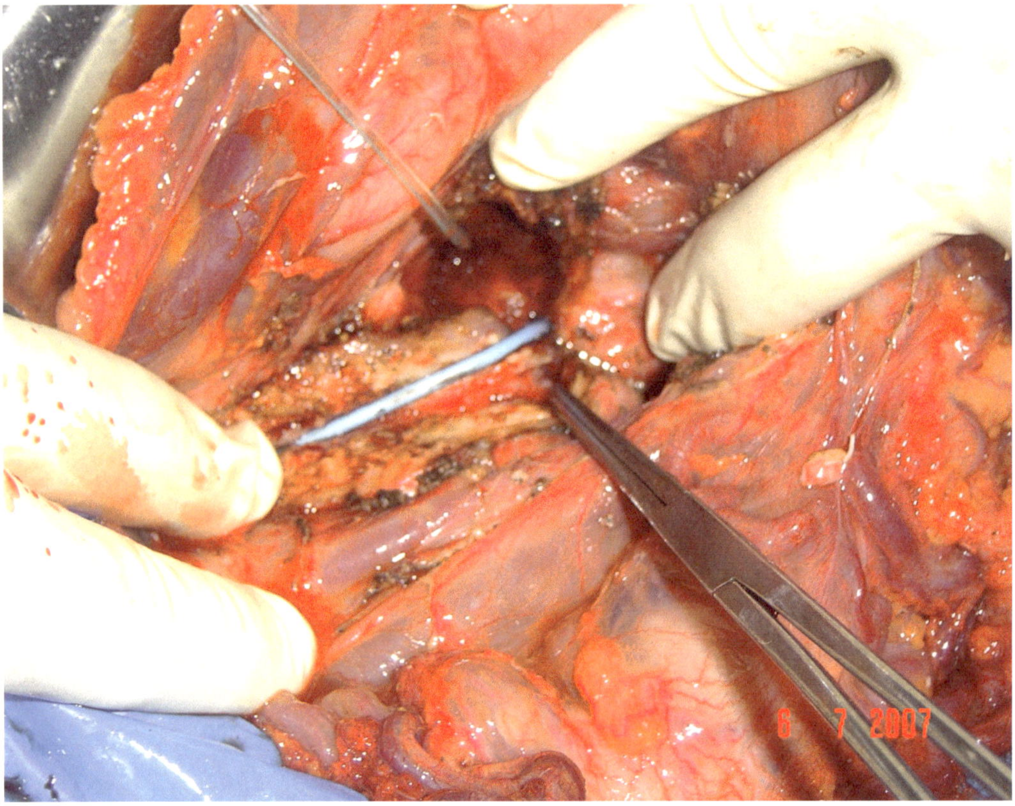

Fig. 2. Operative picture showing disruption of pancreatic duct in the body region with pancreatic stent in situ coming out through the site of disruption.

In those with leak from the neck region Roux -en-Y anastomosis to the fistula site or pancreatogastrostomy has been described. In those patients with disconnected duct syndrome, often secondary to acute pancreatic necrosis, there is often a loss of tissue near the genu with fistula from either distal or proximal duct. A Roux-en-Y anastomosis to the distal duct and closure of the proximal duct or distal pancreatectomy with closure of proximal duct may be performed according to the clinical situation. In patients with long fistulous tract to skin, dissection of fistula and fistula-enterostomy has been reported with varying results[23]. Surgery for pancreatic ascites is often difficult due to the dense inflammatory process in the peripancreatic tissue, mesentery and due to the presence of pseudocysts and often identification of site of leak is difficult and cystojejunostomy to the leaking cyst is also an effective option[24, 25].

9. Conclusion

Pancreatic ascites or pleural effusion are rare complications of acute or chronic pancreatitis wherein there is leakage of pancreatic juice to a serous cavity from a disrupted pancreatic duct or leaking pseudocyst. Preoperative workup should be aimed at the nutritional assessment of the patient and the pancreatic ductal imaging using CT scan or MRI. An algorithmic approach may be adopted in managing this patients using conservative, endotherapy or surgical treatment according to the clinical scenario. A multidisciplinary approach of these modalities is essential for successful management of these patients.

10. References

Barish MA, Soto JA. MR cholangiopancreatography: techniques and clinical applications. AJR Am J Roentgenol 1997; 169:1295–1303.

Bhasin DK. Endoscopic transpapillary nasopancreatic drainage alone to treat pancreatic ascites and pleural effusion. - - J Gastroenterol Hepatol 2006; 21: 1059-64

Bracher GA, Manocha AP, DeBanto JR, Gates LK, Slivka A, Whitcomb DC, et al. Endoscopic pancreatic duct stenting to treat pancreatic ascites. Gastrointest Endosc 1999; 49: 710-5.

Brooks JR. Pancreatic ascites. In: Brooks JR, editor. Surgery of the pancreas. Philadelphia: WB Saunders; 1983, p. 230-2.

Cameron JL. Chronic pancreatic ascites and pancreatic pleural effusions. Gastroenterology 74:134, 1978.

da Cunha JE, Machado M, Bacchella T, Penteado S, Mott CB, Jukemura J, et al. Surgical treatment of pancreatic ascites and pancreatic pleural effusions. Hepatogastroenterology 1995; 42: 748-51.

Dhar P, Tomey S, Jain P, Azfar M, Sachdev A, Chaudhary A. Internal pancreatic fistulae with serous effusions in chronic pancreatitis. Aus N Z J Surg 1996; 66: 608-11.

Eckhauser F, Raper SE, Knol JA, Mulholland MW. Surgical management of pancreatic pseudocysts, pancreatic ascites, and pancreatopleural fistulae. Pancreas 1991; 6: 566-75.

Francois E, Kahaleh M, Giovannini M, Matos C, Deviere J. EUS-guided pancreaticogastrostomy. Gastrointest Endosc 2002; 56: 128-33.

Fulcher AS, Capps GW, Turner MA. Thoracopancreatic fistula: clinical and imaging findings. J Comput Assist Tomogr 1999; 23: 181-7.

Kozarek RA, Ball TJ, Patterson DJ, Freeny PC, Ryan JA, Traverso LW. Endoscopic transpapillary therapy for disrupted pancreatic duct and peripancreatic fluid collections. Gastroenterology 1991; 100: 1362-70.

Kurumboor P, Varma D, Rajan M, Kamlesh NP, Paulose R, Narayanan RG, Philip M. Outcome of pancreatic ascites in patients with tropical calcific pancreatitis managed using a uniform treatment protocol. Indian J Gastroenterol. 2009; 28: 102-6.

Lipsett PA, Cameron JL. Internal pancreatic fistula. Am J Surg 163:216, 1992.

MacLauren IF. Pancreatic ascites. In: Howard JM, Jordan GL, Reber HA, editors. Surgical diseases of the pancreas. Philadelphia: Lea and Febigor; 1987. p. 591-602.

Martineau P, Shwed JA, Denis R. Is octreotide a new hope for enterocutaneous and external pancreatic fistulas closure? Am JSurg 1996; 172: 386-395.

Materne R, Vranckx P, Pauls C, Coche EE, Deprez P, Van Beers BE.. Pancreaticopleural Fistula. Diagnosis with magnetic resonance pancreatography. Chest 2000; 117:912–914.

Moosa AR. Surgical treatment of chronic pancreatitis: an overview. Br J Surg 1987; 74: 661-7.

Oktedalen O, Nygaard K, Osnes M. Somatostatin in the treatment of pancreatic ascites. Gastroenterology 1990; 99: 1520-1.

O'Toole D, Vullierme MP, Ponsot P, Maire F, Calmels V, Hentic O, Hammel P, Sauvanet A, et al. Diagnosis and management of pancreatic fistulae resulting in pancreatic ascites or pleural effusions in the era of helical CT and magnetic resonance imaging. Gastroenterol Clin Biol. 2007; 31:686-93.

Pai CG. Endoscopic treatment as first-line therapy for pancreatic ascites and pleural effusion. - - J Gastroenterol Hepatol 2009; 24: 1198-202.

Parekh D, Segal I. Pancreatic ascites and effusion: risk factors for failure of conservative therapy and role of octreotide. Arch Surg 1992; 127: 707-12.

Qin HL, Su ZD, Zou Y, Fan YB. Effect of parenteral and enteral nutrition combined with octreotide on pancreatic exocrine secretion of patients with pancreatic fistula. World J Gastroenterol 2004; 10: 2419-2422.

Sankaran S, Walt AJ. Pancreatic ascites, recognition and management. Arch Surg 1976; 111: 430-4.

Smith EB. Hemorrhagic ascites and hemothorax associated with benign pancreatic disease. Arch Surg 1953; 67:52-6.

Voss M, Ali A, Eubanks WS. Surgical management of pancreaticocutaneous fistula.J Gastrointest Surg 2003;7:542–6

14

Emphysematous Pancreatitis

Audrius Šileikis
Vilnius University,
Lithuania

1. Introduction

Emphysematous (gas-forming) infections of the abdomen and pelvis

Emphysematous (gas-forming) infections of the abdomen and pelvis represent potentially life-threatening conditions that require aggressive medical and often surgical management. The initial clinical manifestation of these entities may be insidious, but rapid progression to sepsis will occur in the absence of early therapeutic intervention. Conventional radiography and ultrasonography are often the initial imaging modalities used to evaluate patients with abdominopelvic complaints. However, when a differential diagnosis remains, or if further localization or confirmation of tentative findings is needed, computed tomography (CT) should be considered the imaging modality of choice. CT is both highly sensitive and specific in the detection of abnormal gas and well suited to reliable depiction of the anatomic location and extent of the gas. Of equal importance may be the capability of CT to help reliably identify benign sources of gas, because treatment (if any) varies dramatically depending on the source. Knowledge of the pathophysiologic characteristics, common predisposing conditions, and typical imaging features associated with gas-forming infections of the gall-bladder, stomach, pancreas, and genitourinary system will help make early diagnosis and successful treatment possible. In addition, such knowledge will aid in further diagnostic work-up, surveillance of potential complications, and evaluation of therapeutic response. The presence of gas within the parenchyma of solid organs or the walls of hollow viscera may be due to a variety of pathologic or benign entities. Besides infection with gas-forming bacteria, other possible sources include bland tissue infarction with necrosis, enteric fistula formation, and reflux from an adjacent hollow viscus. Gas should be differentiated from atmospheric air introduced at recent instrumentation or surgery. Gas associated with infection is generally thought to consist of carbon dioxide and nitrogen secondary to the fermentation of glucose by some species of bacteria. Poor glycolysis at the tissue level in diabetic patients results in increased glucose concentrations within the interstitial fluid. Other clinical factors that contribute to the increased production or slowed removal of gas include a depressed cell-mediated immune response, local tissue necrosis, and the presence of arteriosclerosis. The increased pH of bile associated with gallbladder inflammation and the focal tissue ischemia seen in gynecologic neoplasms are examples of specific underlying processes that help optimize bacterial culture media. In addition to broad-spectrum antimicrobial therapy and possible surgery, correction of associated underlying conditions such as urinary outflow obstruction, acid-base and electrolyte imbalances, hypovolemia, and hyperglycemia is imperative. In the setting of gas-forming infections, clinical outcome will, in large part, depend on whether early diagnosis and treatment are achieved. The presence of comorbid conditions and equivocal physical examination findings may prevent rapid diagnosis or delay appropriate initial therapy. Consequently, appropriate radiologic imaging with prompt, accurate interpretation plays an important role in the diagnosis and management of these diseases.

2. Main heading, emphysematous pancreatitis

The most common causes of acute pancreatitis are the passage of gallstones and alcohol abuse. An overall mortality rate of 4% rapidly escalates to more than 50% when complications (eg, abscess formation, superinfection with gas-forming bacteria) occur. The infecting organisms are usually coliform bacteria and may reach the pancreatic bed by way of the bloodstream or lymphatic channels, a fistula from adjacent bowel, transmural passage from the transverse colon, or reflux of enteric organisms into the pancreatic duct or biliary tree via a patulous ampulla of Vater. Gas may be detected in up to 22% of pancreatic abscesses; however, its presence alone is not specific for the diagnosis of infection. Other sources of intraductal or parenchymal pancreatic gas include reflux from the duodenum following sphincterotomy, endoscopic instrumentation, enteric fistula (commonly involving the transverse colon), and end-organ infarction. Patients with emphysematous pancreatitis are usually debilitated and often have underlying immunocompromised conditions such as poorly controlled diabetes or chronic renal failure, atherosclerosis, tuberculosis, HIV infected individuals.

2.1 Secondary heading

Retrospective review of literature, and our one experience of treatment 8 patients with emphysematous pancreatitis in our department from 2003 to 2011.

2.1.1 Tertiary heading, left justified

Early radiographic detection of retroperitoneal gas is critical in the evaluation of superimposed emphysematous infection of the pancreas. Conventional abdominal radiography may demonstrate mottled gas overlying the midabdomen (Fig 1).

This finding is not specific for pancreatitis because abscesses involving the lesser sac or perinephric space may also have this appearance. Diagnostic US is often of limited value in the evaluation of acute pancreatitis or its complications secondary to an adjacent air-filled small bowel loop from ileus. When identified, pancreatic gas will manifest as multiple irregular echogenic foci, often with posterior dirty acoustic shadowing. A significant volume of gas may limit the detection of adjacent fluid collections. CT is the modality of choice for detecting parenchymal gas as well as evaluating its extent and location (Fig 2, 3).

Fluid collections or portal venous air are readily identified, and, although intravenously administered contrast material is not necessary for the visualization of air, it is useful for evaluating potential complications including parenchymal necrosis and abscess formation. The prognosis for emphysematous pancreatitis is grave, and successful treatment requires

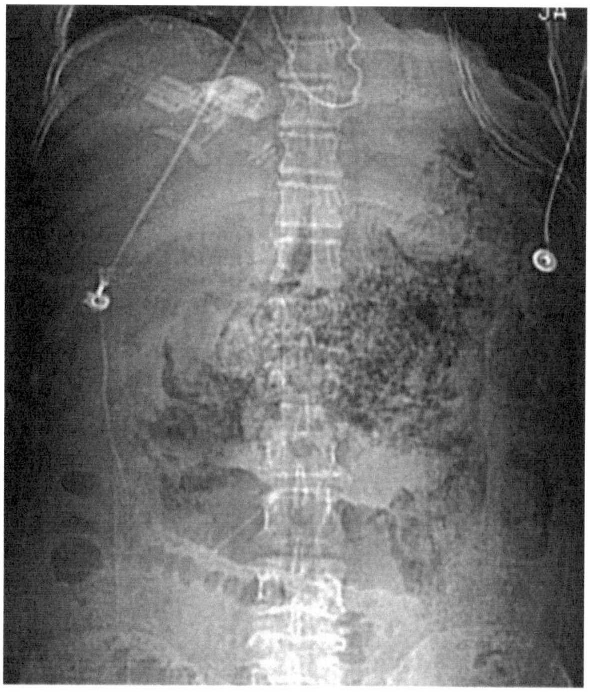

Fig. 1. Emphysematous pancreatitis in a 66-year-old woman. Digital scout image from a CT scan demonstrates a mottled collection of gas bubbles in the midportion of the upper abdomen and extending into the left upper quadrant.

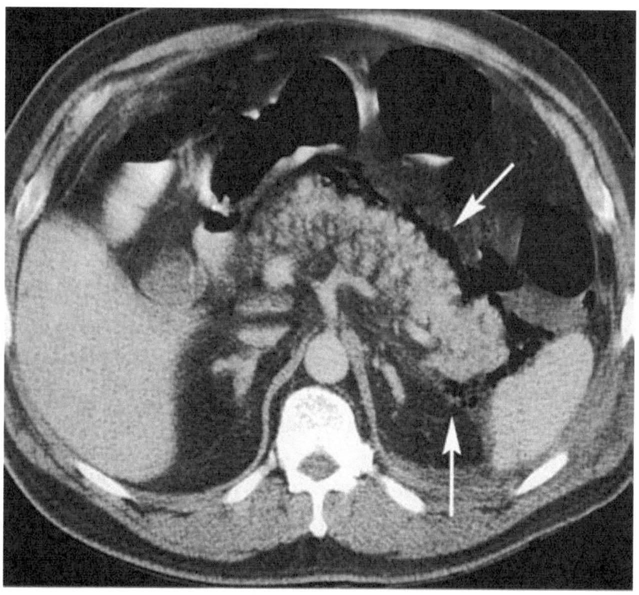

Fig. 2. Emphysematous pancreatitis in a 66-year-old woman. Contrast-enhanced CT scans obtained at the same level as a show gas surrounding the body and tail of the pancreas (white arrows) and extending more cephalic within the anterior pararenal space.

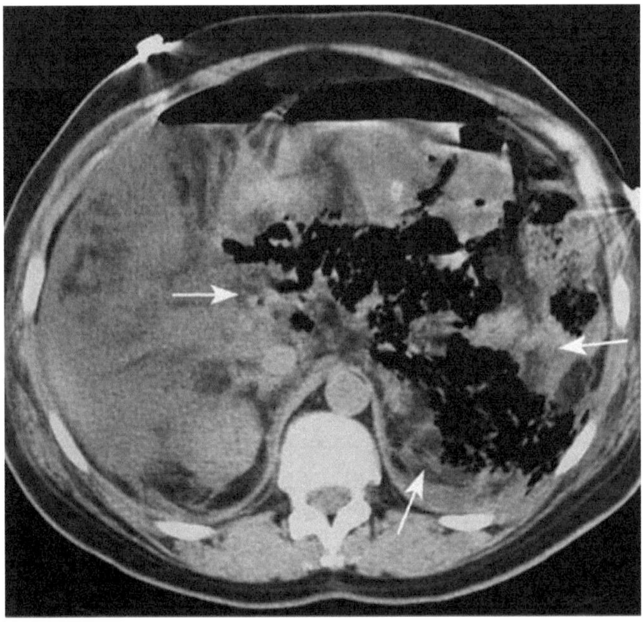

Fig. 3. Contrast-enhanced CT scans in a 66-year-old woman with emphysematous pancreatitis. There are extensive inflammatory changes involving the surrounding fat (white arrows).

aggressive management of the infection with systemic antimicrobial therapy and control of septic shock. Usually emphysematous pancreatitis occurs at the onset of the disease - first week of the illness, but some times it can manifest later on. There is at present a tendency to operate patients with infected necrosis as soon as the diagnosis is made, regardless of the clinical status. It is well known that pancreatic abscesses represent a distinct clinical entity and that they are treatable by nonoperative management, including percutaneous drainage. Similarly, selected patients with localized infected necrosis amenable to endoscopic, transgastric drainage can be managed with this interventional technique. There are some patients with retroperitoneal gas in the setting of severe acute pancreatitis who were treated with focused long-term (3–7 weeks) antibiotics; allegedly the infected necrosis resolved without any interventional drainage or necrosectomy. The emergence of a few cases treatable medically, though small in number, may be due in part to better intensive care and in part to improved antibiotic therapy. However, the lesson learnt from these cases is that some patients may improve without intervention. The above observations suggest the need to correlate clinical versus imaging and bacteriologic findings in acute pancreatitis with infected pancreatic necrosis. Not all patients with infected pancreatic necrosis may need intervention. 368 patients with severe acute necrotic pancreatitis were treated in our department from year 2003 to 2011, including 8 (2%) patients who had developed emphysematous pancreatitis. The data of these patients are presented in Table 1.

The patient's age averaged was 73,9 ± 4,8 years. All of them had manifestation of atherosclerosis (ischemic stroke, myocardial infarction, ischemic heart disease) four had metabolic syndromes such as hyperglycemia, one gastric and another one prostate cancer.

Parameter	Case 1	Case 2	Case 3	Case 4	Case 5	Case 6	Case 7	Case 8
Age, years	72	66	74	67	79	80	80	73
Sex	female	male	male	female	male	male	male	female
Appache II	18	23	16	8	17	22	10	18
CT evidence of necrosis degree	30-50%	30-50%	<30%	<30%	<30%	>50%	<30%	30-50%
Necrosis localization	head	head	head	tail	head	tail	head	head
Glucose during admission mmol/l	12,5	10,2	7,0	11,3	6,9	11,7	6,0	5,8
Comorbid illnesses	IS	IS	MI	ISH	ISH; CaV	MI; CaP	ISH	IS; ISH
Time of gas CT detection*	7	3	3	4	2	2	11	6
Time of the operation**	15	4	3	-	3	3	13	7
Type of the operation	closed	open	open	-	open+G	open	open	open
Number of debridment	2	1	1		3	0	1	1
Hospital stay, days	114	60	78	22	14	3	41	43
Outcome	recovery	recovery	recovery	recovery	dead	dead	recovery	recovery
Cultures of necrotic pancreas tissue	E. coli	E. coli; Pr	E. coli	-	E. coli; Bf	Ef	E. coli	E. coli

Table 1. Patients data treated in our department. IS - ischemic stroke; MI - myocardial infarction; ISH - ischemic heart disease; CaV - gastric cancer; CaP - prostate cancer; *Time of intrapancreatic gas CT detection, days from the onset of the disease; **Time of the operation, days from the onset of the disease; closed - closed lavage; open - open packing; G - gastrectomy; Pr - Providentia rettgeri; Bf-Bacteroides fragilis; Ef - Enterococcus faecalis;

The trigger of the development of emphysematous pancreatitis in all cases was passage of gallstones. All of these patients had calculous cholecystitis and choledocholithiasis. Most of them CT scan showed pancreatic necrosis, retroperitoneal and intrapancreatic gas trapping in the first week of the disease. Necrosis with intrapancreatic gas trapping occurred more frequently in pancreatic head (six cases), less in pancreatic tail (two cases). Six patients, for whom vasopressor-noradrenaline doses were increased to 0,4 μg/kg/min to provide sustainable hemodynamics due to bacteremic shock, had been successfully treated by extensive pancreatic necrosectomy, open packing with debridement immediately after CT diagnosis of emphysematous pancreatitis. One female patient was treated with antibiotics (ciprofloxacin and metronidazole), oxygen therapy, fluid and electrolyte correction and nasojejunal feeding for 9 days, followed by necrosectomy and continued lavage due to failure of organs. One patient at the same time had emphysematous pancreatitis and cholecystitis. All operated on patients had infected pancreatic necrosis which was confirmed bacteriologically. Escherichia coli infection was present in six patients, additionally Bacteroides fragilis, Providentia retgeri and Enterococcus faecalis were cultured respectively. Emphysematous pancreatitis requires urgent surgical management at the onset of disease due to multisystem organ failure and patient instability. Ordinarily early surgical interventions mortality rates are reported as at least 50%, and morbidity can approach 100%. Ideally, surgery should be delayed at the earliest of 3rd or 4'th week of illness until the necrosis has demarcated and organized. At that time, the necrosectomy is technically easier, and there is generally improved mortality and morbidity. However, we found that in cases of emphysematous pancreatitis, pancreatic necrosis is already demarcated and organized at the first week, which is enough to repeat one or two additional necrosectomies for the patient full recovery. The hospital stay was significantly shorter too. In comparison for the other our patients with open packing: an average of time of the operation from the onset of the disease was 29 days, overall hospital stay - 93 days and 4,2 additional necrosectomies for the patient full recovery. We also found that minimally invasive procedures in patients with emphysematous pancreatitis are not available, since fluid collections are absent. One patient (case 4) with overt inflammatory indices - C-reactive protein 177,7 mg/l, white blood cells $16x10^9$, febrile temperature 38,7 C° - on first presenting presenting, underwent conservative treatment regimen after radiological detection of emphysematous pancreatitis (fig.4.).

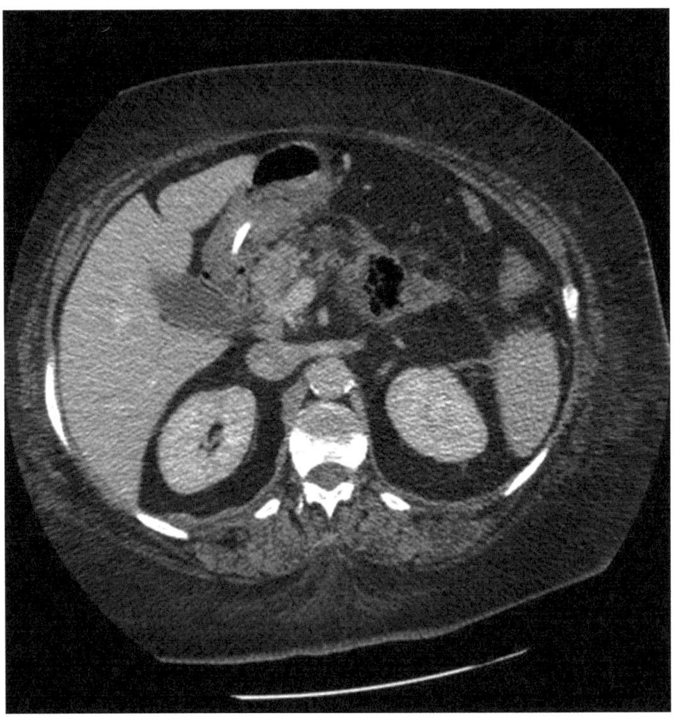

Fig. 4. CT scan showing less than 30% pancreas tail necrosis with intrapancreatic and retroperitoneal gas.

This patient did not undergo a puncture for the bacteriological proof of infection based on the supposition of the possibility to confirm the radiological suspicion of infected pancreatic necrosis during the operation. Since no surgical interventions were performed on the non-operated patient previously, there was no enteric fistula, and pancreatic necrosis was localized in the middle of parenchyma, we therefore considered clinical and CT data to be sufficient in this case for the proof of infection of pancreatic necrosis. Following successful conservative treatment, however, the patient avoided the operation, and, therefore, the causative agent of the infected pancreatic necrosis was not verified. CT follow-up for this female patient was performed in 8 weeks and in 3 months respectively showing complete intrapancreatic and retroperitoneal gas disappearing (fig. 5).

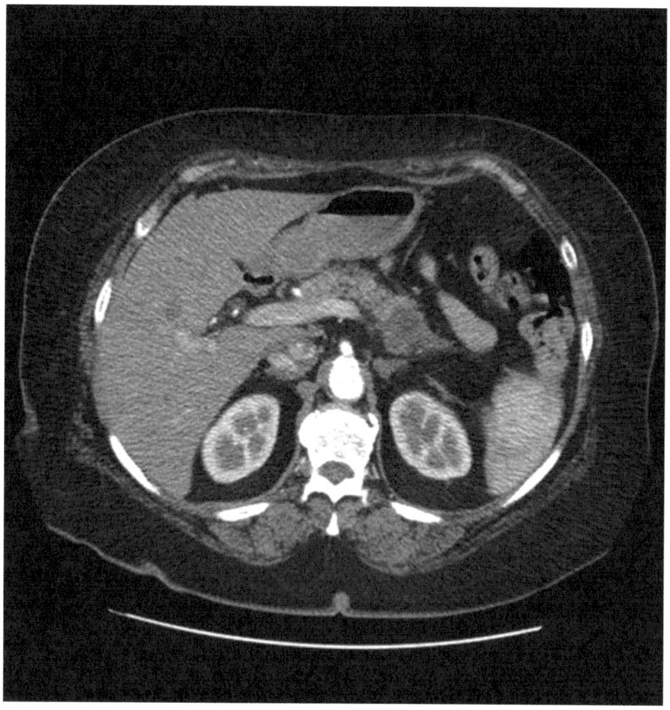

Fig. 5. CT scan showing resolution of intrapancreatic and retroperitoneal gas after 8 weeks

We suggest that the main factor determining such different outcomes of emphysematous pancreatitis in patients of similar age and with similar comorbidities and extend of the necrosis is the varying localization of necrosis in the pancreas. Necrosis in the pancreas head showing higher vascularization than the pancreatic tail is associated with a lower frequency of massive intoxication and organ failure necessitating surgical intervention. Other authors reported some cases of successful antibiotic treatment of infected pancreatic necrosis located in the pancreatic tail as well. In these cases, however, infected pancreatic necrosis was identified later on, not at the onset of the disease, and the number of the cases is too small to draw valid conclusions.

3. Conclusions

Emphysematous pancreatitis is a potentially life-threatening condition. The initial clinical manifestation may be insidious, but rapid progression to sepsis will occur in the absence of early therapeutic intervention. Conventional radiography and ultrasonography are often the initial imaging modalities used to evaluate patients with abdominopelvic complaints. These modalities should be considered complementary, each with strengths and limitations. When a differential diagnosis re-mains, CT should be considered the imaging modality of choice. CT is both highly sensitive and specific in the detection of abnormal gas and well suited to reliable depiction of the anatomic location and extent of the gas. Therefore, with regard to emphysematous pancreatitis, appropriate radiologic evaluation combined with accurate interpretation of findings will help to ensure rapid diagnosis and optimal treatment planning. In addition, knowledge of the pathophysiologic characteristics and common predisposing conditions associated with gas-forming infections of the gallbladder, stomach, pancreas, and genitourinary system will aid in further diagnostic work-up, surveillance of potential complications, and evaluation of therapeutic response. The prognosis for emphysematous pancreatitis is grave, and successful treatment requires aggressive management of the infection with systemic antimicrobial therapy and control of septic shock. Early surgical debridement is usually performed, and recovery is typically prolonged.

4. Acknowledgment

Emphysematous pancreatitis is a rare and life-threatening necrotizing infection of the pancreas - 2% of all acute necrotic pancreatitis. CT is the modality of choice for detecting parenchymal gas as well as evaluating its extent and location. Ordinarily emphysematous pancreatitis requires urgent surgical management, which in most cases is successful, at the onset of disease due to multisystem organ failure and patient instability. In cases of emphysematous pancreatitis, pancreatic necrosis is already demarcated and organized at the first week, which is enough to repeat one or two additional necrosectomies for the patient full recovery. If the patient's condition is stable, aggressive broad-spectrum antibiotic coverage, nutritional support, and routine correlation of clinical progression with radiological evaluation must be taken. As demonstrated by our experience, if the patient's condition is stable, antibiotic treatment could be undertaken without any surgical intervention despite the evidence of pancreatic infection. General physical condition of the patient is an important factor for choosing a treatment rather than bacteriological or radiological findings of the infection. Aggressive broad-spectrum antibiotic coverage, nutritional support, and routine correlation of clinical progression with radiological evaluation were assets.

5. References

Adler, D. et al. (2003). Conservative management of infected necrosis complicating severe acute pancreatitis. *American journal of Gastroenterology*, Vol. 98, No. 1, (January, 2003), pp. 98-103, ISSN 0002-9270.

Anderson, C. et al. (2004). Pneumoretroperitoneum in two patients with Clostridium perfringens necrotizing pancreatitis. *The American surgeon*, Vol. 70, No.3, (March, 2004), pp. 268-271, ISSN 0003-1348.

Barreiro-Pardal, C. et al. (2011). Therapeutic management of emphysematous pancreatitis. *Revista Española de Enfermedades Digestivas*, Vol. 103, No. 5, (May 2011), pp. 282-283, ISSN 1130-0108.

Bazan, HA. Kim, U. (2003). Images in clinical medicine. Emphysematous pancreatitis. *The New England Journal of Medicine,* Vol. 25, No.12, (December 2003), pp. 349, ISSN 0958-3165.

Birgisson, H. et al. (2001). Emphysematous pancreatitis. *European Journal of Surgery*, Vol. 167, No.12, (December 2001), pp. 918-920, ISSN 1741-9271.

Buckley, O. et al. (2006). A case of emphysematous pancreatitis. *British journal of Hospital Medicine*. Vol. 67, No.9, (September 2006), pp. 495, ISSN 1750-8460.

Camps, I. et al. (2009). VAC (vacuum-assisted closure) "covered" laparostomy to control abdominal compartmental syndrome in a case of emphysematous pancreatitis. *Cirurgia Espanola*, Vol. 86, No.4, (October 2009), pp. 250-251, ISSN 0009-739X.

Choi, HS. et al. (2010). Simultaneous emphysematous cholecystitis and emphysematous pancreatitis: a case report. *Clincal Imaging* , Vol. 34, No. 3, (May-Jun 2010), pp. 239-241, ISSN 0899-7071.

Daly. JJ. Et al. (1995). Emphysematous pancreatitis. *Radiographics*, Vol. 15, No.2, (March 1995), pp. 489-492, ISSN 0271-5333.

Holdsworth, RJ. Parratt, D. (1996). The potential role of Clostridium perfringens alpha toxin in the pathogenesis of acute pancreatitis. *Journal of Clinical Pathology,* Vol. 49, No.4, (April 1996), pp. 500-503, ISSN 0021-9746.

Ikegami, T. et al. (2004). Primary gas gangrene of the pancreas: report of a case. *Surgery Today*, Vol. 34, No.1, (January, 2004), pp. 80-81, ISSN 0941-1291.

Fischer, MG. Geffen A. (1959). Emphysematous Necrotizing Pancreatitis. *Archives of surgery*, Vol. 79, No.10, (October 1959), pp. 567-569, ISSN 0004-0010.

Ghidirim, G. et al. (2005). Emphysematous necrotizing pancreatitis. *Chirurgia (Bucur),* Vol. 100, No.3, (May-Jun 2005), pp. 293-296, ISSN 1221-9118.

Grayson, DE. Et al. (2002). Emphysematous infections of the abdomen and pelvis: a pictorial review. *Radiographics*, Vol. 22, No.3, (May-Jun 2002), pp. 543-561, ISSN 0271-5333.

Kvinlaug, K. et al. (2009). Emphysematous Pancreatitis: A Less Aggressive Form of Infected Pancreatic Necrosis? *Pancreas*, Vol. 38, No. 6, (August, 2009), pp. 667-671, ISSN 1727-3048.

Ku, YM. Et al , (2007). Medical management of emphysematous pancreatitis. *Journal of Gastroenterology and Hepatology*, Vol. 22, No.3, (March 2007), pp. 455-456, ISSN 1440-1746.

Levy, P. et al. (1999). Spontaneous gas gangrene of the pancreas caused by Clostridium perfringens. *Gastroentérologie clinique et biologique*, Vol. 23, No.2, (March 1999), pp. 1223-1248, ISSN 0399-8320.

Morris, DL. et al. (1993). Case report: emphysematous tuberculous pancreatitis diagnosis by ultrasound and computed tomography. *Clinical radiology*, Vol. 48, No.4, (October 1993), pp. 286-287, ISSN 0009-9260.

Noorda, EM. Et al. (2002). A particular case of acute necrotizing pancreatitis. *Surgery*, Vol. 131, No.5, (May 2002), pp. 589-590, ISSN 1528-8242.

Novellas. S. et al. (2009). CT imaging features and significance of gas in the pancreatic bed. *Journal de Radiologie*, Vol. 90, No. 2, (February 2009), pp. 191-198, ISSN 0221-0363.

Porter, NA. Lapsia, SK. (2010). Emphysematous pancreatitis: a severe complication of acute pancreatitis. *Oxford journal of Med*icine, Vol. 10, No.8, (August 2010), pp. 1093 ISSN 1460-2725.

Ramesh, H. et al. (2003). Are some cases of infected pancreatic necrosis treatable without intervention? *Digestive surgery*, Vol. 20, No. 4, (April, 2003), pp. 296-299, ISSN 0253-4886

Sadeghi-Nejad, H. al. (1994). Spontaneous gas gangrene of the pancreas. *Journal of Clinical Gastroenterology*, Vol. 18, No.1, (February 1994), pp. 136-138, ISSN 0192-0790.

Sodhi. KS. Et al. (2010). Emphysematous pyelonephritis with emphysematous pancreatitis. *The Journal of Emergency Medicine,* Vol. 39, No.12, (July 2010), pp. 85-87, ISSN 0736-4679.

Stockinger, Z. et al. (2004). Pneumoperitoneum from gas gangrene of the pancreas: three unusual findings in a single case. *Journal of Gastrointestinal Surgery*, Vol. 8, No.4, (April, 2004), pp. 489-492, 1091-255X.

Šileikis, A. et al. (2007). Experience of the Treatment of Emphysematous Necrotizing Pancreatitis. *Chirurgische gastroenterology*, Vol. 23, No. 2, (April, 2007), pp. 195-198, ISSN 0177-9990.

Šileikis, A. et al. (2007). Three cases of emphysematous necrotizing pancreatitis treated by different methods. *Acta medica Lituanica*, Vol. 14, No. 2, (April 2007), pp. 108–110, ISSN 1392-0138.

Verbeeck, N. et al. (2011). Exceptional, potentially fatal combination of emphysematous pancreatitis and gas-forming cholecystitis: successful multidisciplinary conservative treatment supported by repeated CT-staging. *Journal Belge de Radiologie - Belgisch Tijdschrift voor Radiologie*, Vol. 94, No. 2, (March-April 2011), pp. 71-74, ISSN 0302-7430.

Velasco Guardado, A. et al. (2009). Emphysematous pancreatitis: Conservative or surgical treatment? *Journal of Gastroenterology and Hepatology*, Vol. 32, No.93, (November 2009), pp. 605-609, ISSN 1440-1746.

Wig, JD. et al. (2008). Emphysematous pancreatitis. Radiological curiosity or a cause for concern? *Journal of the pancreas*, Vol. 8, No.2, (March 2008), pp. 160-166, ISSN 1590-8577.